ISSUES IN KIDNEY DISEASE SERIES

ISSUES IN KIDNEY DISEASE

TRANSPLANTATION

ISSUES IN KIDNEY DISEASE SERIES

Stephen Z. Fadem – Series Editor

SELZMAN INSTITUTE FOR KIDNEY HEALTH, SECTION OF NEPHROLOGY,
AND MICHAEL E. DEBAKEY VETERANS AFFAIRS MEDICAL CENTER,
BAYLOR COLLEGE OF MEDICINE, HOUSTON, TX, USA;
KIDNEY ASSOCIATES, HOUSTON, TX, USA

Issues in Kidney Disease – Transplantation
Bhamidipati V. R. Murthy and Stephen Z. Fadem (Editors)
2021. ISBN: 978-1-53619-960-4 (Hardcover)

Issues in Kidney Disease – Dialysis
Stephen Z. Fadem and José A. Moura-Neto (Editors)
2021. ISBN: 978-1-68507-000-7 (Hardcover)

Issues in Kidney Disease – Acute Kidney Injury
Stephen Z. Fadem and Ahmed Arslan Yousuf Awan (Editors)
2021. ISBN: 978-1-68507-002-1 (Hardcover)

Issues in Kidney Disease – Chronic Kidney Disease
Stephen Z. Fadem and Samaya Javed Anumudu (Editors)
2021. ISBN: 978-1-68507-001-4 (Hardcover)

ISSUES IN KIDNEY DISEASE SERIES

ISSUES IN KIDNEY DISEASE

TRANSPLANTATION

BHAMIDIPATI V. R. MURTHY
AND
STEPHEN Z. FADEM
EDITORS

nova
Medicine & Health
New York

DOI: https://doi.org/10.52305/HHIR2325

NOTICE TO THE READER

Additional color graphics may be available in the e-book version of this book.

Library of Congress Cataloging-in-Publication Data

Names: Fadem, Stephen Z., editor. | Murthy, Bhamidipati V. Ramana, editor.
Title: Issues in kidney disease : transplantation / Bhamidipati V. Ramana Murthy, MD, Medicine -- Nephrology, Baylor College of Medicine, Houston, Texas, USA, Stephen Z. Fadem, MD, FASN Medicine-Nephrology, Baylor College of Medicine, Houston, Texas, USA; Kidney Associates, PLLC, Houston, Texas, USA, editors.
Description: New York : Nova Science Publishers, [2021] | Series: Issues in kidney disease series | Includes bibliographical references and index. |
Identifiers: LCCN 2021043738 (print) | LCCN 2021043739 (ebook) | ISBN 9781536199604 (hardcover) | ISBN 9781685071288 (adobe pdf)
Subjects: LCSH: Kidneys--Transplantation. | Transplantation of organs, tissues, etc.
Classification: LCC RD575 .I87 2021 (print) | LCC RD575 (ebook) | DDC 617.4/610592--dc23
LC record available at https://lccn.loc.gov/2021043738
LC ebook record available at https://lccn.loc.gov/2021043739

Published by Nova Science Publishers, Inc. † New York

To my dear wife, Sujatha, and to my children, Harini, and Pranav

Bhamidipati V. R. Murthy

To my lovely wife, Joyce

Stephen Z. Fadem

CONTENTS

FOREWORD

A Prince once requested a much-respected artist to draw up his kingdom to scale; the project, of course, became unwieldy by its sheer size. I have taken this lesson to heart in writing this Foreword!

Transplantation has advanced from a high risk, experimental procedure to a safe, life-saving therapy. While reviews capture the spectacular advances in a particular area, a textbook should offer a panoramic view of the progress, challenges, and opportunities. This book on transplantation, superbly edited by Dr. Bhamidipati V. R. Murthy and Dr. Stephen Fadem, meets and exceeds these expectations.

Editors pick and choose! The 17 chapters, authored by dedicated transplant professionals selected by Dr. Murthy, provide us the needed lens to understand the complexities and appreciate the nuances in our chosen field. The book correctly starts with a scholarly overview of kidney transplantation and delves into the importance of careful selection of the transplant recipient before addressing the complexities associated with the noble act of organ donation including the risks of living donation - an issue of increasing importance as the net has been widened by paired kidney donation and altruistic donors.

Our genetic endowments impose barriers to transplantation, and these critical issues are dealt with in chapters on histocompatibility, immunology and on the pesky problem of pre-sensitized recipients. The need for multipronged immunosuppressive therapy and the fine line the transplant clinicians need to toe to avoid the twin evils of infection and malignancy are addressed in successive chapters. The Banff classification, a truly living document, has helped us view allograft rejection in fine detail, and both these topics find their rightful place in this book.

The spectacular progress in short-term outcomes has brought to focus long-term care including the Damocles' sword of recurrent disease. The chapters dedicated to these areas are highly informative.

Almost 20% of patients on the kidney transplant wait list are repeat transplants, and much needs to be learned about the management of the unfortunate patient returning to dialysis after a failed transplant. A chapter on this thorny issue and one on the benefits and challenges surrounding multi-organ transplantation are timely and much needed.

The biological complexity of transplantation is only rivaled by the psychosocial issues and ethics. Thoughtful chapters on these topics round up this book.

"Medicine is a passionate mistress and brooks no rivals" and transplantation medicine more so. I commend the Editors for undertaking the arduous task of developing a textbook that surely will be useful to Fellows in Nephrology and Transplantation, and Nephrologists and Transplant Physicians, practicing in a community or in an academic setting. Indeed, all involved in the care transplant patients would be well-served by this erudite, comprehensive book on transplantation.

Manikkam Suthanthiran, MD
Stanton Griffis Distinguished Professor of Medicine
Chief, Division of Nephrology and Hypertension
Weill Cornell Medical College

Chief, Department of Transplantation Medicine
New York-Presbyterian Hospital/Weill Cornell Medical Center
New York, NY, USA

PREFACE

On December 23, 1954, Joseph E. Murray, a plastic surgeon interested in skin grafting related to battle casualties, performed the history -making first successful living donor kidney transplantation between identical twins at the Peter Bent Brigham Hospital in Boston, Massachusetts. This started a series of events that revolutionized the field of nephrology. The first kidney transplant would precede the first successful dialysis for chronic kidney failure by 6 years. Today, kidney transplantation has become commonplace therapy for patients with end-stage kidney disease (ESKD); however, it is severely limited by a shortage of available kidneys.

Kidney transplantation, more than any other specialty, is a multidisciplinary field, bringing together transplant surgeons, nephrologists, immunologists, urologists, infectious diseases specialists, and many others. It sometimes involves a surgical procedure on perfectly healthy living donors. In recognition of the creativity and innovation in kidney transplantation, the Nobel Prize in Physiology or Medicine was awarded to Drs. Joseph E. Murray and E. Donnall Thomas in 1990. There have been others who have received the Nobel Prize for their contributions to transplantation or to the theories and algorithms that led to kidney transplant allocation [1], [2]. The successes in kidney transplantation and advances in transplant immunosuppression have opened the door to the transplantation of other organs.

As transplantation developed over the past 67 years, it fulfilled a gap in medical care, and is now a major discipline in medicine. Thus, it was necessary to create a book in the Issues in Kidney Disease series completely dedicated to kidney transplantation. This book was a two-year effort orchestrated by frequent dialogs and exchange of ideas that would make it more useable and relevant to renal fellows and all members of the disciplines caring for kidney transplant patients. We assembled a national group of renowned authors, each highly respected for his or her expertise and skill. The result is a collection of 17 chapters, each timely addressing challenges and controversies, which has collectively become our knowledge-base for transplantation. We hope you find this book valuable for navigating this complex field.

Issues in Kidney Disease–Transplantation is a collection of seventeen independent chapters written by renowned authors, covering a wide range of topics in the spectrum of this vast discipline.

This book will appeal to renal fellows, nephrologists, transplant surgeons, urologists, transplant coordinators, social workers, and all other physicians and allied professionals involved with the care of kidney transplant patients, and those interested in the advancement of science. It brings timely and updated reviews and addresses trends, challenges, and controversies of topics and issues related to transplantation .

REFERENCES

[1] Rutkowski P, Ostrowski J, Debska-Slizien A, Rutkowski B. Nobel Prize Winners Who Contributed To Transplantation. *G Ital Nefrol.* 2018;35(Suppl 70):55-60.

[2] Andersson T, Lyttkens CH. [Economic matching theory in renal transplantation. Sveriges Riksbank Prize in Economic Sciences in Memory of Alfred Nobel 2012]. *Lakartidningen.* 2012;109(49-50):2276-7.

ACKNOWLEDGMENTS

We would like to thank those contributors who spent hours researching and refining their chapters. Our publisher, Nova Science, was very helpful in giving us guidance and support.

Moving a manuscript into a format that is readable and understandable, yet with appropriate use of punctuation, correct spelling, and grammar that is exact and precise takes a highly skilled person. We are so grateful for Michelle (Misha) L. Nguyen, our Master Copy Editor, who reads every word of each manuscript and makes certain that the writing is clear and free of errors. She has made a major positive impact on the quality of this work.

We would also like to acknowledge our families. Work of this proportion requires time outside of our busy clinical responsibilities - late into the evenings, early in the mornings, and each weekend. The passionate support and patience of our wives to bear with our erratic hours is deeply appreciated and cherished.

Finally, we would like to acknowledge each of our patients. We have learned much from you; your well-being is our ultimate goal. The gratification we gain from caring for you drives the motivation behind this effort.

EDITORS' CONTACT INFORMATION

Bhamidipati V. R. Murthy, MD, DM
Selzman Institute for Kidney Health, Section of Nephrology,
and Division of Abdominal Transplantation, Department of Surgery,
Baylor College of Medicine, Houston, TX, USA
Email: bvmurthy@bcm.edu.

Stephen Z. Fadem, MD, FACP, FASN
Selzman Institute for Kidney Health, Section of Nephrology,
and Michael E. DeBakey Veterans Affairs Medical Center,
Baylor College of Medicine, Houston, TX, USA;
Kidney Associates, Houston, TX, USA
Email: fadem@fbcm.edu.

List of Contributors

Nidhi Aggarwal, MD
Selzman Institute for Kidney Health, Section of Nephrology,
and Michael E. DeBakey Veterans Affairs Medical Center,
Baylor College of Medicine, Houston, TX, USA

Medha Airy, MD
Selzman Institute for Kidney Health, Section of Nephrology,
Baylor College of Medicine, Houston, TX, USA

Joseph Alge, MD
Division of Nephrology, Department of Pediatrics,
Baylor College of Medicine, Houston, TX, USA

Mauricio A. Amaya, AGACNP-BC2
Division of Abdominal Transplantation, Department of Surgery,
Baylor College of Medicine, Houston, TX, USA

Ahmed A. Awan, MD, FASN
Selzman Institute for Kidney Health, Section of Nephrology,
and Division of Abdominal Transplantation, Department of Surgery,
Baylor College of Medicine, Houston, TX, USA

Enrico Benedetti, MD
Departments of Surgery and Pharmacy, University of Illinois at Chicago,
Chicago, IL, USA

Sadhna Dhingra, MD
Department of Pathology and Immunology, Baylor St Luke's Medical Center,
Baylor College of Medicine, Houston, TX, USA

Pierpaolo Di Cocco, MD
Departments of Surgery and Pharmacy, University of Illinois at Chicago,
Chicago, IL, USA

Angelina Edwards, MD
Division of Kidney Diseases, Hypertension & Transplantation, Department of Medicine,
Houston Methodist Hospital, Houston, TX, USA

Elizabeth Godfrey, MD
Division of Abdominal Transplantation, Department of Surgery,
Baylor College of Medicine, Houston, TX, USA

Marion Hemmersbach-Miller, MD, PhD
Section of Infectious Diseases, Department of Medicine,
Baylor College of Medicine, Houston, TX, USA

Peter Jindra, PhD, D(ABHI)
Division of Abdominal Transplantation, Department of Surgery,
Baylor College of Medicine, Houston, TX, USA

Bruce Kaplan, MD
Colorado Center for Transplant Care, Research and Education,
University of Colorado, Aurora, CO, USA

Pascale Khairallah, MD
Selzman Institute for Kidney Health, Section of Nephrology,
and Michael E. DeBakey Veterans Affairs Medical Center,
Baylor College of Medicine, Houston, TX, USA

Taquiuddin Khaja MD
Selzman Institute for Kidney Health, Section of Nephrology,
Baylor College of Medicine, Houston, TX, USA

Tyler M. Lambing, MD
Section of Infectious Diseases, Department of Medicine,
Baylor College of Medicine, Houston, TX, USA

Bhamidipati V. R. Murthy, MD, DM
Selzman Institute for Kidney Health, Section of Nephrology,
and Division of Abdominal Transplantation, Department of Surgery,
Baylor College of Medicine, Houston, TX, USA

Mohanram Narayanan, MD
Division of Nephrology and Hypertension, Department of Medicine,
Texas A&M Health Science Center College of Medicine,
Baylor Scott & White Medical Center, Temple, TX, USA

Jenny S. Pan, MD
Selzman Institute for Kidney Health, Section of Nephrology,
and Michael E. DeBakey Veterans Affairs Medical Center,
Baylor College of Medicine, Houston, TX, USA

Vishnu Parvathareddy, MD
Selzman Institute for Kidney Health, Section of Nephrology,
Baylor College of Medicine, Houston, TX, USA

Abbas Rana, MD
Division of Abdominal Transplantation, Department of Surgery,
Baylor College of Medicine, Houston, TX, USA

Manikkam Suthanthiran, MD
Division of Nephrology and Hypertension, Weill Cornell Medical College,
New York, NY USA; Department of Transplantation Medicine,
New York-Presbyterian Hospital, New York, NY USA

Stephen Blake Tanner, MD
Division of Nephrology and Hypertension, Department of Medicine,
Texas A&M Health Science Center College of Medicine,
Baylor Scott & White Medical Center, Temple, TX, USA

Luan D. Truong, MD
Department of Pathology and Genomic Medicine, Houston Methodist Hospital,
Houston, TX, USA

Charles T. Van Buren, MD
Department of Surgery, McGovern School of Medicine, University of Texas Health,
Houston, TX, USA

Patricia West-Thielke, Pharm D
Departments of Surgery and Pharmacy, University of Illinois at Chicago,
Chicago, IL, USA

In: Issues in Kidney Disease – Transplantation
Editors: B. V. R. Murthy and S. Z. Fadem
ISBN: 978-1-53619-960-4

Chapter 1

AN OVERVIEW OF KIDNEY TRANSPLANTATION

Charles T. Van Buren*, MD
Department of Surgery, McGovern School of Medicine, University of Texas Health, Houston, TX, USA

ABSTRACT

The field of transplantation originated from Nobel Prize winning investigations into the technical and immunological challenges of transplanting vascularized organs into living beings. Once the technical feat of sewing the organ into the new host was achieved, the nature of specific immune responsiveness needed to be understood, as well as the means of limiting this host response with medications. As the effectiveness of immunosuppressive drugs improved, means of allocating and preserving this limited resource of transplantable organs was developed. This chapter outlines the successes and the challenges of clinical transplantation over the years, as well as the scope for the future.

Keywords: kidney transplantation, history, immunosuppression

INTRODUCTION

The science of transplantation has developed in the pursuit of a quest for relieving human suffering because of organ failure. The human body's response to a foreign tissue, the central theme of organ transplant rejection, has been the biggest hurdle to overcome for success of organ transplantation. This has led to the understanding of the rejection process, the development of drugs targeting the important steps to mitigate this reaction, and efforts to prolong the rejection-free survival of the allograft by maintaining the

---

* Corresponding Author's Email: chasvb@sbcglobal.net.

immunosuppression at an optimal level. This field is thus led by both innovative experimental and clinical investigations. Simultaneously, surgical techniques needed to be developed and refined for organ perfusion and easy access for biopsies for recognition of complications. The concepts of brain death and brain-stem death, and the enactment of the organ transplantation act have led to increasing the scope and safe retrieval of organs from potential deceased donors. Then came the challenge of equitable allocation of a scarce resource for an increasing demand of organs. This chapter will outline these developments in the challenging field of kidney transplantation.

The field of renal transplantation is based upon both innovative experimental and clinical investigations resulting in international recognition of the innovators. Alexis Carrel in 1912 received the Nobel Prize in Medicine for his technique of suturing blood vessels and auto-transplantation [1]. He noted that transplantation of organs between animals of the same species inevitably led to atrophy of the transplanted organ, for unknown reasons. The same observation was noted for non-vascularized transplants such as skin grafts. Gibson and Medawar noted in a patient who received graft of her own skin (autologous skin graft) was accepted and expanded; the skin donated from her brother (heterologous) was initially vascularized but failed to proliferate. It was eventually rejected by a process that histologically was marked by a mononuclear infiltrate and eventual necrosis of the transplanted skin. A second skin graft from the brother degenerated within 3-4 days, a so-called "second set phenomenon" [2]. Medawar then tested the basis of this phenomenon observed in man in skin grafting experiments in rabbits. The rejection of skin grafts from a second rabbit was increased if a larger amount of skin was grafted, occurring 4-5 days earlier than in animals bearing a lower burden of a foreign tissue. Second skin grafts from the same donor animal were rejected rapidly within 4 to 5 days. The blood vessels that extended into the second skin grafts showed endothelial disruption and engorgement of the vessels [3]. Thus, Medawar documented the histological differences in man and rabbits of primary and secondary skin graft rejection, and the importance of the load of foreign antigen on the rate of immunization against the foreign tissue. Medawar's later experiments injecting neonatal cells into fetal inbred mice and then later successfully grafting these mice with skin from the same donor strain proved the possibility of establishing specific tolerance to a given donor, while maintaining the recipient animal's ability to reject a third-party skin graft [4]. Due to the results of these experiments, the Nobel Prize in Medicine was awarded to Medawar in 1960. This experimental achievement of specific transplantation tolerance has been the aspiration of clinical transplant physicians ever since.

Because of the possibility of rejection, most early work in renal transplantation had resulted in only temporary success. In 1946, a patient was referred with acute renal failure due to massive hemolysis to the Peter Bent Brigham Hospital (PBBH), Boston, MA. After several days of conservative medical therapy that failed to result in a recovery of the patient's own renal function, Dr. David Hume transplanted a kidney from a recently deceased accident victim attaching the kidney vessels to the brachial artery and median cubital vein under local anesthesia. The kidney remained outside the patient's body, covered with a moist gauze, while the ureter dripped urine into a flask. A few days later, the patient's own kidneys began to function, and the cadaver donor kidney could be removed [5]. A series of renal transplants from unrelated donors were then performed by Dr. Hume, with most kidneys being placed in the thigh of the patient and the ureter draining urine externally. The longest success from this series was 175 days of function, with little to no immunosuppression given [6]. Jean Hamburger, another pioneer in the field of transplantation, collaborating with the surgeon Rene Kuss, had transplanted patients with kidneys from executed prisoners. His transplantation of a living donor kidney from a mother into her son in 1952 resulted in function of the kidney for three weeks before it was rejected. The biopsy of the rejecting kidney had pathologic features paralleling those observed by Medawar in his homologous skin transplants from living related donors [7]. Hamburger also predicted the usefulness of corticosteroids in treatment of rejection episodes.

With these frustrations in overcoming the rejection response to the donor tissue, an opportunity appeared when a 22-year-old patient with glomerulonephritis was referred to Dr. John Merrill at the PBBH for treatment. Fortunately, the patient had an identical twin brother. At his time, there was no laboratory test to confirm that the brothers were in fact twins. In the potential transplant recipient, the protein malnutrition, causing both hair thinning and as well as reddish discoloration, along with change in stature due to renal rickets, made the siblings different in physical appearance. To confirm genetic identity, skin grafts were transferred between the twins [8]. The grafts were not rejected, and it confirmed the twins were identical. The kidney transplant was performed at the PBBH on December 23, 1954, with Dr. Joseph Murray performing the kidney transplant. With prompt functioning of the transplant, the patient's hypertension resolved, and the patient was discharged with a new functioning kidney [9]. In 1990, Dr. Murray shared the Nobel Prize in Medicine with E. Donnell Thomas for their pioneering work in solid organ and bone marrow transplant ation, respectively.

Unfortunately, even with an identical twin as a donor, without immunosuppression problems occurred. As had been anticipated by Merrill, identical twin recipients with glomerulonephritis as their original disease were prone to recurrence of the disease in the new transplant. One was replacing one target organ with another with the same nephritogenic humoral facts still present in the patient. In fact, Glassock reported that of 17 patients with glomerulonephritis as their original disease, 65% (11/17) had recurrence of the glomerulonephritis and 41% of these patients died due to this recurrence [10]. Among those succumbing to recurrent disease was the first successful identical twin renal transplant, dying 8 years after his historical operation.

New methods of controlling the rejection response or diminishing the damage of autoimmune diseases were needed. Hamburger again led the way with subtotal irradiation of the recipient prior to renal transplantation. Although this case and Merrill's case at the PBBH were both successful with long-term success, the myelosuppression induced by the radiation was unpredictable and often led to neutropenia and sepsis [11].

In 1959, Schwartz and Dameshek noted that 6-mercaptopurine (6MP) was able to reduce antibody responses to foreign protein in rabbits [12]. Roy Calne, a young English surgeon, recognized the opportunity this discovery offered for organ transplantation. In 1960, he reported remarkable prolongation of kidney transplant survival in mongrel dogs using 6MP [13]. Calne noted the difficulty in avoiding fatal bone marrow suppression using 6MP. Collaborating with George Hitchings of Burroughs Wellcome, Calne noted improved efficacy as well as diminished toxicity of an imidazole derivative of 6MP, azathioprine, in a large study of canine renal transplants [14]. George Hitchings, in 1988, shared the Nobel Prize in Medicine with two others for their work developing drugs for transplantation and chemotherapy .

Calne's work in animals stimulated the PBBH group to use azathioprine in transplanting renal failure patients with organs from living or cadaveric donors. Murray and colleagues reported treatment of 13 cases with azathioprine [15]. Although most of the cadaver donor kidneys had survival for over a month, reflecting the relatively poor preservation techniques as well as the kidneys having been retrieved under suboptimal conditions from critically ill donors, there were five allografts with long term survival, including one from a cadaver donor that survived 363 days. A new era began in renal transplantation with the widespread use of azathioprine immunosuppression .

Two further developments expanded the population of patients that could be served by renal transplantation. The first was the definition of the concept of brain death as defined by a Harvard criteria protocol [16]. This, plus the passage of the Uniform Anatomic Gift Act, permitted transplant surgeons to obtain consent from donor families of the altruistic gift of lifesaving organs. These organs could then be removed in controlled conditions in the operating room while the heart was till beating, keeping the organs well-perfused [17].

The increase in organ donors from brain dead individuals necessitated better means of preserving these organs from the time of removal until the time of transplantation. Euro-Collins solution was developed, proving superior to Ringer's lactate for preservation, partially due to both its attempts to duplicate intracellular electrolyte concentrations and its hyperosmolarity, to mimic cellular swelling which occurs under hypoxic preservation conditions [18]. This was the mainstay perfusate for organ preservation until Belzer and his colleagues at the University of Wisconsin developed a solution which proved superior for liver preservation. This solution, called UW solution, was hyperosmolar (320 mOsm), and contained potassium lactobionate (100 mM), potassium phosphate (25 mM), magnesium sulfate (5 mM), raffinose (30 mM), adenosine (5 mM), glutathione (3 mM), allopurinol (1 mM). This solution proved superior to Euro-Collins for preservation of the liver and has consequently displaced Euro-Collins solution as the perfusate of choice for organ preservation [19]. Other perfusates have been developed of varying composition, but none have proven superior to UW solutions.

It was recognized early in clinical transplantation that living donor renal transplants fared better than transplants from cadaveric donors. Hamburger was quick to note the work of Jean Dausset on leuko-agglutinating antisera and febrile transfusion responses might have relevance to immunologic responses to renal transplants. Hamburger and Dausset, retrospectively, examined the outcomes of renal transplants and correlated these results with pretransplant sera compatibilities with the donor leukocyte antigens [20]. Collaboration between Europe and America led to identification and classification of sera from multiparous women or multiple-transfused individuals that were directed against specific human leukocyte antigens (HLA) that became recognized to be associated with the major histocompatibility complex in man. Class I antigens, that evoked vigorous antibody responses, were labeled in the order they were identified. Thus, antigens such as A1 and A2 were both common in the general population and evoked vigorous antibody responses when exposed to individuals who lacked. Transplantation with a kidney bearing an antigen toward which the recipient has an antibody directed can result in hyperacute rejection of the transplant [21]. To avoid such reactions, cytotoxic antibodies in the recipient against the putative donor were screened for by incubating recipient serum against donor lymphocytes in the presence of complement and eosin dye. Dye leaking into the cells revealed damage to the cells by the serum of the recipient amounted to a positive lymphocyte crossmatch and precluded renal transplantation.

In 1978, the PBBH group published their historical experience with renal transplantation [22]. The 1-year mortality rate post renal transplantation in the early to mid-1970s hovered about 15%, without a discernible improvement in transplant success despite vigorous immunosuppression. Once the protocol eliminated seven grams of methylprednisolone for treatment of rejection in favor of 3 grams of the drug, mortality rate of the living related recipients decreased to 2% and those of cadaveric renal transplants to 4%. Graft survival of living donor renal transplants was approximately 80% at one year; the success rates for recipients of cadaveric donor kidneys were approximately 45% at one year. With these types of complications and successes, the demand for renal transplants did not greatly exceed the supply.

Several additional means of immunosuppression were developed in an attempt to make immunosuppression more effective. Both experimentally and in clinical use, the thoracic duct fistula decreased rejection rates in patients receiving corticosteroid and azathioprine immunosuppression [23]. The use of the fistula was optimal when it was placed prior to transplantation in living donor renal transplants. Patients with well-functioning fistulas developed lymphopenia and subsequently had fewer rejection episodes compared to those with poorly functioning fistulas. However, in this report, 45% of the patients had poorly functioning fistulas, and had a high mortality rate. The labor-intensive daily drainage of the patient's lymph combined with the high rate of septic complications limited the application of this technique.

The use of total lymph node irradiation for the treatment of Hodgkin's disease was noted to be associated with lymphopenia. Levin B et al. applied this to organ transplantation, and in their study, 25 patients were treated with total lymph node irradiation prior to cadaveric renal transplant, with weekly boosts of irradiation until transplantation. At the time of transplantation, patients were treated with a brief course of anti-thymocyte globulin, and daily low-dose prednisone [24]. Patients were supplemented with a 3-month course of azathioprine if they had two or more rejection episodes. Graft survival was 76% at two years, with 2 grafts having been lost to rejection. Patient survival was 84%. The problem with this regimen was maintaining radiation treatment over potentially an awfully long time until a transplant was available. A subset of these patients was studied two years post-transplant ation. Nine patients who had only one or no rejection episodes, had a serum creatinine below 2 mg/dl, and who had a mixed lymphocyte culture (MLC) index of 5 or greater against a panel of lymphocytes from four random donors were studied for responsiveness to frozen lymphocytes from the kidney donor. All individuals exhibited donor specific unresponsiveness while maintaining a vigorous response against third party donor lymphocytes [25]. This documents that at least a subset of patients could develop a muted immune response to donor antigens.

An alternative treatment for high-risk living related donor (LRD) haploidentical recipients who manifested high MLC responsiveness to their potential donor was advocated by the group at the University of California at San Francisco. These patients at this center had experienced a kidney transplant success rate scarcely better than achieved by patients with cadaveric renal transplants. Forty five patients were deliberately transfused with three successive units of donor blood prior to LRD renal transplants. At least 29% of patients developed a positive cytotoxic crossmatch with their donor and could not receive the transplant from their living donor. Thirty patients received a transplant from their living donor. The success rate was 94% at one year, with only 44% of patients experiencing rejection episodes. The historical comparators had experienced an 82% rejection episode rate. The kidney transplant success at one year was 94% [26]. The risk of this approach was sensitizing high immune responders with blood transfusion, risking their access to future transplants. Still, as with total lymphoid irradiation, there was a subset of patients who proved susceptible to immune modulation .

Anti-thymocyte globulin (ATG) was used as an adjuvant to azathioprine and prednisone immunosuppression. This polyclonal product, when administered at the time of cadaver donor renal transplant with concomitant azathioprine and prednisone immune suppression, significantly improved the allograft survival of strong immune responders compared to those not treated by ATG. No improvement in outcome was noted for weak immune responders [27]. Once again, tailoring treatment to the immune responder status of the host was necessary to optimize outcomes.

In 1978, Roy Calne, the surgeon who innovated the use of azathioprine, reported improved preclinical and clinical results with a new drug Cyclosporin A [28]. He reported a high degree of success with minimal rejection in these kidney transplant patients. An expanded experience with Calne's group documented excellent graft survival but a disturbing 9% incidence of lymphomas [29]. This was not duplicated in the Phase 2 studies of the drug in the United States and may have been due to the difference in dose administered (25 mg/kg/day by Calne versus 14 mg/kg/day in U.S. trials) [30]. The incidence in lymphoma is not unique to any one agent, but rather due to over immunosuppression of the recipient. As cyclosporine A came into wider clinical use, it improved both LRD and cadaveric donor kidney transplant survival significantly [31, 32]. The risk of rejection decreased remarkably as did the mortality rate post-transplant, even for older patients. This markedly increased the demand for transplantable kidneys .

In 1984, in response to public demand, the Congress passed the National Organ Transplant Act, which called for a national network to be established to coordinate allocation and distribution of transplantable organs. The United Network for Organ Sharing (UNOS) was awarded the contract to provide this service under the auspices of HHS [33]. The matching system for distributing kidneys from cadaveric donors was initially based on blood group, HLA match, and panel reactive antibody (PRA) level. National matching was required for those patients who had a six HLA antigen match with donors anywhere in the country. Although early in its existence it was documented that HLA matching discriminated against African Americans ' access to cadaver donor kidneys, this injudicious allocation priority continued for over twenty years until the points for matching HLA A, B, or C locus antigens was eliminated from the priority matching [34, 35]. After this the waiting time for African American recipients improved compared to non-Hispanic white patients' waiting time on the list.

As outcomes for renal transplants steadily improved, both the list as well as the waiting time until transplantation steadily grew, until at present the waiting list numbers over 99,522 patients. Fewer than 40% of these patients receive a deceased donor kidney transplant within five years of being placed on the transplant waiting list [36, 37]. The interest in living donor renal transplantation increased with the advent of laparoscopic kidney donation [38]. This decreased the postoperative pain and length of hospital stay for living donors and increased donation rates for living donor kidneys. The laparoscopic donor nephrectomy is not without problems. At least 8 donor perioperative deaths and 15 technical graft losses have been reported, which probably underrepresents the actual experience [39].

As the clinical success of live donor transplantation improved with better immunosuppression, the pool of potential donors expanded. Living unrelated donation, most commonly in the form of spousal donation, became more common. The success rate of these living donor renal transplants surpassed that of deceased donor transplants, leading to continued growth of this donor source [40]. In cases of sensitized recipients or those with an ABO incompatibility with their potential donor, paired donation registries have arisen to match pairs of potential donor recipient combinations to facilitate exchange of living unrelated kidneys to the compatible recipient, either synchronously or as chains of donation [41].

Though kidney transplant survival improved with the routine use of cyclosporine therapy, there were still clinical problems that persisted. The routine incidence of rejection episodes was approximately 40%. A poor correlation between trough levels of cyclosporine and the area under the curve (AUC) of the drug following a dose (correlation coefficient or r^2 of 0.71), may have been responsible. With the introduction of the micro-emulsion mixture of cyclosporine in 1992, the stability of the drug levels significantly improved, with a much better correlation between trough levels and the AUC (r^2 of 0·91), and corresponding decrease in acute rejection episodes [42]. In addition, nephrotoxicity of cyclosporine made management of kidneys with delayed graft function difficult.

The introduction of monoclonal antibodies to targets in the immune reaction cascade has started a new era in the immunosuppression management of transplantation. OKT3, a monoclonal antibody against the T cell receptor, was the first to be introduced, and was very effective in treating steroid resistant rejections, as well as popular as an induction agent [43]. This monoclonal led to cytokine storms in a disturbingly large minority of patients, making it difficult to advocate it as a routine induction agent. Basiliximab, a monoclonal antibody against the IL-2 receptor, for induction decreased acute rejection episodes in cyclosporine -treated patients from 49 to 35% [44]. This drug had few side effects and was easy to add to the induction regimen.

The lack of correlation between trough level and AUC with cyclosporine continued to pose a challenge in some patients even with the use of micro-emulsification formulation. Cyclosporine level 2 hours after the dose (C2) was noted to be a better correlate in these patients, but this monitoring was cumbersome in an outpatient clinic setting [45]. A macrolide immunosuppressant, tacrolimus (Tac), had overcome some of the disadvantages of cyclosporine. It had a similar mechanism of action (calcineurin inhibition), but it had a much better correlation between the trough level and the AUC. Tac has a different side effect profile than cyclosporine - less hypertension and lipid metabolism abnormalities, more diabetes and neurotoxicity [46]. It is at least as nephrotoxic as cyclosporine. Because of the ease of regulating drug exposure by monitoring trough levels, there is less rejection using this agent and it has displaced cyclosporine as the mainstay of renal transplant immunosuppression [47]. Both drugs have relatively short half-lives. This makes them both vulnerable to variations in drug exposure on the same dose of drug. The coefficient of variation in AUC on the same dose of drug is directly correlated to increasing creatinine due to chronic rejection [48].

Azathioprine as an adjunct to immunosuppressive maintenance regimens was replaced after 1995 with mycophenolate mofetil, an immunosuppressant which suppressed T lymphocyte proliferation. The initial studies in cyclosporine -treated patients documented a decrease in treated rejection episodes from 46 to 17% compared to patients with placebo [49]. The drug has been less successful when used alone with steroid therapy in the absence of calcineurin inhibitors, with unacceptably high incidence of treated rejection [50]. It requires no drug level monitoring in usual clinical use, and is perhaps the most widely used agent besides corticosteroids in renal transplant maintenance regimens [51].

Attempting to minimize calcineurin -inhibitor exposure, a new class of agents, the mammalian Target Of Rapamycin (mTOR) inhibitors, was tested with low dose calcineurin regimens. Sirolimus, the first of its class to be introduced, could successfully be used to treat patients with low dose cyclosporine [52]. The advantage of this drug for maintenance was its long half-life; little week-to-week variation in drug exposure was seen on a stable dose of drug. The problem with using it as an induction agent was its long half-life. If the patient was a rapid metabolizer, one could not rapidly increase the levels, since no intravenous formulation was available [53]. Its side effects include proteinuria, hyperlipidemia, and wound healing problems. Because of proteinuria, converting patients with chronic rejection to this drug was not very effective [54]. Both this drug and everolimus, the other mToR inhibitor clinically used for renal transplant patients, can reduce calcineurin inhibitor exposure due to a synergistic interaction with cyclosporine, an interaction not observed with tacrolimus [52]. mToR inhibitors appear to be the only immunosuppressants that do not increase the incidence of malignancies in renal transplant recipients [55].

Belatacept was approved by the FDA in 2011 for kidney transplantation. This drug permits the clinician to avoid calcineurin inhibitors (CNI) and results in better long-term kidney transplant function. The incidence of treated rejection was similar between the belatacept and CNI groups. The initial studies revealed a higher incidence of post-transplant lymphoma in the belatacept group, leading to the recommendation to avoid this drug in CMV negative recipients. A better kidney function and less kidney scarring on biopsy were noted with belatacept compared to the CNI treated patients [56]. The optimum setting and accompanying immunosuppression to be used with belatacept remains to be determined.

Steroid withdrawal has been attempted in each era of immunosuppressive therapy. While it is popular with pediatric kidney transplantation, limitations exist with adult kidney transplant recipients. This is covered in more detail elsewhere in the book.

Renal transplantation has continued to be complicated by delayed graft function of the newly transplanted deceased donor kidney. To combat this problem, Dr. Belzer developed a perfusion pump to constantly perfuse the kidney ex vivo rather than storing it in a sterile bag surrounded by ice [57]. While this was an improved function of deceased donor kidneys at the University of Wisconsin, the technology became widely used only in the past 15 years. The multicenter report documented that there was a significant decrease in delayed graft function in the machine perfused kidneys compared to cold storage kidneys. This resulted in an improved kidney transplant survival at one year [58].

Conclusion

Kidney transplant survival, either from a living or from a deceased donor, has improved markedly since the first transplants in the 1950s. The improved outcomes have been due to improved immunosuppression, improved ex-vivo preservation of the kidneys, and improved logistics for matching the appropriate donor and recipient. Further improvements depend upon improved preservation of the transplants to optimize donor recipient matches and achievement of the still unrealized dream of specific tolerance to the donated kidney .

References

[1] Carrel A. *Nobel Lectures. Physiology or Medicine 1901–1921*. Amsterdam: Elsevier Publishing Company, 1967.

[2] Gibson T and Medawar PB. Fate of Skin Homografts in Man, *J Anat*, 1943; 77: 299-308.

[3] Medawar PB. The behavior and fate of skin autografts and homografts in rabbits: A report to the War Wounds Committee of the Medical Research Council. *J Anat*, 1944; 78: 176-99.

[4] Billingham RE, Brent L, Medawar PB. "Actively acquired tolerance" of foreign cells. *Nature*. 1953; 172: 603–06.

[5] Moore FD. "Rejection, Twins, Irradiation" in "A Miracle and a Privilege – Recounting A Half Century of Surgical Advance". Joseph Henry Press, 1995; 159-77.

[6] Hume D, Merril JP, Miller BF. Homologous transplantation of human Kidneys, *J Clin Invest*, 1952; 31: 640-41.

[7] Lengendre C, Kreis H. A Tribute to Jean Hamburger's Contribution to Organ Transplantation, *Am J Transplant*, 2010; 10: 2392-95.

[8] Tilney N. Renal transplant between identical twins: A review. *World J Surg*, 1986; 10: 381-88.

[9] Merril JP, Murray JE, Harrison JH. Successful homotransplantation of the human kidney between identical twins; *JAMA*, 1956; 160: 277-82.

[10] Glassock R, Feldman D, Reynolds E, Dammin G, Merrill J. Human renal isografts: a clinical and pathologic analysis; *Medicine (Baltimore)*, 1968; 47: 411-54.

[11] Merrill J, Murray J, Harrison H, Friedman E, Dealy J, Dammin G. Successful homotransplantation of the kidney between nonidentical twins. *N Engl J Med,* 1960; 262: 1251-60.

[12] Schwartz R, Dameshek W. Drug induced immunologic tolerance. *Nature*, 1959; 183: 1682-83.

[13] Calne R. The rejection of renal homografts inhibition in dogs by 6-Mercaptopurine. *Lancet*, 1960; 1(7121): 417-18.

[14] Calne R. Inhibition of the rejection of renal homografts in dogs by drugs. *Ann R Coll Surg Engl,* 1963; 32: 281-302.

[15] Murray J, Merrill J, Harrison H, Wilson R, Dammin G. Prolonged survival of human kidney homografts by immunosuppressive drug therapy. *N Engl J Med*, 1963; 268: 1315-23.

[16] Anonymous. A Definition of Irreversible Coma: Report of the Ad Hoc Committee of Harvard Medical School to Examine the Definition of Brain Death. *JAMA*, 1968; 205: 337-40.

[17] Uniform Anatomical Gift Act, 1968.

[18] Kreis H. Renal preservation - in "*Renal Transplantation: Theory and Practice*", Eds. Hamburger, J, Crosnier, J, Bach, JF, Kreis, H., 2nd Edn, Williams and Wilkins, 1981: 70-88.

[19] Southard J, Belzer F. Organ preservation. *Annu Rev Med*, 1995; 46: 235-47.

[20] Rapaport F, Dausset J, Hamburger J, Hume D, Dano K, Williams G, Milgrom F. Serologic factors in human transplantation, *Ann Surg*, 1967; 166: 596-608.

[21] Amos D, Sanfilippo F. *Transplantation Antigens and Immune Mechanisms, in Textbook of Surgery*, Ed: Sabiston, D. W.B. Saunders, 1986: 381-93.

[22] Tilney N, Strom T, Vineyard G, Merrill J. Factors contributing to the declining mortality rate in renal transplantation, *N Engl J Med*, 1978; 299: 1321-25.

[23] Tilney N, Murray J. The thoracic duct fistula as an adjunct to human immunosuppression in human renal transplantation, *Transplantation*, 1967; 5 (Suppl 4):1204-08.

[24] Levin B, Collins G, Mark W, Girisnsky T, Hoppe RT, Miller E, Bieber C, Strober S. Treatment of cadaveric renal transplant recipients with total lymphoid irradiation, anti-thymocyte globulin and low dose prednisone, *Lancet*, 1985; 2 (8468): 1321-25.

[25] Chow D, Saper V, Strober S. Renal transplant patients treated with total lymphoid irradiation show specific unresponsiveness to donor antigens, *J Immunol*, 1987; 138: 3746-50.

[26] Salvatierra O, Vincente F, Amend W, Potter D, Iwaki Y, Opelz G, Terasaki P, Duca R, Cochrum K, Hanes D, Stoney R, Feduska N. Deliberate donor specific blood transfusions prior to living donor renal transplantation. A new approach, *Ann Surg*, 1980; 192: 543-52.

[27] Kerman R, Floyd M, Van Buren C, Kahan B. Improved allograft survival of strong immune responder high risk recipients with adjuvant antithymocyte globulin therapy, *Transplantation*, 1980; 30: 450-54.

[28] Calne R, Thiru S, McMaster P, Craddock G, White D, Evans D, Dunn D, Pentlow B, Rolles K. Cyclosporine A in patients receiving allografts from cadaver donors, *Lancet*, 1978; 2 (8104): 1323-27.

[29] Calne R, Rolles K, Thiru S, McMaster P, Craddock G, Aziz S, White D, Evans D, Dunn D, Hernderson R, Lewis P. Cyclosporin A as the only immunosuppressant in 34 recipients of cadaveric organs, *Lancet*, 1979; 2 (8151):1033-36.

[30] Kahan B. Cosmos and Damian in the twentieth century, *N Engl J Med*, 1981; 305: 280-81.

[31] Anonymous. Randomized clinical trial of cyclosporine A in cadaveric renal transplantation - Canadian Multicentre Transplant Study group, *N Engl J Med*, 1986; 314: 1219-25.

[32] Lewis R, Janney R, Golden D, Kerr N, Van Buren C, Kerman R, Kahan B. Stability of renal allograft function associated with long term cyclosporine immunosuppressive therapy - 5 year follow up, *Transplantation*, 1989; 47: 266-71.

[33] *UNOS history* at https://unos.org (UNOS website).

[34] Van Buren C, Lewis R, Kerman R, Kahan B. Exchanging donor kidneys - *N Engl J Med*, 1988; 319: 1092-94.

[35] Roberts J, Wolfe R, Bragg-Gresham J, Rush S, Wynn J, Distant D, Ashby V, Held P, Port F. Effect of changing priority for HLA matching on rates and outcomes of kidney transplantation in minority groups, *N Engl J Med*, 2004; 350: 545-51.

[36] *OPTN* website - https://optn.transplant .hrsa.gov/data/view-data-reports/national-data/ Accessed on 10/16/2020.

[37] Hart A, Smith J, Skeans M, Gustafson S, Wilk A, Castro S, Foutz J, Wainwright J, Snyder J, Kasiske B, Israni A. OPTN/SRTR 2018 Annual Data Report: Kidney. *Am J Transplant*, 2020; 20 (Suppl s1): 20-130.

[38] Ratner L, Ciseck L, Moore R, Cigarroa F, Kaufman H, Kavoussi L. Laparoscopic live donor nephrectomy, *Transplantation*, 1995; 60: 1047-49.

[39] Shokeir A. Open versus laparoscopic live donor nephrectomy: a focus on the safety of donors and the need for a donor registry, *J Urol*, 2007; 178: 1860-66.

[40] Terasaki P, Cecka M, Gjertson D, Takemoto S. High survival rates of kidney transplants from spousal and living unrelated donors, *N Engl J Med*, 1995; 333: 333-36.

[41] Akkina S, Muster S, Steffens E, Kim S, Kasiske B, Israni A. Donor exchange kidney transplantation: rationale and operational details from the North Central Exchange Cooperative; *Am J Kid Dis*, 2011; 57: 152-58.

[42] Kahan B. Therapeutic drug monitoring of cyclosporine – 20 years of progress, *Transpl Proc*, 2004; 36 (Suppl 2): S378-91.

[43] Norman D, Kahana L, Stuart F, Thistlethwaite J, Shield C, Monaco A, Dehlinger J, Wu S, Horn A, Haverty T. Randomized clinical trial of induction therapy with OKT3 in kidney transplantation, *Transplantation*, 1993; 55: 44-50.

[44] Kahan B, Rajagopalan P, Hall M. Reduction of the occurrence of acute cellular rejection among renal allograft recipients treated with basiliximab – a chimeric anti-interleukin-2 receptor monoclonal antibody. *Transplantation*, 1999; 67: 276-84.

[45] Takeuchi H, Matsuno N, Senuma K, Hirano T, Yokoyama T, Taira S, et al. Evidence of different pharmacokinetic relationship among AUC, peak, and trough levels between cyclosporine and tacrolimus in renal transplant patients using new pharmacokinetic parameter- why cyclosporine is monitored by C2 and tacrolimus by trough. *Biol Pharm Bull,* 2008; 31: 90-94.

[46] Hathaway D, Winsett R, Predergast M, Subaiya I. First report from the patient outcomes registry for transplant effects on life (PORTEL): differences in side-effects and quality of life by organ type, time since transplant and immunosuppressive regimens, *Clin Transplant*, 2003; 17: 183-94.

[47] Vincente F, Jensik S, Filo R, Miller J, Pirsch J. A long-term comparison of tacrolimus (FK506) and cyclosporine in kidney transplantation: evidence of improved graft survival at 5 years, *Transplantation*, 2002; 73: 775-82

[48] Kahan B, Welsh M, Schoenberg L, Rutsky L, Katz S, Urbauer D, Van Buren C. Variable oral absorption of cyclosporine: A biopharmaceutical risk factor for chronic rejection, *Transplantation*, 1996; 62: 599-606.

[49] Anonymous. Placebo-controlled study of mycophenolate mofetil combined with cyclosporin and corticosteroids for the prevention of rejection, European Mycophenolate Mofetil Cooperative Study Group; *Lancet*, 1995; 345: 1321-25.

[50] Roodnat J, Hilbrands L, Hene R, Sevaux R, Smak Gregoor P, Kal-van Gestel J, Konjin C, van Zuilen A, van Gelder T, Hoitsma A, Weimar W. 15 year follow-up of a multicenter, randomized, calcineurin inhibitor withdrawal study in kidney transplantation, *Transplantation*, 2014; 98: 47-53.

[51] van Gelder T, Hesselink D. Mycophenolate revisited, *Transpl Int*, 2015; 28: 508-15.

[52] Kahan B. Sirolimus: a comprehensive review, *Expert Opin Pharmacother*, 2005; 2: 1903-17.

[53] Anglicheau D, LeCorre D, Lechaton S, Laurent-Puig P, Kreis H, Beaune P, Legendre C, Thervet E. Consequences of genetic polymorphisms for sirolimus requirements after renal transplant in patients on primary sirolimus therapy, *Am J Transplant*, 2005; 5: 595-603.

[54] Haynes R, Blackwell L, Staplin N, Herrington W, Emberson J, Judge P, Storey B, Landray M, Harden P, Baigent C, Friend P. Campath, calcineurin inhibitor reduction and chronic allograft nephropathy (the 3C Study) - results of a randomized controlled clinical trial, The 3C collaborative Group. *Am J Transplant*, 2018; 18: 1424-34.

[55] Asleh R, Clavell A, Pereira N, Smith B, Briasoulis A, Alnsasra H, Kremers W, Haberman T, Otley C, Li X, Edwards B. Incidence of malignancies in patients treated with sirolimus following heart transplantation, *J Am Coll Cardiol*, 2019; 73: 2676-88.

[56] Masson P, Henderson L, Chapman J, Craig J, Webster A. Belatacept for kidney transplant recipients, *Cochrane Database Syst Rev*, 2014; (11). https://doi.org/10.1002/14651858.CD010699.pub2.

[57] Bonventre J, Weinberg J. Kidney preservation ex-vivo for transplantation, *Annu Rev Med*, 1992; 43: 523-51.

[58] Moers C, Smits J, Maathuis M, Treckmann J, van Gelder F, Napieralski B, Kasterop-Kutz J, et al. Machine perfusion or cold storage in deceased-donor kidney transplantation, *N Engl J Med*, 2009; 360: 7-19.

In: Issues in Kidney Disease – Transplantation
Editors: B. V. R. Murthy and S. Z. Fadem
ISBN: 978-1-53619-960-4

Chapter 2

MEDICAL EVALUATION OF THE POTENTIAL TRANSPLANT RECIPIENT

***Taquiuddin Khaja*[1]*, MD, Mauricio A. Amaya*[2]**
and Ahmed A. Awan*[1,2,*]*, MD, FASN
[1]Selzman Institute for Kidney Health, Section of Nephrology,
Baylor College of Medicine, Houston, TX, USA
[2]Division of Abdominal Transplantation, Department of Surgery,
Baylor College of Medicine, Houston, TX, USA

ABSTRACT

Kidney transplantation offers the best survival advantage to patients with advanced chronic kidney disease (CKD) and End-stage Kidney Disease (ESKD). However, a thorough evaluation prior to transplant is required to identify candidates who can be safely and successfully transplanted. This evaluation consists of a detailed history and physical examination by a transplant nephrologist, extensive laboratory evaluation, and multiple imaging studies to identify major comorbidities that can lead to adverse outcomes in the peri- and post-transplant period. However, it is also important to identify the social determinants, psychiatric tendencies, and financial limitations that might lead to less than optimum results after transplantation. Finally, a coordination among various members of the transplant team, as well as strong rapport with the patient and family, is vital to steer the patient through the long and sometimes frustrating maze of transplant evaluation and waitlisting. This chapter describes the clinical, as well as practical considerations during the evaluation of potential kidney transplant recipients based on the most recent guidelines by Kidney Disease: Improving Global Outcomes (KDIGO). Where a definitive recommendation is not available and decision is left to the individual transplant center, certain protocols are shared to provide a roadmap to the readers taking care of this patient population.

* Corresponding Author's Email: ahmed.awan@bcm.edu.

Keywords: pre-transplant evaluation, kidney transplant recipient, cardiovascular mortality, graft survival

Introduction

Kidney transplantation confers survival benefit to the recipients when compared to patients who remain on dialysis [1, 2]. However, not all patients with End-Stage Kidney Disease (ESKD) benefit uniformly from this major intervention. Evaluation and selection of patients who would benefit from kidney transplantation is a multidisciplinary effort, requiring input from the patient's primary nephrologist, transplant nephrologist, transplant surgeon, social worker, dietician, financial counselor, and transplant coordinators. A close collaboration among all these disciplines is vital to the success of this process. However, the center of the transplant universe is the patient, who has to commit himself/herself to this major undertaking. Without active participation and continued motivation on behalf of the patient and their families, the long and arduous process of transplant evaluation, listing, and waitlist maintenance can easily result in poor patient outcomes and compromise patient safety. Besides the policies and procedures implemented by transplant centers based on scientific models and evidence to improve outcomes (as described later in this chapter), the members of the transplant team also need to -display compassion and care to help the patients navigate this challenging course.

Who Should Be Transplanted?

Kidney transplantation should be considered in all patients with chronic kidney disease (CKD) stage 4 and 5 who are anticipated to initiate dialysis within the next 6-12 months and do not have an absolute contraindication. Early referral would facilitate the work-up for kidney transplantation, allow for the evaluation of a living donor if available, and may preclude the need for dialysis prior to transplantation. Transplantation with a living kidney donor is the preferred treatment for eligible CKD patients. Kidney Disease: Improving Global Outcomes (KDIGO) recommends pre-emptive transplantation in adults when the estimated glomerular filtration rate (eGFR) is <10 ml/min/1.73 m^2 or earlier if patients have symptoms [3].

Who Should Not Be Transplanted?

Absolute contraindications to kidney transplantation alone include decompensated cirrhosis (may be considered for combined liver -kidney transplant), severe irreversible and symptomatic cardiac disease (to be determined by a cardiologist and may be considered for combined heart-kidney transplant), severe irreversible obstructive or restrictive lung disease (may not be eligible for kidney transplantation alone, but may be considered for combined lung-kidney transplant), active malignancy (with rare exceptions described under the section on malignancy), and active untreated infection (except hepatitis C). Patients with hematologic malignancies (e.g., multiple myeloma, light and heavy chain deposition disease, etc.) should only be referred for kidney transplantation once they have received a curative treatment for the primary disorder and after consultation with a hematologist. Patients with amyloid light-chain (AL) amyloidosis with extra-renal involvement are poor candidates for kidney transplantation alone. Patients with unstable psychiatric disorders or ongoing substance use disorders should not be listed for kidney transplantation until they are in remission.

Approach to Pre-Transplant Evaluation of Kidney Transplant Recipients

The Process

The evaluation of candidacy and eligibility of kidney transplant recipient (KTR) is not restricted to the single clinic visit conducted at the time of the initial history & physical (H&P) examination. The evaluation starts before the initial clinic visit and continues even after the visit is complete. The pre-visit evaluation includes receiving patients' records from the primary care physician, primary nephrologist, dialysis center (if patient is on dialysis), as well as records from previous hospitalizations, including any imaging studies performed. As the transplant nephrologist is usually not familiar with the patient prior to these visits, and patients might not remember details of every medical issue in the past, every effort should be made to collect these collateral sources of patients' medical history. Any and all information collected during this process is not only valuable during the pre-transplant evaluation but might prove useful in the post-transplant management, as well. After the patients' visit, members of the transplant team need to stay in touch with the patient to ensure compliance with the recommendations made by the transplant center, assimilate data as it becomes available, and to stay updated regarding new and developing health issues that might affect the transplant status of the patient. Most transplant centers have protocols in place to achieve these goals in a timely and efficient manner with various members of the transplant team working in tandem to expedite the process. After the initial visit, the patient needs to be seen by the transplant team at least once a year while the patient is active on the waitlist to stay abreast of his or her ongoing medical problems.

History and Physical

Of all the patients who receive a kidney transplant, nearly 3% die in the first year after transplant, and 22% die in ten years. Despite the downtrend in mortality in the last 2 decades, a significant percentage of patients die due to cardiovascular disease, infections, and malignancy [4]. Initial evaluation of the patient includes a detailed history and thorough physical exam to gather the relevant data to assess the presence and severity of these ailments. The physician might need to ask specific questions in order to inquire about these conditions, as patients sometimes might not spontaneously offer this information either due to recall problems, or because they might think certain diseases are irrelevant to the transplant evaluation. Collateral history, if possible, must be obtained from family members or partners in order to corroborate the information provided by patients. Further pertinent questions during history taking at initial visit should include the questions about etiology of ESKD, the date of dialysis initiation (as it determines the time on waitlist), dialysis unit (where the transplant center can send or request further information), type of dialysis access, dialysis modality and schedule (important for clinic visits and dialysis planning around the time of transplant), and patients' primary nephrologist (who should be kept involved throughout the process of transplant evaluation). Detailed social history, including patient's occupation, living situation and family support, as well as history of substance abuse should also be obtained and documented. Control of diabetes and hypertension should be assessed and addressed during pre-transplant evaluation. Not only hypertension, but hypotension is also associated with worse graft outcomes that may lead to slow or delayed graft function (DGF). Patients with chronic undiagnosed hypotension or on midodrine (used to treat orthostatic hypotension) should be assessed for adrenal insufficiency.

Physical examination should include thorough examination of all organ systems, including dental exam as well as examination of the entire skin to look for any suspicious lesions. Feet should always be examined, especially in diabetic patients, to assess the distal pulses and skin integrity.

Investigations

Initial laboratory evaluation must include a basic metabolic panel, complete blood count with differential, coagulation testing, urinalysis with microscopy, liver function tests, serum protein level, TSH, B12, folate, iron studies, metabolic bone disease parameters (to assess secondary hyperparathyroidism), and tests for presence of latent TB and other viral infections (as described below). An electrocardiogram, chest x-ray, and abdominal ultrasound (to look for evidence of cirrhosis /ascites and to assess kidneys for suspicious cysts) should be performed on all patients. Doppler of pelvic vessels (sometimes followed by abdominal and pelvic CT angiography) is performed on all candidates to assess target vessels for transplantation. Cardiac risk assessment starts with an electrocardiogram, and an echocardiogram. The need for non-invasive stress test ing such as a dobutamine stress echocardiogram (DSE) or nuclear medicine myocardial perfusion imaging (MPI), or invasive testing such as cardiac catheterization, should be determined on an individual basis and is described in further detail later in the chapter.

Counseling

Physicians and other members of the transplant team should also take the opportunity of a first visit to educate the patient and family regarding the process of transplant evaluation, waitlisting, and follow-up post-transplant. Some transplant centers have formal education sessions for potential transplant recipients prior to initial visits. Patients and family members who are new to transplant might believe this is a panacea to all their medical problems, and transplantation will emancipate them from the tough demands of healthcare interventions. Thus, detailed information should be provided regarding the need for updated work-up during years of waitlisting, need for availability for transplantation at any time should they get an offer, perioperative complications, need for close post-transplant follow-up, and need for immunosuppression medications for the rest of their lives including their potential side-effects. Unrealistic expectations and incomplete information regarding these processes might lead to frustration and exaggerated disappointment if things do not go as planned. Initial visit is also an opportunity to educate patients regarding the benefits of living donor transplantation. Patients should be encouraged to seek living donors to avoid extended dialysis vintage.

Medical Review Board

Once all the data is gathered and studies carried out, the patient is usually presented to a Medical Review Board (MRB), where the candidacy for transplant is discussed among a panel of experts. The panel usually consists of medical director of the transplant program, transplant nephrologist, transplant surgeon, social worker, dietitian, financial counselor, Histocompatibility & Immunogenetics Laboratory (HLA lab) representative and transplant coordinators. After input from all the participants, a decision is made to either list the patient for transplant, conditionally accept with further testing or interventions required, or to deny the patient a kidney transplant. In any case, a letter is sent to both the patient and the primary nephrologist regarding the rationale for the decision. If the patient is denied at a transplant center, he/she should always be given the option to seek a second opinion regarding transplant candidacy elsewhere.

Identifying the Etiology of ESKD

Determining the etiology of ESKD is vital in determining the prognosis post-transplant (e.g., diabetic patients have worse graft outcomes compared to non-diabetic patients), as well as to determine the plan of care in the peri-transplant period (need for plasma exchange in patients with primary focal segmental glomerulosclerosis (FSGS) or complement inhibitors in patients with atypical hemolytic-uremic syndrome HUS). However, delineating the exact etiology of ESKD is sometimes not possible as very few patients with advanced CKD and ESKD that present to the transplant center for evaluation had a kidney biopsy done by primary nephrologists. In patients with long-standing diabetes and hypertension, renal failure is usually attributed to these comorbidities, and a biopsy is not pursued to confirm that renal pathology is in fact secondary to these etiologies and not another primary or secondary renal disorder [5]. In an Italian study of 393 patients with diabetes and CKD who underwent kidney biopsy, only 40% of patients had only diabetic glomerulosclerosis, and 45% of patients had glomerular disease superimposed on diabetic changes [6]. The primary nephrologist should make every effort to identify the cause of ESKD and should have a low threshold for a kidney biopsy especially if the patient is a candidate for kidney transplant in the future.

Identifying a concurrent or primary glomerular disorder is important as most forms of primary glomerulonephritis (GN) may recur in a kidney transplant and affect graft outcomes. Furthermore, certain diseases require a quiescent period prior to transplantation. IgA Nephropathy (IgAN) is the most common recurrent GN and may recur in up to 30-60% of cases post-transplant [7]. Approximately 30% of patients with FSGS have recurrent disease in the first kidney allograft, with risk of recurrence approaching 100% in the second allograft [8]. Membranoproliferative Glomerulonephritis (MPGN), although a pattern of injury and not a disease itself, nonetheless has a risk of recurrence ranging from 27 to 65% [9] and is associated with poor graft outcomes. These statistics highlight the need for diligently exploring the cause of ESKD in pre-transplant evaluation of KTRs. In patients with a history of lupus nephritis, antineutrophil cytoplasmic antibodies (ANCA) vasculitis, or antiphospholipid syndrome (APS), the disease should be clinically quiescent prior to transplantation. Patients with anti-glomerular basement membrane (GBM) disease should not be transplanted until antibody titer is undetectable.

Evaluation and Management of Vascular Disease

Cardiovascular Disease

Patients with advanced CKD and ESKD are at increased risk of cardiovascular mortality due to altered pathophysiology in the setting of pressure and volume overload, and the deleterious effects of uremic milieu, leading to a syndrome commonly known as uremic cardiomyopathy. In addition, there is accelerated vascular calcification in these patients leading to atherosclerosis and reduced compliance of vessels. Although 50% of patients with ESKD may have occult coronary artery disease (CAD) [10], other cardiac diseases like left ventricular hypertrophy (LVH) and dysfunction, pulmonary hypertension, and valvular disorders are also very common. One study showed that the best predictor of mortality after kidney transplantation is ejection fraction (EF), with mortality increasing by 2.7% for each 1% decrease in EF [11]. Therefore, initial evaluation with 2D-echocardiogram is part of transplant evaluation for nearly all transplant candidates without exception. The need and frequency of follow-up exams can be determined by the findings on initial echocardiogram. For example, a finding of mitral annular calcification (MAC) requires monitoring for progression (some centers do yearly echocardiograms), whereas a normal echocardiogram on initial evaluation is reassuring and requires less frequent follow-up unless there is a change in clinical status. Figure 1 shows a proposed algorithm for initial and follow-up echocardiogram evaluation currently used at our institution. Pulmonary hypertension is not an infrequent finding on echocardiogram in ESKD patients. The predominant cause of pulmonary hypertension is volume overload in these patients. So, the first step is aggressive volume management. With the help of the patient's primary nephrologist, a dialysis prescription change with lowering the "dry weight" and subsequently documenting improvement of pulmonary hypertension is important. If reducing dry weight does not lead to improvement in findings on echocardiogram, referral to cardiology is recommended for a right heart catheterization and further delineation of the cause of pulmonary hypertension.

The high prevalence of coronary artery disease in CKD /ESKD population theoretically dictates the need for ischemic work-up prior to transplant, and transplant centers are reluctant to operate on patients with unknown CAD status. High prevalence of atypical presentation of acute coronary syndrome (ACS) in ESKD patients [12], majority being diabetic [13], provides a justification for universal screening in this patient population. However, various societies differ in their recommendations regarding the frequency and intensity of work-up for underlying ischemic heart disease [14]. The abnormal non-invasive testing for CAD (usually a dobutamine stress echocardiogram or nuclear medicine myocardial perfusion imaging study) is usually followed by referral to a cardiologist for further evaluation and treatment prior to listing for transplant.

The recently published ISCHEMIA-CKD trial has challenged the paradigm of treating stable CAD with revascularization instead of optimal medical treatment (OMT). The trial enrolled 777 patients with advanced CKD and evidence of moderate to severe ischemia on non-invasive testing. Patients were assigned to either initial invasive strategy (consisting of coronary angiography and revascularization) or initial conservative strategy (consisting of medical therapy with intervention only in patients with who failed medical therapy). There was no difference in primary outcome (a composite comprising fatal or nonfatal myocardial infarction (MI)) between the two groups at a median follow-up of 2.2 years. However, there was higher incidence of stroke and death, as well as dialysis in the invasive strategy group [15]. This conclusion was also supported by another prospective observational study from the UK that followed 2,572 KTRs across 18 transplant centers [16]. Propensity-matched analysis did not show any association between screening for asymptomatic coronary artery disease and major adverse cardiac events (MACE) up to 5-years post-transplant. Based on these results, there are calls to rethink the strategy of requiring "stenting for every obstruction " due to potential for more harm than good [17].

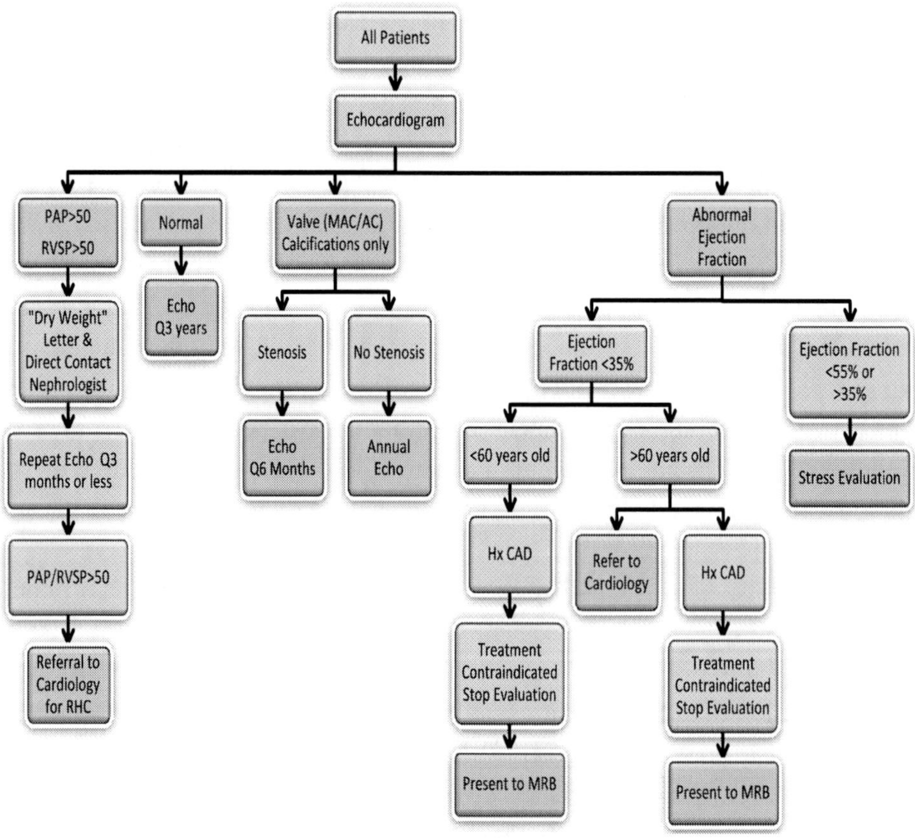

Figure 1. Legend: MAC- Mitral Annular Calcification, AC- Aortic Calcification, Hx – History of, CAD – Coronary Artery Disease, RHC- Right Heart Catheterization, MRB – Medical Review Board.

KDIGO recommends evaluating all candidates for cardiac disease using history, physical examination, and electrocardiogram. Asymptomatic candidates who have been on dialysis for 2 years, or with risk factors for pulmonary hypertension, should undergo echocardiography. Asymptomatic candidates for high risk of CAD (e.g., diabetes, prior CAD) should undergo non-invasive CAD screening. Patients with left ventricular dysfunction (EF < 30%) should be excluded from kidney transplantation alone [3]. Figure 2 shows the screening algorithm used at our institution for detecting and managing ischemic heart disease.

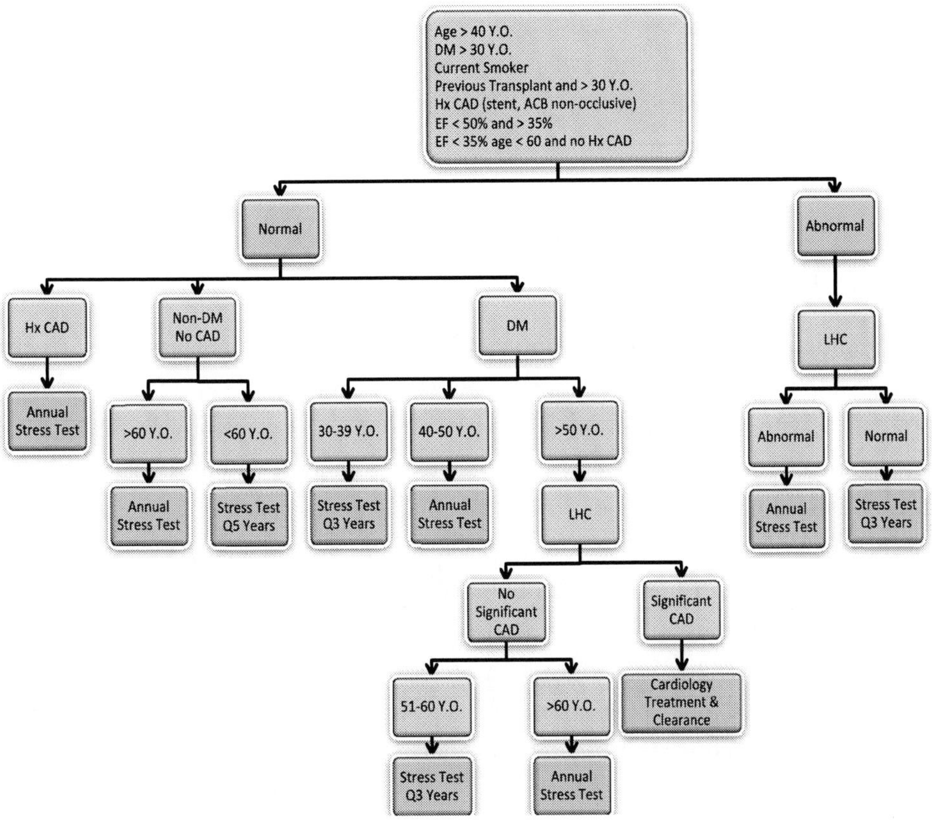

Figure 2. Legend: DM – Diabetes Mellitus, LHC – Left heart Catheterization, EF – Ejection Fraction, Q-Every, CAD – Coronary Artery Disease.

The Canadian Australasian Randomized Trial of Screening Kidney Transplant Candidates for Coronary Artery Disease (CARSK) (ClinicalTrials.gov No: NCT03674307) will test the hypothesis that eliminating the regular use of non-invasive screening tests for CAD after waitlist activation is not inferior to regular (i.e., annual) screening for CAD during waitlisting for the prevention of Major Adverse Cardiac Events. Secondary analyses will assess the impact of screening on the rate of transplantation, and the relative cost -effectiveness of screening. The trial is estimated to finish enrollment in 2023.

Cerebrovascular Disease

Kidney transplant recipients are at a higher risk for stroke and case fatality [18]. Risk factors include diabetes, systemic hypertension, age, anemia, and prior stroke. Eliciting a history of prior stroke and residual functional and cognitive deficits is important in making decisions regarding transplantation. KDIGO recommends a wait time of 6 months after stroke and 3 months after transient ischemic attack (TIA) prior to transplantation [3].

Screening for asymptomatic carotid artery stenosis is not recommended. In patients with autosomal dominant polycystic kidney disease (ADPKD), screening for intracranial aneurysms is only recommended if patients have a prior personal or family history of subarachnoid hemorrhage.

Peripheral Vascular Disease

All candidates for kidney transplant should be evaluated for presence and severity of peripheral arterial disease (PAD). Patients who have symptomatic PAD should be managed in consultation with a vascular surgeon. If a patient has lower extremity non-healing ulcers with active infection due to PAD, transplant should be delayed until infection has resolved. In patients with clinical evidence of PAD, KDIGO recommends non-contrast computed tomography (CT) of abdomen and pelvis to evaluate for presence of vascular calcifications and to guide operative planning. Although the presence of severe aorto-iliac disease or distal arterial disease does not preclude transplantation, there is a risk for progression after transplant that needs to be considered and discussed with the patient. Diabetic patients with peripheral vascular disease spend more time in the hospital post-transplant and undergo more non-graft related operations than graft-related procedures [19].

Evaluation and Management of Infectious Diseases

Infections are a common cause of morbidity and mortality in KTRs [4]; every effort should be made to detect and treat latent and active infections during the pre-transplant evaluation. Transplantation should not be done unless active infections are treated, as post-transplant immunosuppression makes it more difficult to control these infections. Post-transplant infections also lead to disruption of immunosuppressive medications, leading to increased risk for graft rejection. During the initial interview, detailed history of prior infections and treatments received should be obtained. Social history, including history of travel to endemic areas of infection, should be acquired. Identifying increased risk behavior for transmission of infection is an important part of transplant evaluation. A detailed physical examination, including dental examination, should be performed to look for any areas suspicious for active infections. Latent tuberculosis (TB) should be investigated using chest x-ray and Purified Protein Derivative (PPD) or Interferon Gamma Release Assay. If detected, latent TB should be treated prior to, or immediately after transplantation.

Table 1 details the recommended screening tests prior to transplantation. Table 2 lists the recommended vaccinations prior to transplant .

Table 1. Recommended screening tests for infection in pre-transplant

All Candidates
Latent Tuberculosis (TB)
Syphilis (Treponema Pallidum)
Hepatitis B Virus (HBV)
Human Immunodeficiency Virus (HIV)
Hepatitis C virus (HCV)
Cytomegalovirus (CMV)
Herpes-Simplex Virus (HSV)
Epstein-Barr Virus (EBV)
Varicella-Zoster Virus (VZV)
Measles, Mumps and Rubella (MMR)
Candidates from Endemic Areas
Human T-Cell Lymphotropic Virus (HTLV)
Malaria
Chagas Disease
Strongyloides

Table 2. Recommended vaccinations for kidney transplant candidates

Hepatitis B vaccination if seronegative
MMR – at least 4 weeks prior to transplantation
VZV – at least 4 weeks prior to transplantation
Influenza Vaccination
Pneumococcal vaccination (especially if history of splenectomy)
Hemophilus (if history of splenectomy)
Meningococcal vaccination (if history of splenectomy or requiring complement inhibitors)
Ensure that Diphtheria, Pertussis, Tetanus, Polio, HiB vaccinations are up-to-date
In rare individual circumstances (based on age, travel history, endemic area exposure):
Rabies
Tick-Borne Meningoencephalitis
Japanese Encephalitis
Yellow Fever
Salmonella Typhi (inactivated)

Selected Infections

HIV

Candidates with human immunodeficiency virus (HIV) can be evaluated and listed for kidney transplantation. Patients should be listed if they demonstrate compliance with treatment and their infection is controlled, as evidenced by a CD4 count > 200 cells/mm^3 and HIV viral load < 20 copies/ml. These patients are better managed in collaboration with the treating infectious disease specialist.

HBV

As prevalence of hepatitis B virus (HBV) might be as high as 7% in dialysis population [20], a positive hepatitis B surface antigen (HBsAg) or hepatitis B core antibody (anti-HBc) requires further evaluation. Although it does not preclude transplantation, hepatology consultation to determine treatment plan and to rule our liver cirrhosis or hepatocellular carcinoma is mandatory prior to transplantation.

HCV

Due to the emergence of direct-acting antivirals (DAAs), treatment of hepatitis C virus (HCV) has become quite simple and effective. Candidates with HCV infection can be treated before or after kidney transplantation, depending on the time to transplantation. If transplant is imminent in the next 24 weeks, HCV treatment should be delayed until after the transplantation. However, if wait time to transplant is longer than 24 weeks, or is unknown, HCV should be treated to prevent decompensated liver disease [21]. If patients with HCV demonstrate evidence of cirrhosis or portal hypertension, they should be evaluated for simultaneous kidney-liver transplant (SKLT) in conjunction with hepatology. Due to emergence of DAAs, kidney transplant from HCV-positive donors to HCV-negative recipients is also being successfully performed at this time with treatment of HCV in the post-transplant period [22, 23].

CMV

Cytomegalovirus (CMV) is the most common opportunistic infection in kidney transplant recipients [24]. Risk factors that place potential recipients at a disadvantage include donor seropositivity, use of induction immunosuppression with T-Cell depleting antibodies, simultaneous kidney-pancreas transplant ation, older donor, and concurrent infection from other viruses. Transplant candidates who are CMV negative at initial evaluation should be tested again at the time of transplantation.

BKV

On the other hand, testing for BK virus (BKV) is not recommended prior to transplant as it is unclear if pre-transplant *BK viremia* or viruria affects graft outcomes [25]. KDIGO does not recommend excluding patients for repeat transplantation if they have a history of graft loss due to BK nephropathy [26].

Follow-Up Testing

If negative at initial screening, serology for HIV, HCV, and HBV should be repeated annually while on the waitlist and at the time of transplantation. For other viruses such as

CMV, EBV, HSV, MMR, and VZV, if initial serology is negative, then testing should be repeated at the time of transplantation [3].

EVALUATION AND MANAGEMENT OF MALIGNANCY

Screening

Overall risk of cancer is at least 2-2.5-fold higher in KTRs compared to age and gender matched general populations [27], with a greater risk for virally related cancers like Kaposi sarcoma (20-fold), cervical cancer (5-10 fold), and post-transplant lymphoproliferative disease (PTLD). Although the mortality due to cardiovascular and infectious causes has been trending down over the past 20-years, mortality due to malignancy has not declined [4]. Therefore, detection of an undiagnosed malignancy and appropriate management and follow-up of a known malignancy is an important task during the pre-transplant evaluation.

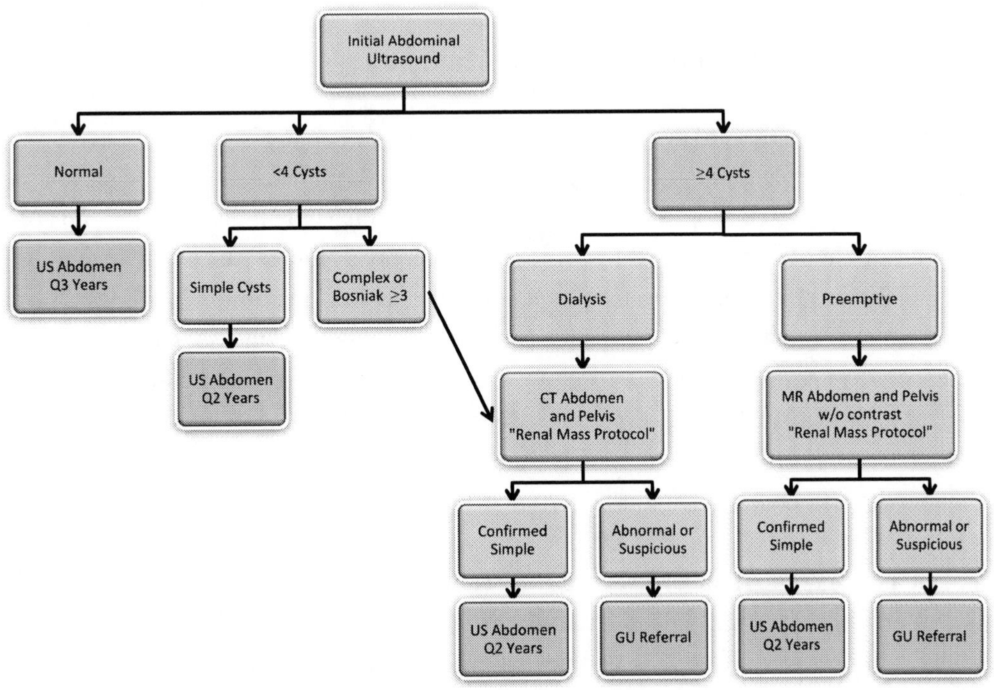

Figure 3. Legend: US – Ultrasound, MR – Magnetic Resonance, GU – Genitourinary, CT – Computed tomography.

Trials have reported at least 20% reduction in solid-organ cancer (like colorectal cancer) related mortality in screened vs. unscreened patients [28]. Age-appropriate cancer screening is recommended during the transplant evaluation. Women should undergo mammogram and Papanicolaou (PAP) smear according to the guidelines for the general population. Both men and women should undergo colonoscopy if they are aged 50 or above. However, the United States Preventive Services Task Force (USPSTF) has recently recommended to start screening for colorectal cancer at the age of 45 (Grade B recommendation) [29]. Some transplant centers (including our center) have already adopted this approach for early detection of colorectal malignancy. Recommendation for prostate cancer screening is also same as for the general population, i.e., men between the ages of 55 to 69 should be offered screening using prostate specific antigen (PSA) if they wish to do so after understanding risks and benefits [3].

Chest imaging is recommended in all candidates prior to transplantation. Patients with ≥30 pack-year history of smoking should undergo a chest CT. Patients with cirrhosis should undergo screening to rule out hepatocellular carcinoma. It has been suggested that high-risk individuals (e.g., with history of dialysis for more than 3 years) should undergo screening for renal cell carcinoma using ultrasonography (followed by CT abdomen and pelvis if needed) and urinary cytology /cystoscopy [30, 31]. Figure 3 shows the approach used at our transplant center for evaluation and management of kidney cysts.

Approach to Patients with a History of Malignancy

Although guidelines are available regarding the recommended waiting times between remission and transplantation (Table 3), these are only recommendations - the patients are better managed by a close collaboration between patients' oncologist and the transplant team. Waiting times of two to five years are recommended for most cancers as several large registry analyses suggested that risk of cancer recurrence was maximum in the first 5 years after transplant. Input from oncologists is extremely valuable in assessing the risk of recurrence after transplant and to determine the approach to cancer screening post-transplant. Although the long-term risk of recurrence is not very high (ranging from 5-10%), the prognosis after recurrence is poor in KTRs (32).

Kidney transplantation should be avoided in patients with acute leukemia and high-grade lymphoma (including PTLD) until they have achieved remission after curative treatment and a certain time has elapsed (see Table 3). This duration is best determined in consultation with a hematologist. Hematologists can also aid in the decision to transplant a patient with myelodysplasia, as certain lesions may have higher risk of progression or transformation after the transplant.

Table 3. KDIGO Recommended waiting times between cancer remission and transplantation (3)

No Wait Time	At least 2 years	2 to 5 years	At least 5 years
	Early Breast Ca		*Advanced Breast Ca*
	Colorectal Duke A/B	Colorectal Duke C	Colorectal Duke D
	Invasive Bladder Ca		
Kidney Incidentaloma (<3cm)	*Kidney early*		*Kidney large & invasive*
		Lung localized	
	Uterine localized		Uterine invasive
	Cervical localized		*Cervical invasive*
	Testicular localized	*Testicular invasive*	Melanoma localized
Prostate Gleason < 6	Gleason 7		Gleason 8-10
Papillary/Follicular/ Medullary Thyroid Stage 1	Stage 2		Stage 3
	Hodgkin's Lymphoma Localized	Regional (3-5 yrs.)	Distant
	Non-Hodgkin's Lymphoma Localized	Regional (3-5 yrs.)	Distant
	Post-Transplant Lymphoproliferative disorder Nodal		Extranodal and Cerebral

Monoclonal Gammopathy of Unknown Significance (MGUS) is a condition at the lower end of the spectrum of plasma cell dyscrasias. While it can progress to multiple myeloma (MM), such progression is extremely uncommon. Unlike MM, systemic involvement like anemia, lytic bone lesions, kidney involvement, and hypercalcemia is not present in patients with MGUS. Patients with MGUS should not be excluded from transplantation as there is no conclusive evidence to suggest increased progression to MM in KTRs, compared to patients without MGUS. Although the risk of PTLD may be increased, the risk of graft failure and patient survival is not different [33]. For patients with smoldering MM, the risk of progression to MM ranges from 8-10% in the first 5 years of diagnosis. KDIGO recommends not excluding these patients from transplant listing, but the higher risk should be discussed with the patient.

MISCELLANEOUS ISSUES

Tobacco Use

Current smokers have increased risk of respiratory complications perioperatively and risk depends on the duration of smoking and presence of chronic lung disease. Long-term increased risk of cardiovascular disease, malignancy, and death in these patients are all well known. All candidates should be counseled to avoid tobacco products before and indefinitely after transplantation. Referral to tobacco cessation programs should be considered for interested patients. Smoking cessation even 4 weeks prior to transplantation may reduce the risk of post-operative complications [34].

Obesity

Obesity is defined as a Body Mass Index (BMI) of greater than 30 kg/m^2 or a waist-to-hip ratio of greater than 0.85 in women and 0.9 in men. Obesity at the time of transplantation is correlated with delayed wound healing, increased duration of hospitalization, increased readmission rate in first year, presence of post-transplant diabetes, and lower graft survival rates [35]. Although obesity is not a contraindication for transplant and there is no defined cutoff at which transplantation cannot be performed, patients with obesity (especially if BMI > 35 kg/m^2) should be referred to the weight-management clinic for dietary and exercise counseling and possibly considered for bariatric surgery if needed. Surgeons should evaluate these patients for operative suitability, and risk of impaired wound healing should be discussed with the patients. Pretransplant panniculectomy may be useful in reducing BMI and improving wound healing after transplant [36].

Psychosocial Evaluation

Psychosocial assessment is performed by a trained transplant social worker in most centers. Some centers also use a psychologist, psychiatrist, or a psychiatric nurse practitioner. Social barriers to a successful transplant should be elicited, and sources of social support should be assessed during this evaluation. History and risk for substance abuse is also ascertained. Patients' compliance and adherence to medical advice is usually assessed by an interview and records from the patient's dialysis unit. However, physicians should keep in mind that it is not known if non-compliance with dialysis treatments predicts non-adherence to medications after transplant. Most common reason for missed dialysis treatments is lack of transportation [37], whereas the most common reason for nonadherence to transplant medications is inability to afford the medications [38]. However, as nonadherence to medication regimen is the major cause of kidney transplant rejection, every effort should be made to address the factors that might contribute to future non-adherence after transplant. Patients should have an identified support plan in place prior to transplantation if they are unable to care for themselves.

Anxiety and depression are the leading factors to non-adherence in ESKD and KTRs [39] and are associated with major morbidity and mortality. If suspected or diagnosed, these patients should be referred for further evaluation and management by a psychiatrist. Patients with unstable psychiatric disorders or ongoing substance use disorders that affect decision-making should not be transplanted until these conditions are under adequate control [3].

Assessment of Functional Status

Objective measures are available to assess the functional status of a patient, including measurement tools such as the Timed Get Up and GO test (TGUG), Karnofsky Performance Score, Short Physical Performance Battery and Frailty Score [40]. In addition, clinical data such as history of serious falls [41] and admissions to hospitals also predict post-transplant mortality. Worse scores in these objective assessments are associated with worse outcomes post-transplant. However, it is not clear if these patients should be outright denied kidney transplantation or should be enrolled in rehabilitation programs in order to improve their functional status prior to transplantation [42]; these decisions should be individualized.

Clinically, the frailty index is assessed in all patients above the age of 70, as well as in younger patients with apparent poor functional status. Frailty is characterized by loss of function in 5 domains, including muscle mass, muscle strength, endurance, gait, and physical activity. Patients determined to be frail at the time of transplant have higher incidence of delayed graft function (DGF), higher length of stay (LOS), as well as graft loss and mortality (36). Referral for rehabilitation and training for conditioning might be helpful in these patients, although there is no strong evidence to support this approach.

Conclusion

Transplantation gives hope not only to the patient, but also to the healthcare team members taking care of that patient. Transplant physicians and surgeons are eager to accept any and all candidates for kidney transplantation as every successful transplant provides an impetus to this motivation. It is important to create, update, and follow the protocols for evaluation of transplant candidates, tailored to the patient population catered to by the transplant center. All members of the transplant team should strictly and proactively follow these protocols in order to avoid missing the clues that might lead to complications around and after the transplantation. Every member of the team, whether a physician or ancillary staff, has a vital role to play in order to make this endeavor successful. No member of the team should ignore a significant finding, assuming some other team member might have already reviewed and addressed it. Any of the above steps that is not adequately addressed during pre-transplant evaluation could lead to disastrous consequences post-transplant. Also, it should be noted that navigating the transplant world, and patiently waiting for a transplant for years is a monumental task that patients perform every day of their lives with impressive fortitude and perseverance. These patients deserve all the respect, attention, and care to make this seemingly insurmountable task a little less uncomfortable.

References

[1] Wolfe RA, Ashby VB, Milford EL, Ojo AO, Ettenger RE, Agodoa LY, et al. Comparison of mortality in all patients on dialysis, patients on dialysis awaiting transplantation, and recipients of a first cadaveric transplant. *N Engl J Med.* 1999;341(23):1725-30.

[2] Gill JS, Tonelli M, Johnson N, Kiberd B, Landsberg D, Pereira BJ. The impact of waiting time and comorbid conditions on the survival benefit of kidney transplantation. *Kidney Int.* 2005;68(5):2345-51.

[3] Chadban SJ, Ahn C, Axelrod DA, Foster BJ, Kasiske BL, Kher V, et al. KDIGO Clinical Practice Guideline on the Evaluation and Management of Candidates for Kidney Transplantation. *Transplantation.* 2020;104(4S1 Suppl 1): S11-S103.

[4] Awan AA, Niu J, Pan JS, Erickson KF, Mandayam S, Winkelmayer WC, et al. Trends in the Causes of Death among Kidney Transplant Recipients in the United States (1996-2014). *Am J Nephrol.* 2018;48(6):472-81.

[5] Gonzalez Suarez ML, Thomas DB, Barisoni L, Fornoni A. Diabetic nephropathy: Is it time yet for routine kidney biopsy ? *World J Diabetes.* 2013;4(6):245-55.

[6] Mazzucco G, Bertani T, Fortunato M, Bernardi M, Leutner M, Boldorini R, et al. Different patterns of renal damage in type 2 diabetes mellitus: a multicentric study on 393 biopsies. *Am J Kidney Dis.* 2002;39(4):713-20.

[7] Ponticelli C, Glassock RJ. Posttransplant recurrence of primary glomerulonephritis. *Clin J Am Soc Nephrol.* 2010;5(12):2363-72.

[8] Newstead CG. Recurrent disease in renal transplants. *Nephrol Dial Transplant.* 2003;18 Suppl 6:vi68-74.

[9] Lorenz EC, Sethi S, Leung N, Dispenzieri A, Fervenza FC, Cosio FG. Recurrent membranoproliferative glomerulonephritis after kidney transplantation. *Kidney Int.* 2010;77(8):721-8.

[10] Ohtake T, Kobayashi S, Moriya H, Negishi K, Okamoto K, Maesato K, et al. High prevalence of occult coronary artery stenosis in patients with chronic kidney disease at the initiation of renal replacement therapy: an angiographic examination. *J Am Soc Nephrol.* 2005;16(4):1141-8.

[11] Hage FG, Smalheiser S, Zoghbi GJ, Perry GJ, Deierhoi M, Warnock D, et al. Predictors of survival in patients with end-stage renal disease evaluated for kidney transplantation. *Am J Cardiol.* 2007;100(6):1020-5.

[12] Sosnov J, Lessard D, Goldberg RJ, Yarzebski J, Gore JM. Differential symptoms of acute myocardial infarction in patients with kidney disease: a community -wide perspective. *Am J Kidney Dis.* 2006;47(3):378-84.

[13] Jacoby RM, Nesto RW. Acute myocardial infarction in the diabetic patient: pathophysiology, clinical course and prognosis. *J Am Coll Cardiol.* 1992;20(3):736-44.

[14] Sandal S, Chen T, Cantarovich M. The Challenges with the Cardiac Evaluation of Liver and Kidney Transplant Candidates. *Transplantation.* 2020;104(2):251-8.

[15] Bangalore S, Maron DJ, O'Brien SM, Fleg JL, Kretov EI, Briguori C, et al. Management of Coronary Disease in Patients with Advanced Kidney Disease. *N Engl J Med.* 2020;382(17):1608-18.

[16] Nimmo A, Forsyth JL, Oniscu GC, Robb M, Watson C, Fotheringham J, et al. A propensity score-matched analysis indicates screening for asymptomatic coronary artery disease does not predict cardiac events in kidney transplant recipients. *Kidney Int.* 2021;99(2):431-42.

[17] Georgianos PI, Agarwal R. Every obstruction does not need a stent: an important lesson from the ISCHEMIA-CKD trial for kidney -transplant surgeons. *Nephrol Dial Transplant.* 2021;36(1):4-8.

[18] Findlay MD, Thomson PC, MacIsaac R, Jardine AG, Patel RK, Stevens KK, et al. Risk factors and outcome of stroke in renal transplant recipients. *Clin Transplant.* 2016;30(8):918-24.

[19] Lubetzky M, Kamal L, Ajaimy M, Akalin E, Kayler L. Hospital readmissions in diabetic kidney transplant recipients with peripheral vascular disease. *Clin Transplant.* 2018;32(6): e13271.

[20] Burdick RA, Bragg-Gresham JL, Woods JD, Hedderwick SA, Kurokawa K, Combe C, et al. Patterns of hepatitis B prevalence and seroconversion in hemodialysis units from three continents: the DOPPS. *Kidney Int.* 2003;63(6):2222-9.

[21] Awan AA, Jadoul M, Martin P. Hepatitis C in Chronic Kidney Disease: An Overview of the KDIGO Guideline. *Clin Gastroenterol Hepatol.* 2020;18(10):2158-67.

[22] Goldberg DS, Abt PL, Blumberg EA, Van Deerlin VM, Levine M, Reddy KR, et al. Trial of Transplantation of HCV-Infected Kidneys into Uninfected Recipients. *N Engl J Med.* 2017;376(24):2394-5.

[23] Durand C, Brown D, Wesson R, Bhair N, Naqvi F, Ostrander D, et al. EXPANDER-1: exploring renal transplants using hepatitis - C infected donors for HCV negative recipients [abstract 2]. *Am J Transplant.* 2017;17(Suppl. 3):207.

[24] Brennan DC. Cytomegalovirus in renal transplantation. *J Am Soc Nephrol.* 2001;12(4):848-55.

[25] Bicalho CS, Oliveira RR, Pierrotti LC, Fink MC, Urbano PR, Nali LH, et al. Pre-transplant shedding of BK virus in urine is unrelated to post-transplant viruria and viremia in kidney transplant recipients. *Clin Transplant.* 2016;30(7):796-801.

[26] Chadban SJ, Ahn C, Axelrod DA, Foster BJ, Kasiske BL, Kher V, et al. Summary of the kidney disease: Improving Global Outcomes (KDIGO) Clinical Practice Guideline on the Evaluation and Management of Candidates for Kidney Transplantation. *Transplantation.* 2020;104(4):708-14.

[27] Vajdic CM, McDonald SP, McCredie MR, van Leeuwen MT, Stewart JH, Law M, et al. Cancer incidence before and after kidney transplantation. *JAMA.* 2006;296(23):2823-31.

[28] Atkin W, Wooldrage K, Parkin DM, Kralj-Hans I, MacRae E, Shah U, et al. Long term effects of once-only flexible sigmoidoscopy screening after 17 years of follow-up: the UK Flexible Sigmoidoscopy Screening randomised controlled trial. *Lancet.* 2017;389(10076):1299-311.

[29] USPSTF recommends expansion of colorectal cancer screening. *Lancet Gastroenterol Hepatol.* 2021;6(1):1.

[30] Sarasin FP, Wong JB, Levey AS, Meyer KB. Screening for acquired cystic kidney disease: a decision analytic perspective. *Kidney Int.* 1995;48(1):207-19.

[31] Singanamala S, Brewster UC. Should screening for acquired cystic disease and renal malignancy be undertaken in dialysis patients? *Semin Dial.* 2011;24(4):365-6.

[32] Viecelli AK, Lim WH, Macaskill P, Chapman JR, Craig JC, Clayton P, et al. Cancer-Specific and All-Cause Mortality in Kidney Transplant Recipients With and Without Previous Cancer. *Transplantation.* 2015;99(12):2586-92.

[33] Alfano G, Fontana F, Colaci E, Messerotti A, Bettelli F, Potenza L, et al. Monoclonal Gammopathy of Undetermined Significance After Kidney Transplantation: Single-Center Experience. *Transplantation.* 2017;101(11): e337-e42.

[34] Thomsen T, Villebro N, Moller AM. Interventions for preoperative smoking cessation. *Cochrane Database Syst Rev.* 2014(3):CD002294.

[35] Erturk T, Berber I, Cakir U. Effect of Obesity on Clinical Outcomes of Kidney Transplant Patients. *Transplant Proc.* 2019;51(4):1093-5.

[36] Troppmann C, Santhanakrishnan C, Kuo JH, Bailey CM, Perez RV, Wong MS. Impact of panniculectomy on transplant candidacy of obese patients with chronic kidney disease declined for kidney transplantation because of a high-risk abdominal panniculus: *A pilot study. Surgery.* 2016;159(6):1612-22.

[37] Brar A, Babakhani A, Salifu MO, Jindal RM. Evaluation of non-adherence in patients undergoing dialysis and kidney transplantation: United States transplantation practice patterns survey. *Transplant Proc.* 2014;46(5):1340-6.

[38] Nevins TE, Nickerson PW, Dew MA. Understanding Medication Nonadherence after Kidney Transplant. *J Am Soc Nephrol.* 2017;28(8):2290-301.

[39] Cukor D, Rosenthal DS, Jindal RM, Brown CD, Kimmel PL. Depression is an important contributor to low medication adherence in hemodialyzed patients and transplant recipients. *Kidney Int.* 2009;75(11):1223-9.

[40] McAdams-DeMarco MA, Olorundare IO, Ying H, Warsame F, Haugen CE, Hall R, et al. Frailty and Postkidney Transplant Health-Related Quality of Life. *Transplantation.* 2018;102(2):291-9.

[41] Lynch RJ, Patzer RE, Pastan SO, Bowling CB, Plantinga LC. Recent History of Serious Fall Injuries and Posttransplant Outcomes Among US Kidney Transplant Recipients. *Transplantation.* 2019;103(5):1043-50.

[42] McAdams-DeMarco MA, Ying H, Van Pilsum Rasmussen S, Schrack J, Haugen CE, Chu NM, et al. Prehabilitation prior to kidney transplantation: Results from a pilot study. *Clin Transplant.* 2019;33(1):e13450.

In: Issues in Kidney Disease – Transplantation
Editors: B. V. R. Murthy and S. Z. Fadem
ISBN: 978-1-53619-960-4

Chapter 3

EVALUATION OF THE LIVING KIDNEY DONOR, AND KIDNEY PAIRED DONATION

***Stephen Z. Fadem**[*,1], MD, FACP, FASN*
***and Bhamidipati V. R. Murthy**[2], MD, DM*
[1]Selzman Institute for Kidney Health, Section of Nephrology,
and Michael E. DeBakey Veterans Affairs Medical Center,
Baylor College of Medicine, Houston, TX, USA;
Kidney Associates, Houston, TX, USA
[2]Selzman Institute for Kidney Health, Section of Nephrology,
and Division of Abdominal Transplantation, Department of Surgery,
Baylor College of Medicine, Houston, TX, USA

ABSTRACT

There are approximately 112,000 dialysis patients who are awaiting a kidney transplant, yet only 20% will be fortunate enough to receive one. A living donor transplant can make a huge difference in the quality and longevity of the potential recipient, particularly those who are on dialysis. The donor nephrectomy must be done with safety as the primary concern. The donor must be well-informed about the risks before being assessed for eligibility and compatibility. The potential of having a reduced renal mass should be weighed and understood before agreeing to donate one's kidney. Tests for renal function and underlying medical conditions are necessary. Donors who are not candidates because of potentially modifiable conditions such as obesity or tobacco use should be counseled. Transmissibility of infectious or malignant diseases must be taken into consideration. Of special importance is the female donor of childbearing age who might wish to conceive in the future.

Keywords: living donor, transplantation, organ donation, paired kidney donation

* Corresponding Author's Email: fadem@bcm.edu.

Introduction

There are approximately 112,000 patients awaiting a kidney transplant based on the latest United Network of Organ Sharing (UNOS) database, yet many of these patients will need to wait for several years. According to the last available figures, there were 23,404 kidney transplant surgeries performed in the USA (Source: UNOS https://unos.org) in 2019. UNOS reported that 17 people die each day awaiting a transplant. Many of these patients could be saved if a living donor transplant is performed. In the past, live donor transplants were largely limited to donation from a living related donor, but this has changed dramatically. Now, innovations in immunosuppression and donor-matching processes have expanded living donor transplant program to receiving a transplant from one who is unrelated, and from those with incompatible blood group s, and to recipients with high immunological risk .

Guidelines for Living Kidney Donors

In 2017, the Kidney Disease Improving Global Outcomes (KDIGO) group published comprehensive guidelines for the evaluation and management of living donors [1]. While these guidelines serve as guidance for the physician wishing to assess a prospective living donor, they must be considered along with other guidelines, such as The British Transplantation Society (BTS), the Canadian Kidney Paired Donation (KPD) Program, and the European Renal Best Practice (ERBP). The KDIGO Guidelines emphasize that it is essential to first assure that candidates are suitable, and then provide them with an estimate of the short- and long-term risks of donating a kidney. Using the same criteria for all prospective donors, transplant centers should evaluate donor candidates for health characteristics and medical comorbidities, surgical risks, psycho-social risks, and histocompatibility. Candidates must understand the risks of surgery and the potential lifelong consequences of living with a solitary kidney. The transplant centers must establish the threshold for acceptable risk, as well as decline candidates' requests who are above their designated post-donation risk. In the end, transplant candidates must completely understand the evaluation and donation procedure and also consent that they have been informed. Support is recommended for donors who have been declined. Moreover, a plan should be formulated to include alternative ways of helping the intended recipient or offering a chance for a second opinion.

After ABO blood group typing and crossmatching, the prospective donor's renal function is determined, and the donor is risk assessed and also evaluated for underlying medical conditions and transmissible disease risks. Once the patient and the donor are acceptably matched, a detailed medical and psycho-social evaluation of the donor is performed. A surgical evaluation is also performed to determine that the donor can safely undergo a nephrectomy, and the anatomy of the kidney has an acceptable risk profile, especially the vascular anatomy. If the donor and recipient are not acceptably matched, but the donor is otherwise eligible to donate, a kidney paired exchange should be considered. Donors who are not surgical candidates because of potentially modifiable conditions such as obesity or tobacco use should be counseled.

ABO Typing and Compatibility

Prior to any other assessment, one must determine ABO type and histocompatibility. ABO typing must be performed on two separate occasions. For purposes of kidney transplantation, only ABO typing is considered for compatibility because Rhesus (Rh) antigens are not expressed on the renal tissue. A lymphocyte crossmatch is then performed. A positive crossmatch indicates a significant level of anti-HLA antibodies in the recipient against the donor tissue antigens. Donors and patients who are incompatible have the option to consider transplant exchange programs, or transplantation across ABO-incompatible groups in centers that pursue this option. Human leukocyte antigen (HLA) typing may be performed for both classes I (A, B, C) and II (DP, DQ, DR) antigens, but outcomes have been acceptable even in HLA-incompatible donor and recipient pairs in the current era with improved immunosuppression regimens. HLA typing and matching are undergoing significant changes with availability of better molecular techniques. The standard HLA matching of Class I and II antigens may be replaced in the future by epitope matching and may include a matching score as opposed to the current numerical match of the antigens [2]. In situations where there are donor-specific antibodies in lower titers such that the lymphocyte crossmatch is negative, transplantation could be performed in some cases using desensitization protocols in the recipient.

Factors That Impact Risk

This section discusses the factors that one should take into consideration when assessing the risk to the donor, as well as the health of the kidney to be transplanted prospectively.

Donor Age

While the donor age is not limited by any of the guidelines, it is worth noting that age-related kidney function is variable from person to person and depends upon many factors that also determine well-being and general health [3]. Thus, an assessment of kidney function will most likely reflect donor suitability than age. Many elderly patients who are undergoing dialysis therapy but wish to receive a kidney transplantation are limited from receiving a deceased donor allograft because of the long waiting period. For them, a living donor transplant from a healthy contemporary is more realistic. A case report of an 87-year old healthy grandfather donating a kidney reveals its value in expanding donor possibilities [4]. It appears that using older individuals as transplant donor candidates does not have worsened outcomes for either the donor or the recipient [5, 6].

A systemic review of renal functional reserve (RFR) in living donors after donation evaluated 16 studies that demonstrated RFR was preserved in young healthy donors but was significantly reduced in older donors [7].

Evaluation of Kidney Function

The exact estimation or calculation of the kidney function is the cornerstone for kidney donor evaluation. Significant advances have been made over the years in the quest for a good measure of kidney function. A detailed discussion of various measures of kidney function, including their pros and cons, are out of scope for this chapter; however, a brief discussion is worthwhile. The Cockcroft-Gault formula (a calculation used to estimate creatine clearance based on such factors as age, weight, serum creatinine, and gender) is the first basic method of renal function estimation but is unreliable particularly in individuals with higher GFR as in kidney donors. The serum creatinine may vary based on simple analytic variation or on variation based on biologic fluctuations. The analytic variation for a serum creatinine measured with the enzymatic method is 13% (CI 0.87 to 1.13 mg/dL) for a serum creatinine of 1.0 [8]. Biologic variation includes muscle mass differences, creatine supplements containing ethyl esters, or cooked meat ingestion within a few hours of testing. A common class of medications, the cephalosporins, interfere with the picric acid assay, falsely elevating the value. A small amount of the creatinine is secreted by the tubules; this may vary, or even be transiently altered by medications such as trimethoprim or dronedarone. Acute medical conditions, such as an acute upper respiratory infection or a urinary tract infection, can affect serum creatinine, as can hydration status or the recent administration of iodinated contrast agents.

The traditional method of a 24-hour creatinine clearance is still one of the standard methods adopted by most transplant centers. However, it lacks reproducibility as errors in urine collection are inherent problems with this method. While designed to assess the value of dietary protein restriction, the Modification of Diet in Renal Disease (MDRD) trial required highly accurate measurements of glomerular filtration. Its byproduct was a creatinine-based mathematical estimate of glomerular filtration, the MDRD study equation that was internally corroborated using the more accurate measured glomerular filtration rate (GFR) [9]. GFR estimating equations are only relevant in the populations for which they have been validated. To better validate estimating equations across multiple populations, the estimated glomerular filtration rate (eGFR) is calculated using the 2009 Chronic Kidney Disease Epidemiology Collaboration (CKD -EPI) equation. It also follows a best fit analysis, factoring age, race, and gender into the estimate for GFR (http://mdrd.com). The CKD-EPI creatinine equation uses a 2-slope spline to model the relationship between estimated GFR and serum creatinine and performed with less bias than the MDRD study equation in patients with a higher GFR. The CKD-EPI GFR equation and other predictive models are available as free, web -based downloadable apps from the author (http://touchcalc.com/predictors - http://touchcalc.com/predictors/epi_resources).

Cystatin C is an alternate marker that does not depend upon muscle metabolism. A cross-sectional analysis was used to develop estimating equations both alone and in combination with the serum creatinine. Renal function is somewhat difficult to assess in the elderly as muscle mass may decline. Cystatin C and serum creatinine is a reasonable combination for assessing kidney function in the aged kidney patient [10]. Although dependent upon creatinine, the Cockcroft-Gault equation with ideal body weight performs better than the MDRD and CKD -EPI GFR in persons over 70 years old [11]. The Berlin Initiative Study (BIS) equation is also creatinine-based but has been internally validated against iohexol and performed well in older patients [12]. The BIS formula is available online by this author at http://touchcalc.com/bis.

After the age of 40 years, the GFR declines 6.5 mL/min/1.73m^2 for men and 7.9 mL/min/1.73m^2 per decade for women. A donor nephrectomy will reduce the renal mass by 50%; but because of compensation, the loss is generally only 30% of the pre-donation GFR. An adequate level of renal function is necessary, and accurate measurement of the GFR is thus essential. The standard estimated glomerular filtration rate (eGFR) is currently the Chronic Kidney Disease Epidemiology Collaboration (CKD -EPI) creatinine equation [13]. The eGFR is recommended by KDIGO as the preliminary step, to be followed by confirmatory GFR measurements using either the measured GFR using an exogenous filtration marker, an eGFR calculated with combined values of the serum cystatin C and serum creatinine (http://mdrd.com), a measured creatinine clearance or a repeat eGFR from a follow-up serum creatinine (See Table 1).

While there is no cut-off GFR value for accepting donors, most centers require eGFR to be > 80 ml/min, and some centers require > 90 ml/min. Those with values greater than 80 mL/min/1.73m^2 are acceptable provided other transplantation parameters have been successfully met. Donors whose eGFR is below 60 mL/min/1.73 m^2 should be declined. Those with eGFR between 60 and 79 mL/min/1.73m^2 should have confirmatory GFR studies by other methods. Based upon these results, a long-term kidney failure risk assessment should be undertaken using predictive models. (http://transplantmodels.com/esrdrisk) [14]. Those with an unacceptable risk should be declined.

The BTS Guidelines first recommend an eGFR using plasma creatinine. These guidelines also mandate a measured GFR, as well as a normal and adequate result in order to remain normal for the future life of the donor. The BTS recommends using an age - related GFR with different thresholds for men and women. A minimum GFR of 90 mL/min/1.73m^2 is recommended for donors under the age of 30. Age adjusted GFRs are also recommended for European Renal Best Practice (ERBP).

Table 1. Initial kidney function evaluation

GUIDELINE	eGFR	Measured GFR ^{99m}Tc-DTPA, Iothalamate or ^{51}Cr-EDTA
KDIGO (2017)	eGFR first	Confirm w Measured GFR or eGFR$_{cys\ cr}$, Measured creatinine clearance (CrCl), follow up eGFR
Canadian KPD Program (2015)		Required on one occasion and/or 24 h CrCl, on two separate occasions
ERBP (2013)	First line	Recommended
BTS (2011)		Mandate

The renal ultrasound is an important tool for imaging and is recommended for prospective living donors.

CKD /ESRD Risk

Studies published in the last decade have shown advanced understanding of donor risks over the long term in terms of renal function deterioration [15]. The first of such long-term studies [16] analyzed health -related quality of life (HRQol) using the 36-item Short Form Health Survey (SF-36) in approximately 2,500 adult kidney donors with a mean follow-up of 17 years. Gross and colleagues concluded that the donors had better health than their age - and sex -matched controls in the general population. Better outcomes probably reflected a select group who are motivated and have a better understanding and control of lives compared with the general population. Factors associated with lower scores of HRQoL included donors who were obese, less educated, had prior psychiatric difficulties, non-white, or not first-degree relatives of the recipient. African Americans and Hispanics had lower outcome scores.

While it was encouraging to see that donors did better than their counterparts in the population, risks of renal function deterioration over time were concerning. Two studies published around the same time: a Norwegian study [17], and a US study [18] raised alarms about future ESRD in this population. The Norwegian study included 1,904 individuals who donated a kidney with a median follow-up of 15 years. These donors were compared with a control group of 32,621 potentially eligible kidney donors in the population. The hazard ratio (HR) for all primary endpoints significantly increased - all-cause mortality among donors to 1.30 (95% confidence interval or CI 1.11 to 1.52), cardiovascular death 1.40 (CI 1.03 to 1.91), and risk of ESRD 11.38 (CI 4.37 to 29.6) [17]. Published around the same time was the US study by Muzaale et al. who compared 96,217 kidney donors with an equal number of healthy non-donors for a median follow-up of 7.6 years. ESRD developed in 99 individuals after donation compared with only 36 in healthy non-donors. The risk of ESRD developing 15 years after donation was 30.8/10,000 (CI 24.3 to 38.5) in kidney donors but only 3.9/10,000 (CI 0.8 to 8.9) in healthy non-donors ($p < .001$). The difference in risk of ESRD between donors and non-donors was observed regardless of race, with a risk of 74.7/10,000 black donors (CI 47.8 to 105.8) vs. 23.9/10,000 among black non-donors (CI, 1.6 to 62.4), and an estimated risk of 22.7/10,000 for white donors (CI, 15.6 to 30.1) vs. 0.0/10,000 (CI 0.0-0.0) for white non-donors developing ESRD ($P < .001$). The lifetime risk of developing ESRD was 90 per 10,000 for donors, and 14 per 10,000 for healthy non-donors [18]. These studies raised significant unease in the transplant community and led to a decrease in living donor transplants in the next couple of years.

Studies also showed risk of CKD among living donors. One study of nearly 4,000 predominantly white kidney donors found that 36% had eGFR < 60 ml/min per 1.73 m^2 (corresponding to CKD stage 3 or higher) at a median time of 9.2 years post-donation, and 2.6% had eGFR< 30 ml/min per 1.73 m^2 (corresponding to CKD stage 4 or higher) at a median of 23.9 years [19].

While the relative risk of ESRD is higher among living donors over time, the absolute risk is very small. These risks are well-analyzed by Lentine and Segev [15], such that they concluded the risks justify the practice of living donation. However, individual programs should identify donors at higher risk of developing CKD /ESRD in the future; these include younger age, African American race [20], high BMI, degrees of proteinuria, and hypertension. Particularly, African Americans with variants of APOL1 gene are at much higher risk. In this context, risk-projection models designed by Grams et al. [14], Massie et al. [21], and Ibrahim et al. [19] are available online and can be used to quantify individual risks. While these are helpful, it should be realized that none of these provide estimates risk for identical twin donors, or biological relatives vs. non-related donors. Liyanage et al. [22] point out that stratification based on familial risk by race cannot be conducted using these calculators because they do not take into account the genetic susceptibility that is based on APOL1 variants. In such cases, the individual program team, along with the patient, has to make an informed decision whether to proceed with the donation.

Hematuria and Proteinuria

The presence of protein in the urine dictates that the proteinuria to be quantified. According to the KDIGO and BTS guidelines, the urine albumin excretion rate or albumin-to-creatinine ratio (ACR) should also be determined. The Canadian KPD and ERBP guidelines support quantifying proteinuria or albuminuria. The ERBP suggests the protein excretion to be used as a screening test, and the ACR used for proteinuria levels under 300 mg/day. The ERBP considers albuminuria between 30 to 300 mg/day as high risk for donation, and an ACR > 30 mg/mmol as an absolute contraindication.

KDIGO accepts albuminuria below 30 mg/day as suitable, given other factors are also acceptable. However, BTS considers an ACR between 3 and 30 mg/mmol as a relative contraindication, and an ACR over 30 mg/mmol as an absolute contraindication. The CKPD is the most stringent with regard to microalbuminuria, declining those with an ACR greater than 3 mg/mmol.

This contrasts with KDIGO guideline recommendations that candidates between 30 and 100 mg/day should be individualized, and that the cutoff for declining transplant donor candidates should be an albuminuria over 100 mg/day.

Hematuria is also a factor that determines eligibility of a prospective kidney donor. While reversible causes are generally accepted, those with irreversible causes, especially those secondary to underlying glomerulonephritis, should be declined. Urologic disorders, particularly bladder cancer, should be excluded by cystoscopy and imaging procedures, especially in donors greater than 35 to 40 years of age. Kidney stones and urinary tract infections must be excluded. The presence of thin basement membrane disease is not a contraindication for donating a kidney. This benign disease is the cause of microscopic hematuria in 1% of the population and is characteristically a disorder of type 4 collagen. However, a kidney biopsy might be necessary to exclude other glomerular disorders associated with microscopic hematuria; i.e., 3 or more red blood cells per high power field (RBC /HPF). This is predominantly true if the hematuria is associated with proteinuria, or if upon examination of the urine sediment, the red blood cells are accompanied by red blood cell casts. Candidates diagnosed with primary or secondary glomerular disorders diagnosed on biopsy should be categorically declined.

Kidney Stones

Kidney stones occur in 11% of men and 7% of women in the United States, and the incidence is rising [23]. Patients with kidney stones should be evaluated with respect to the risk for recurrence. The Canadian KPD Program excludes donation candidates under 40 years of age who have had stones. A history of kidney stones should be given special attention considering there is a high risk of acute kidney injury in solitary kidney patients who develop a kidney stone. The donor candidate should be screened with imaging studies to assure unobstructed stones are present. Metabolic conditions, recurrent stones, and the presence of bilateral stones are contraindications for donation. Idiopathic hyperuricosuria patients are considered candidates. With respect to uric acid stones, a low urine pH is the most likely cause. One must consider that while gastrointestinal anion absorption is a strong determinant of urine pH, uric acid stone formation is seen more commonly in those with obesity, insulin resistance, and diabetes. Metabolic acidosis is associated with insulin resistance and may be present with microalbuminuria [24]. Most of these conditions will be screened during the evaluation. However, patients with idiopathic uric acid nephrolithiasis may have a lower ammonium excretion response to acid loading, suggesting that donor candidates with a history of uric acid stones and no systemic cause should have an acid-loading test performed as part of the evaluation [25]. Donor candidates should be aware of the possibility that a change in their renal function may put them at a higher risk for developing hyperuricemia or gout and may also put them at risk for metabolic bone disease. A reduction in renal mass could also accelerate a rise in hypertension and the need for antihypertensive therapy .

If a donor with isolated kidney stone is approved, the guidelines support that the kidney affected with the stone be selected for donation. In general, when asymmetry in GFR, parenchymal abnormalities, vascular abnormalities, or urological abnormalities are present but do not preclude donation, the more severely affected kidney should be used for donation [1].

Hypertension, Diabetes and Obesity

Hypertension

Hypertension should be assessed during the donor evaluation and should be measured on two separate occasions. Although essential hypertension is most common, there are several secondary causes. Candidates with possible secondary hypertension should be referred to their primary physicians for evaluation, and the secondary causes should be addressed before considering the patient for donation. White coat hypertension is characterized by an elevated blood pressure reading during the clinical encounter that may not occur in the home setting. Therefore, 24-hour ambulatory monitoring may be valuable to exclude it. Patients who have blood pressure readings below 140/90 mm Hg in office (<135/85 mmHg home readings) are acceptable as candidates for donation. Patients with hypertension but controlled blood pressure readings as previously mentioned with use of one or two antihypertensive medications are also candidates so long as they do not have target organ damage [1]. The decision to approve donor candidates with hypertension should be individualized based on demographic, health profile and family history, and the transplant program's acceptable risk threshold [1]. In a meta-analysis of pooled studies, the effect of kidney donation on blood pressure showed an increase of 6 mmHg in systolic pressure and 4 mmHg in diastolic pressure after 7 years of follow-up [26]. These were predominantly white men. The prevalence in African Americans is higher and follows same demographics as in the general population [20, 27].

Hypertension increases systemic resistance and causes endothelial damage. It disrupts the autoregulatory mechanisms of the kidney and potentiates glomerular damage. Thus, it can worsen kidney function over time unless appropriately managed. The risks of CKD and ESRD after donation as seen in the Norwegian and the US studies have been discussed previously.

Living donors of African American ancestry who have the high-risk APOL1 genotype are at greater risk. In a study of 19 two risk allele and 117 one risk allele donors the high-risk group had a lower GFR (57±18 versus 67 ± 15 ml/min per 1.73 m2; P=0.02) at a median of 12 years after surgery. Two of the high-risk donors developed ESRD. The high-risk group had a lower mean pre-donation GFR. The authors suggest the study to be interpreted with caution, as the study sample was small [28]. Several other studies have also shown a strong association of APOL1 gene variant and future CKD and hypertension particularly in African Americans. A large National Institutes of Health (NIH) study is now ongoing, assessing the risks of APOL1 gene variant and hypertension and kidney disease in kidney donors – the APOLLO study.

Diabetes

Age, body mass index, presence of diabetes, proteinuria or cardiovascular disease, increases the natural rate of kidney disease progression. Living donor candidates need to be screened for diabetes using a fasting blood sugar and follow-up glucose tolerance studies as needed. The hemoglobin A1c (HbA1c) is recommended as part of the lab panel for donor testing. The presence of type 1 diabetes is an absolute contraindication to donating a kidney. In contrast, type 2 diabetes is not a contraindication for either the BST or the KDIGO Guidelines. The CKPD and the ERBP guidelines do exclude type 2 diabetes. The risk of donors with type 2 diabetes developing ESRD is low, but diabetes is a leading cause among those donors who do develop ESRD. The decision to accept a donor candidate with type 2 diabetes or pre-diabetes should be individualized depending on the acceptable risk threshold of the transplant program [1].

Obesity

It is incumbent to evaluate the patient's body mass index (BMI), assess for diabetes and hyperlipidemia, and determine if the patient is using tobacco. A BMI over 35 kg/min^2 is an absolute contraindication in the ERBP, BST, and CKPD guidelines while the KDIGO guidelines recommend individualizing donor candidates with a BMI greater than 30 kg/m^2. KDIGO recommends evaluating the patient based on the presence of diabetes, tobacco use, and lipid profile. Lifestyle measures to control body mass index, cease cigarette smoking, and incorporate a regular exercise routine into one's routine activities should be emphasized. Active smokers are encouraged to cease the use of cigarettes for at least 4 weeks prior to surgery, and to commit to attempting to permanently stop tobacco use.

Assessing Cardiac Risk

Perioperative cardiovascular complications rarely occur among living donors, but the cardiovascular outcomes related to long-term reduction in GFR remain unknown. In a follow-up period of 6.5 years (median), ranging up to 17.7 years, 2,028 living kidney donors followed between 1992 and 2009 had a lower risk of death or major cardiovascular disease than healthy, matched controls (HR 0.66 CI 0.48 to 0.90) [29]. The survival curves are similar for the first decade but may converge in the second. After a median 15.1-year follow-up period, the risk of all-cause mortality and cardiovascular death were higher among living donors than their non-donor counterparts (HR 1.3 CI 1.1 to 1.5 HR 1.4 CI 1.0 to 1.9, respectively) [17].

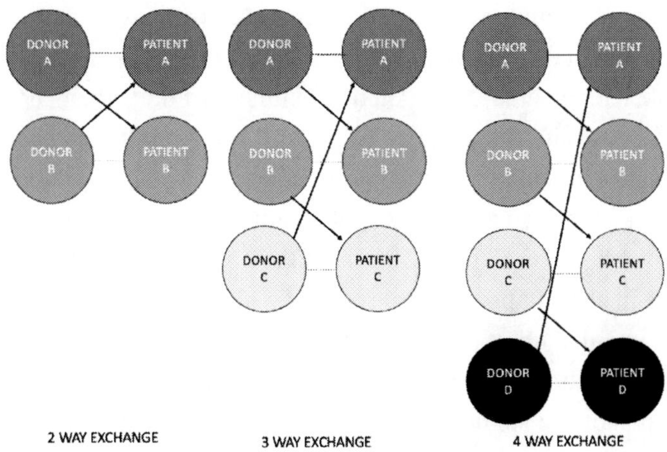

Figure 1. Scheme of kidney paired exchanges.

Although an electrocardiogram and chest x-ray are standard recommendations, there is no evidence thus far that demonstrates more rigorous cardiac testing would decrease either the short- or long-term risk but may serve as a baseline for future follow-up. Further testing such as echocardiography and stress test should be individualized. As this chapter goes to press, a prospective study is underway in Norway. The Cardiovascular rEmodelling in liviNg kidney donorS (CENS) study will evaluate 60 living kidney donors and 60 age - and sex -matched controls and follow them for 10 years. In addition to echocardiography and blood pressure monitoring, the study will look at numerous other factors, including bone density, microbiota, inflammation, calcium -phosphorus metabolism, nailfold capillaroscopy, and cardiac magnetic resonance imaging [30].

KIDNEY PAIRED DONATION (KPD)

Kidney paired donation (KPD) was originally proposed by Rapaport in 1986; it has expanded in every country and has increased the number of patients who are able to receive a kidney transplant [31]. Originally, this exchange was limited to two incompatible pairs to overcome ABO incompatibility or incompatibility due to sensitization. They could thus overcome immunological barriers to transplantation. Subsequently, they expanded to include more pairs as shown in Figure 1. The more the number of pairs, the more complicated it became for organizing and implementing the exchange, hence needing sophisticated software programs. Local, national, and even international registries have cropped up all over the world to make these transplants possible. These transplants have become reliable, convenient, result in good outcomes, and to some extent solved the dilemma of ABO incompatibility and sensitization that precluded living donors to help their loved ones or friends. It became evident that this domino-paired donation that had to be performed simultaneously limited the ability to scale upwards. Using an altruistic donor to donate a kidney to an unknown but compatible recipient whose family member then donates to another recipient started a chain that could expand to endless number of pairs. Still, a logistical barrier existed that limited the number of transplants because of the need for transplants to occur simultaneously. The use of non-simultaneous extended altruistic donor (NEAD) chains created the bridge donor concept. The bridge donor is the donor at the end of the chain. Although a person might decide not to donate, it was shown to be rare in actuality [32], as shown in Figure 2. Some of these concepts were based upon the game theory developed in the 1950s, the Gale-Shapley algorithm. In 2012, a Nobel Prize in Economics was awarded to Alvin Roth and Lloyd Shapley for the theory of stable allocations and the practice of market design. Non-simultaneous kidney exchange cycles (NSKEC) are chains of transplants that involve many donors and recipients. Pairs are co-registered, and backup deceased donor criteria offset the chance of reneging. A cohort study of 17 NSKECs culminated in 67 living-donor kidney transplants, some of which were sensitized and difficult to match. The study found the programs to be successful as a means to increase living-donor kidney transplants in developing countries [33]. Another strategy that has been adopted is inclusion of ABO/HLA compatible pairs for exchange with incompatible pairs such that an incompatible pair could be benefited; i.e., unbalanced KPD. This altruism of the compatible pair should be weighed against potential delay in the transplant for the compatible pair waiting to find a match with an incompatible pair [22]. Lastly, a voucher program could be used in which a donor could donate at his/her convenience in exchange for a voucher to the recipient when he/she needs it. This is particularly useful when donors have constraints on donation time. This "out-of-sequence' surgery allows flexibility for operating rooms and surgeons in scheduling the surgeries.

Prior to the implementation of KPD, living donors generally traveled to the recipient's destination, or vice versa. The success at being able to ship a kidney from one site to another revolutionized this process and set into motion the ability for recipients to find a match through a swap program across geographical zones. The first shipped living donor kidney was arranged by the National Kidney Registry (NKR) in 2008.

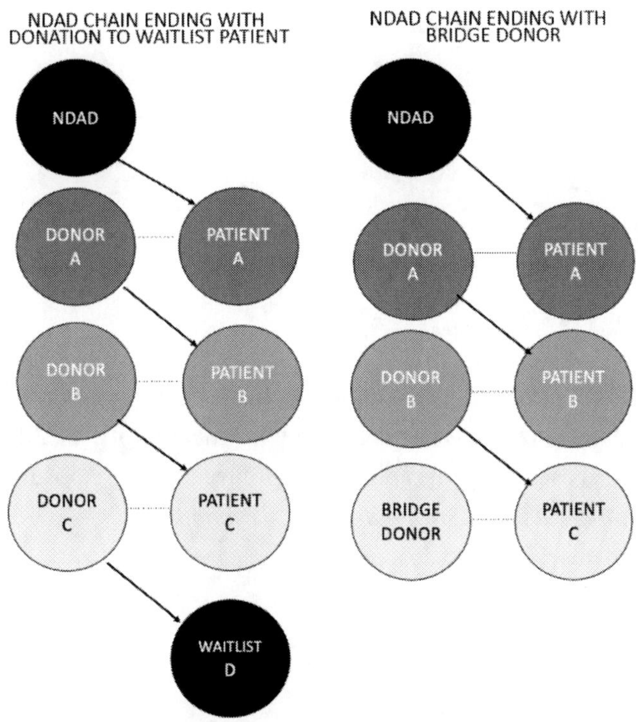

Figure 2. The concept of a chain started by a non-directed altruistic donor and ending with a bridge-donor. NDAD – non-directed anonymous donor (Good Samaritan donor).

Another innovation was the development of cryopreservation (2014 NKR Press Release - Cryo.docx - kidneyregistry.org – accessed 4/4/2021). This was implemented in 2015 by the National Kidney Registry and enabled more rapid completion of the crossmatch procedure. It also decreased the need for the donor to have blood drawn at multiple times for crossmatch for highly sensitized patients where there is a higher chance of unacceptable crossmatches. Desensitization was once a familiar way to confront the problems of a high calculated Panel Reactive Antibody (cPRA) level when an acceptable match was not possible. With a larger donor/recipient pool, acceptable histocompatibility matching has become more possible thus reducing the reliance on desensitization. Consequently, the graft survival of these transplants has also improved [34].

Risks of Transmissible Disease

Infection

The donor candidate should undergo a thorough history that inquires about past infections and risk factors. Based on KDIGO Guidelines, patients should be screened for the following transmissible infections.

- Human immunodeficiency virus
- Hepatitis B virus
- Hepatitis C virus
- Cytomegalovirus
- Epstein-Barr virus
- Syphilis (*Treponema pallidum)*
- Urinary tract infection

Geography and travel will play a role in determining the appropriateness of screening. The transplant centers should also coordinate with local public health authorities. Other potential infections (based on geographical or environmental exposure) include risks for *Mycobacterium tuberculosis, Strongyloides*, *Trypanosoma cruzi*, West Nile virus, histoplasmosis, and coccidiodomycosis.

Malignancy

Donors should also be screened for cancer, and those with active malignancy excluded from participation. The concerns with respect to malignancy are that occult disease may be transmitted to an immunosuppressed patient, and that the disease may recur in the donor. Those with a past history of cancer that have a low risk for transmission or recurrence may be acceptable on an individualized basis.

Genetics

There are many genetic disorders that need to be considered when evaluating a prospective donor. These include apolipoprotein-Ll (APOL1) variant, autosomal dominant polycystic kidney disease (ADPKD), atypical hemolytic uremic syndrome (aHUS), Alport syndrome, Fabry disease, familial focal segmental glomerulosclerosis (FSGS), and hereditary interstitial nephritis. Disease histories of autosomal recessive diseases are generally not considered contraindications. The risks of either the donor or recipient acquiring kidney disease after the transplantation should be assessed and fully explained to the donor. Genetic testing has been simplified in the past few years and should be considered. Those of sub-Saharan Africa n ancestry should be offered tests for APOL1 risk alleles. The presence of two copies of the APOL1 allele variant increases the chance of developing kidney failure in the donor irrespective of donating. The consequence of donating a kidney with 2 copies of the APOL1 allele variant is not known, and studies are in progress currently.

CHILDBEARING DONORS

The female donor of childbearing potential should be confirmed as not being pregnant by the human chorionic gonadotropin pregnancy test prior to donating a kidney. Those within a year of giving birth should be considered with respect to the psychological as well as general health needs of both the mother and the child. All female donor candidates should be asked about the prior history of hypertension or other disorder of pregnancy. They should not be excluded based on a desire to have children. But donors should be aware of the potential consequences donation may have on pregnancy in the future, such as mild degree of proteinuria, and a slightly increased frequency of hypertension during pregnancy. Neither of these affect the mother or the baby during pregnancy or after birth, but prospective mothers need to be aware of these risks. The long-term post donation risks on women with a history of preeclampsia or other hypertensive disorder should be considered.

PSYCHOSOCIAL EVALUATION

Donor candidates should have a face-to-face psychosocial evaluation. A detailed discussion of psychosocial evaluation of the donors and implications for donation are covered in the chapter on “Psychosocial Aspects of Kidney Transplantation in Kidney Transplant Recipients and Living Donors”. Donor autonomy should be respected, and transplantation services should follow all local laws and regulations. In the event that a living donor develops kidney failure and requires renal replacement therapy, there should be a process to assure suitable care. Candidates should be made aware of certain benefits that are available for donors. The current deceased donor allocation system allows a ‘safety net’ for such patients to elevate them to the top of the list for a kidney transplant when listed.

Surgical Approach

The current surgical approaches now most often suggested are the "mini-open" laparoscopy or hand-assisted laparoscopic technique. Post-operative recovery time is greatly reduced with laparoscopy. On occasion of mitigating circumstances, such as extensive previous surgery or adhesions, an open donor nephrectomy may be necessary. Since the publication of the most recent living donor recommendations (BTS 2018), progress with robotic living donor nephrectomy has been made using the da Vinci SI robotic platform in a three-arm configuration, in which the procedure is both safe and feasible with no conversion to an open nephrectomy procedure. The warm time ranged from 140 to 255 seconds and the median eGFR at 24months was 57.4 mL/min/1.73m^2. The level of experience with robotic surgery will influence outcomes [35].

Follow-Up Evaluation

The kidney donor should be monitored for CKD, followed in the clinic post donation, and should receive age -appropriate healthcare. KDIGO recommends that an annual follow-up visit include:

1. Blood pressure assessment
2. Body mass index
3. Serum creatinine and eGFR
4. Urine albumin determination
5. Review and promotion of a healthy lifestyle (eating habits, exercise routine, smoking abstinence)
6. Review as well as support of psychosocial health needs

Conclusion

The appropriate evaluation of the potential donor candidate must be done in the interest of safety and well-being for the donor while at the same time assuring the recipient receives a healthy kidney and a chance for an improved quality of life. Setting up a checklist for the evaluation, care, and follow-up of the living donor is advisable.

REFERENCES

[1] Lentine KL, Kasiske BL, Levey AS, Adams PL, Alberú J, Bakr MA, et al. KDIGO Clinical Practice Guideline on the Evaluation and Care of Living Kidney Donors. *Transplantation*. 2017;101(8S Suppl 1):S1-s109.

[2] Kim JJ, Fuggle SV, Marks SD. Does HLA matching matter in the modern era of renal transplantation ? *Pediatr Nephrol*. 2021;36(1):31-40.

[3] Weinstein JR, Anderson S. The aging kidney: physiological changes. *Adv Chronic Kidney Dis*. 2010;17(4):302-7.

[4] Kesimci E, Erkilic E, Kilinc I, Kilic M. Is an 87-Year-Old Grandfather Too Marginal for Being a Kidney Donor? The View of Anesthesiologists. *J Clin Med Res*. 2016;8(9):680-2.

[5] Hirano H, Maenosono R, Matsunaga T, Uehara H, Nomi H, Ichihashi A, et al. Safety of Elderly Living Kidney Donors: 2 Cases of Donors Older Than 80 Years: A Case Report. *Transplant Proc*. 2018;50(8):2569-71.

[6] Ivanovski N, Masin J, Kolevski P, Stojceva-Taneva O, Popov Z. Use of elderly living kidney donors: twenty years' experience in the Balkans. *Transplant Proc*. 2011;43(9):3415-7.

[7] Figurek A, Luyckx VA, Mueller TF. A Systematic Review of Renal Functional Reserve in Adult Living Kidney Donors. *Kidney Int Rep*. 2020;5(4):448-58.

[8] MacGregor MS, Boag DE, Innes A. Chronic kidney disease: evolving strategies for detection and management of impaired renal function. *QJM*. 2006;99(6):365-75.

[9] Levey AS, Stevens LA, Schmid CH, Zhang YL, Castro AF, 3rd, Feldman HI, et al. A new equation to estimate glomerular filtration rate. *Ann Intern Med*. 2009;150(9):604-12.

[10] Werner K, Pihlsgård M, Elmståhl S, Legrand H, Nyman U, Christensson A. Combining Cystatin C and Creatinine Yields a Reliable Glomerular Filtration Rate Estimation in Older Adults in Contrast to β-Trace Protein and β2-Microglobulin. *Nephron*. 2017;137(1):29-37.

[11] Drenth-van Maanen AC, Jansen PA, Proost JH, Egberts TC, van Zuilen AD, van der Stap D, et al. Renal function assessment in older adults. *Br J Clin Pharmacol*. 2013;76(4):616-23.

[12] Raman M, Middleton RJ, Kalra PA, Green D. Estimating renal function in old people: an in-depth review. *Int Urol Nephrol*. 2017;49(11):1979-88.

[13] Levey AS, Stevens LA. Estimating GFR using the CKD Epidemiology Collaboration (CKD-EPI) creatinine equation: more accurate GFR estimates, lower CKD prevalence estimates, and better risk predictions. *Am J Kidney Dis*. 2010;55(4):622-7.

[14] Grams ME, Sang Y, Levey AS, Matsushita K, Ballew S, Chang AR, et al. Kidney-Failure Risk Projection for the Living Kidney-Donor Candidate. *N Engl J Med.* 2016;374(5):411-21.

[15] Lentine KL, Segev DL. Understanding and Communicating Medical Risks for Living Kidney Donors: A Matter of Perspective. *J Am Soc Nephrol.* 2017;28(1):12-24.

[16] Gross CR, Messersmith EE, Hong BA, Jowsey SG, Jacobs C, Gillespie BW, et al. Health-related quality of life in kidney donors from the last five decades: results from the RELIVE study. *Am J Transplant.* 2013;13(11):2924-34.

[17] Mjøen G, Hallan S, Hartmann A, Foss A, Midtvedt K, Øyen O, et al. Long-term risks for kidney donors. *Kidney Int.* 2014;86(1):162-7.

[18] Muzaale AD, Massie AB, Wang MC, Montgomery RA, McBride MA, Wainright JL, et al. Risk of end-stage renal disease following live kidney donation. *Jama.* 2014;311(6):579-86.

[19] Ibrahim HN, Foley RN, Reule SA, Spong R, Kukla A, Issa N, et al. Renal Function Profile in White Kidney Donors: The First 4 Decades. *J Am Soc Nephrol.* 2016;27(9):2885-93.

[20] Lentine KL, Schnitzler MA, Xiao H, Saab G, Salvalaggio PR, Axelrod D, et al. Racial variation in medical outcomes among living kidney donors. *N Engl J Med.* 2010;363(8):724-32.

[21] Massie AB, Muzaale AD, Luo X, Chow EKH, Locke JE, Nguyen AQ, et al. Quantifying Postdonation Risk of ESRD in Living Kidney Donors. *J Am Soc Nephrol.* 2017;28(9):2749-55.

[22] Liyanage L, Muzaale A, Henderson M. The true risk of living kidney donation. *Curr Opin Organ Transplant.* 2019;24(4):424-8.

[23] Tundo G, Vollstedt A, Meeks W, Pais V. Beyond Prevalence: Annual Cumulative Incidence of Kidney Stones in the United States. *J Urol.* 2021:101097ju 0000000000001629.

[24] Souto G, Donapetry C, Calviño J, Adeva MM. Metabolic acidosis -induced insulin resistance and cardiovascular risk. *Metab Syndr Relat Disord.* 2011;9(4):247-53.

[25] Maalouf NM, Cameron MA, Moe OW, Sakhaee K. Novel insights into the pathogenesis of uric acid nephrolithiasis. *Curr Opin Nephrol Hypertens.* 2004;13(2): 181-9.

[26] Boudville N, Prasad GV, Knoll G, Muirhead N, Thiessen-Philbrook H, Yang RC, et al. Meta-analysis: risk for hypertension in living kidney donors. *Ann Intern Med.* 2006;145(3):185-96.

[27] Doshi MD, Goggins MO, Li L, Garg AX. Medical outcomes in African American live kidney donors: a matched cohort study. *Am J Transplant.* 2013;13(1):111-8.

[28] Doshi MD, Ortigosa-Goggins M, Garg AX, Li L, Poggio ED, Winkler CA, et al. APOL1 Genotype and Renal Function of Black Living Donors. *J Am Soc Nephrol.* 2018;29(4):1309-16.

[29] Garg AX, Meirambayeva A, Huang A, Kim J, Prasad GV, Knoll G, et al. Cardiovascular disease in kidney donors: matched cohort study. *BMJ* 2012;344: e1203.

[30] Blom KB, Bergo KK, Espe EKS, Rosseland V, Grøtta OJ, Mjøen G, et al. Cardiovascular rEmodelling in living kidNey donorS with reduced glomerular filtration rate: rationale and design of the CENS study. *Blood Press.* 2020;29(2):123-34.

[31] Rapaport FT. The case for a living emotionally related international kidney donor exchange registry. *Transplant Proc.* 1986;18(3) Suppl. 2):5-9.

[32] Ashlagi I, Gilchrist DS, Roth AE, Rees MA. Nonsimultaneous chains and dominos in kidney - paired donation-revisited. *Am J Transplant.* 2011;11(5):984-94.

[33] Kute VB, Patel HV, Modi PR, Rizvi SJ, Shah PR, Engineer DP, et al. Non-simultaneous kidney exchange cycles in resource-restricted countries without non-directed donation - a prospective single-center cohort study. *Transpl Int.* 2021.

[34] D'Alessandro T, Veale JL. Innovations in kidney paired donation transplantation. *Curr Opin Organ Transplant.* 2019;24(4):429-33.

[35] Serni S, Pecoraro A, Sessa F, Gemma L, Greco I, Barzaghi P, et al. Robot-Assisted Laparoscopic Living Donor Nephrectomy: The University of Florence Technique. *Front Surg.* 2020;7:588215.

In: Issues in Kidney Disease – Transplantation
Editors: B. V. R. Murthy and S. Z. Fadem
ISBN: 978-1-53619-960-4

Chapter 4

HISTOCOMPATIBILITY IN RENAL TRANSPLANTATION, AND IMMUNOLOGY OF TRANSPLANT REJECTION

Peter Jindra**, PhD, D(ABHI)
Division of Abdominal Transplantation, Department of Surgery,
Baylor College of Medicine, Houston, TX, USA

ABSTRACT

The study of human leukocyte antigen (HLA) molecules and their role in kidney transplant has evolved over the years to provide clinicians with enhanced diagnostic testing for pre-transplant evaluation of patients awaiting kidney transplant and post-transplant monitoring. High resolution HLA typing combined with single antigen bead (SAB) anti-HLA antibody detection ensure a highly accurate interpretation of donor-recipient histocompatibility. This chapter will define and highlight the essential role of histocompatibility in renal transplantation, explain the immunologic mechanisms of rejection and present the classification schema used with specific criteria to define various types of renal transplant rejections.

Keywords: histocompatibility, kidney transplantation, transplant rejection, immunology

INTRODUCTION

The human alloimmune response provides a complexity and range to ensure a host is protected from any foreign material that might pose a risk to its survival. This response is

* Corresponding Author's Email: Peter.Jindra@bcm.edu.

multifactorial which includes cellular responses (i.e., T cell s, Natural Killer cells, Macrophages), humoral responses (B cells), immune response genes, cytokines, and chemokines. Many additional factors including a host's genetics, ethnicity, nutrition, and viral infections can further act as modifiers to either enhance or inhibit the effectiveness of this response.

HLA Loci, Structure, and Function

The most essential genes involved in an alloimmune response are the human leukocyte antigen (HLA) genes located on chromosome 6. These highly polymorphic genes encode for major histocompatibility complex (MHC) molecules which function to present peptides to initiate the adaptive immune response. There are two classical HLA antigens, HLA class I (A, B, C) and HLA class II (DRB1, DRB3, DRB4, DRB5, DQA1, DQB1, DPA1, DPB1) shown in Figure 1. An HLA haplotype refers to the collection of these HLA genes inherited on the same chromosome. Each individual will therefore have two HLA haplotypes comprising two alleles at each locus. The polymorphic nature of HLA ensures a great amount of heterogeneity at each locus; however, some individuals can inherit two copies of the same allele at a specific HLA locus, hence considered homozygous. Interestingly, in HLA class II haplotypes, DRB1 alleles are linked to specific DRB3, DRB4, and DRB5 loci, while some have no DRB3/4/5 linkage association. Within the human population, having more or fewer HLA class II molecules creates an additional phenotype of diverse expression profiles on the cell surface to present peptides. Most individuals will not match another's HLA profile at all HLA specific loci; however, within siblings there is a 25% chance they will be HLA identical inheriting the same haplotypes from their parents.

Major histocompatibility complex (MHC) class I structure originated from a single heavy chain in association with β2 microglobulin; conversely, MHC class II has two chains (α-chain and β-chain) [1]. The expression level of HLA molecules is different between the loci and can be upregulated if induced with inflammatory stimuli. Regarding HLA class I molecules, HLA-A and B are more polymorphic and expressed 10 times higher than HLA-C antigens [2]; furthermore, HLA-DR is expressed higher than HLA-DQ and HLA-DP antigens. HLA class I molecules are expressed on all nucleated cells loaded with peptides limited to 9-10 amino acids from proteins found within the cell [3]. This provides a mechanism for the adaptive immune system to survey all nucleated cells for potential non-self peptides and react accordingly. Within the kidney graft, all nucleated cells express HLA class I molecules, which provides a mechanism for host effector $CD8^+$ T cells to recognize allopeptides. In contrast, MHC class II molecules are loaded with peptides, 13-25 amino acids in length, that are generated by proteolysis of self and non-self proteins in endosomes and lysosomes. This allows the APCs (antigen presenting cells) to collect antigen from the surrounding environment for presentation. HLA class II is expressed on interstitial dendritic cells and macrophages in healthy kidneys. When focusing on the glomerulus, MHC class II expression is less prominent only on some intrinsic glomerular cells. MHC class II antigens may also be present on the tubular epithelial cells and patrolling intravascular B cells and monocytes. Once inflamed, MHC class II expression can additionally be found on endothelial cells and podocytes in glomeruli [4].

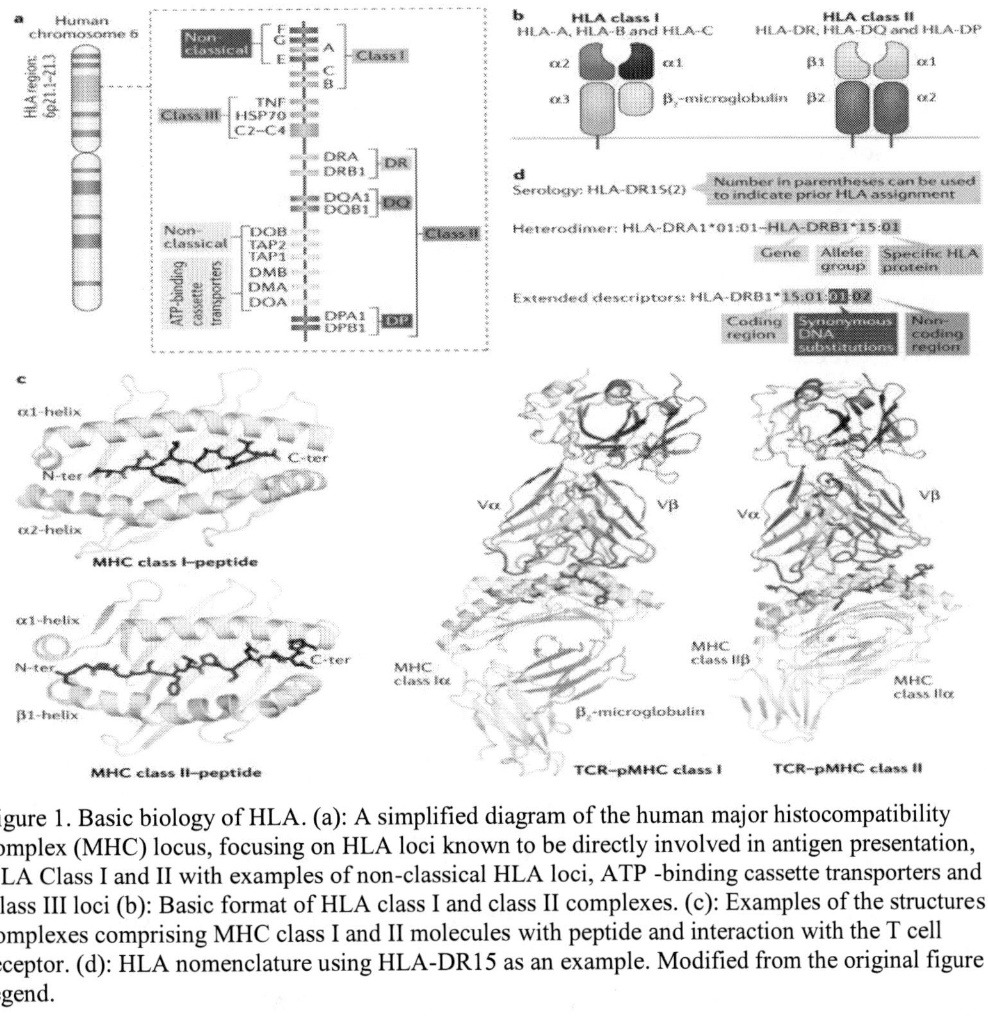

Figure 1. Basic biology of HLA. (a): A simplified diagram of the human major histocompatibility complex (MHC) locus, focusing on HLA loci known to be directly involved in antigen presentation, HLA Class I and II with examples of non-classical HLA loci, ATP -binding cassette transporters and Class III loci (b): Basic format of HLA class I and class II complexes. (c): Examples of the structures of complexes comprising MHC class I and II molecules with peptide and interaction with the T cell receptor. (d): HLA nomenclature using HLA-DR15 as an example. Modified from the original figure legend.

The expressed HLA class I and II molecules on the surface of antigen -presenting cells (APCs) present peptide to a T cell receptor (TCR) on $CD8^+$ or $CD4^+$ T cells, respectively [4]. The engagement of the TCR by the peptide-MHC complex is essential for the activation of $CD4^+$ and $CD8^+$ T cells, thereby leading to a robust cellular immune response, which includes the subsequent activation of B cells. B cells in turn are able to specifically bind native protein antigens and differentiate into plasma cells that secrete high amounts of antibody directed against the immunizing antigen. Activated effector $CD8^+$ T cells, Th1 phenotype $CD4^+$ T cells which secrete IFN -γ and Th17 $CD4^+$ T cells, can injure the renal allograft.

Advances in HLA Typing Methods

Typing of HLA antigens for renal transplant began using serology trays able to define HLA-A, B, Cw, DR, DRw and DQ antigens. This method uses antibodies in sera that recognize HLA complexes on the plasma membrane of the cell used for the test. HLA typing was more ambiguous without the ability to split some parent antigens. The expression levels of some HLA antigens were too low for detection by serology methods, leading the field to focus on molecular methods to HLA type all HLA loci A, B, C, DRB1, DRB3,4,5 DQA1, DQB1, DPA1, and DPB1. Molecular methods themselves have various levels of resolution depending on their primer designs and methods for amplifying HLA loci. They are able to achieve low resolution first field data from all 11 loci. Hybridization with sequence specific oligonucleotide probes (SSOP) and PCR with sequence specific primers (SSP) can provide low- and high-resolution HLA typing results. Optimally, with the advent of high throughput Next Generation Sequencing (NGS), recipient and confirmatory donor samples are able to be batched in order to obtain a high-resolution sequence in 3-5 days with minimal ambiguities/need for additional testing.

Physical Crossmatch Assessment

The gold standard assay for assessment of donor and recipient compatibility is the physical crossmatch assay. It was found early on that a positive cytotoxic crossmatch was associated with allograft failure [5]. The first crossmatch assay developed was based on the principle of assessing complement -dependent cytotoxicity. The complement-dependent cytotoxicity crossmatch (CDC -XM) is performed within a 72-well tray in which donor cells are plated and mixed with recipient serum at a variety of concentrations and dilutions. Following incubation, complement is added to all the wells. At this time in the assay, if there is a donor-specific anti-HLA antibody present and bound at high titer, this will cause antibody cross-linking and complement binding, which leads to cell death; this is visualized using a viability dye in all cells plated in the well. In order to increase the sensitivity of the CDC-XM assay following recipient serum incubation, anti-human globulin (AHG) is quickly added for a brief period of time that increases the crosslinking potential of anti-HLA antibodies. Deceased donors who were negative using the standard CDC-XM crossmatch, yet positive with AHG enhancement, displayed a significantly reduced kidney graft survival [6]. The CDC-XM can be performed on isolated T cell s, which is a measure of anti-HLA antibodies to class I antigens or isolated B cells expressing class I and II antigens on their cell surface. A measure of anti-HLA antibodies to class II antigens would be a positive B cell CDC-XM result in conjunction with a negative T cell CDC-XM result. CDC-XM assays performed solely on isolated lymphocytes in whole blood would mainly provide the detection of strong anti-HLA class I antibodies due to the lower percentage of B cells, less than 10% compared to T cells. With few cells expressing HLA class II antigen in a lymphocyte mixture isolated from whole blood, it is imperative to further isolate donor B cells if there is a concern for anti-HLA class II antibodies.

There are situations in which the CDC -XM can be positive and needs to have additional tests performed to confirm the reason for positivity. At initial kidney transplant evaluation, it's important to perform an auto CDC-XM by combining recipient serum with recipient lymphocytes, specifically in patients with a history of autoantibody. The presence of autoantibodies can lead to a false positive CDC-XM when on a single antigen bead panel since there are no anti-HLA antibodies detected. Auto reactivity can be acquired over time and there may be cases in which an auto XM is required at the time of transplant with the patient's pre-transplant serum drawn within the last 30 days. Another factor which could cause a false positive CDC-XM is the presence of anti-CD20 monoclonal antibody drug Rituximab in the patient serum. The presence of this drug in the recipient serum will bind to donor B cells, recruit complement, and lead to cell death. Residual serum Rituximab can induce false positive B cell crossmatches more than 6 months post-infusion emphasizing the importance of obtaining a detailed log of all transplant candidate's medication history [7]. Donors have also been documented to be taking Rituximab. For deceased donors, whole blood will be void of B cells; requesting donor lymph nodes or spleen is required to perform B cell crossmatches.

As we focus on which antibodies are detrimental to kidney allograft survival, IgG isotype antibodies are the main drivers of allograft loss, whereas IgM isotype antibodies are not contraindicated for kidney transplantation and are commonly found during crossmatch evaluation. To inactivate IgM, yet preserve IgG activity in the CDC -XM assay, recipient serum treatment with dithiothreitol (DTT) or Heat inactivation 63° for 10-13 mins are two validated methods. Performing the CDC-XM testing with and without one of these serum treatments provides accurate assessment of IgM and IgG antibody responses. IgM antibodies have not been shown to be deleterious to renal allograft transplantation, which some have attributed this to the IgM isotype low affinity [8, 9]. Furthermore, IgM antibodies may provide a protective role in organ transplantation inhibiting the pathological function of IgG autoantibodies and phagocytosis of apoptotic cells through activation of complement [10].

Flow cytometry crossmatch (FCXM) was developed as more of a sensitivity test to detect the binding of IgG isotype anti-HLA antibodies. Recipients with a positive FCXM experience more acute rejection episodes and have diminished long term survival [11]. FCXM requires no separation of T cells and B cells as each lymphocyte population is identified with specific antibodies directed against distinguishable cell surface markers CD3 for T cells and CD19 for B cells. Selection of a negative control serum using a variety of control samples with no detectable anti-HLA antibodies sets the background upon which 2 or 3 standard deviations define the positive cutoff values in the assays. Recipient serum and a negative control serum are incubated independently with donor lymphocytes. During this setup, if anti-HLA antibodies are present in the recipient serum, they will bind and the following step will be to detect this binding with an anti-human IgG secondary antibody, typically F(ab')2 fragment to eliminate non-specific binding between the Fc portions of the IgG secondary antibody and Fc receptors on lymphocytes. A fluorescence shift is calculated between the donor cells incubated with recipient serum and donor cells mixed with negative control serum. This channel shift difference in fluorescence is compared to the labs established positive cutoff as described previously. Any channel shift above this pre-determined cutoff is considered positive and any shift below is considered negative. Because there are anti-HLA antibodies binding at various strengths, the FCXM assay helps to quantitate the total sum of all anti-HLA antibodies binding to specific T cells or B cells. The amount of channel shift will increase with more anti-HLA antibody-bound. Therefore, small to borderline shifts can be detected at low titer or when a single anti-HLA antibody is present. Observing channel shift over this dynamic range highlights the sensitivity of FCXM over CDC -XM.

FCXM positivity exclusively on B cells is indicative of anti-HLA antibodies to class II antigens, whereas FCXM positivity on T cells and B cells, which both express class I antigen, is characterized as binding of anti-HLA class I antibodies. There are situations in which a T cell FCXM is positive in the absence of a B cell FCXM. This type of positive result requires further testing because if an anti-HLA antibody to MHC class I exists, one would expect to see both a T cell and B cell positive FCXM. One of these reasons why a T cell FCXM is positive in the absence of B cell FCXM positivity is related to how the lymphocytes are treated in the FCXM. The enzyme pronase is typically incubated with lymphocytes in order to eliminate the interference by the non-specific immunoglobulin binding by the Fc receptors with B cell surface immunoglobulins. As a side effect, pronase can denature additional proteins on the cell surface creating new epitopes for antibodies to bind. In the presence of pronase, kidney patients on Highly Active Antiretroviral Therapy (HARRT) due to HIV infection produce antibodies against epitopes exposed on donor T cells which leads to a false positive T cell FCXM. In these cases, running a FCXM without pronase confirms that channel shifts for T cells are significantly decreased and the T cell FCXM interpretation is truly negative which correlates with no anti-HLA class I antibodies detected. Like the CDC -XM, autoimmunity can also play a significant role in the result interpretation of a FCXM. In the absence of donor-specific anti-HLA antibodies, a positive T cell and/or B cell FCXM requires comparison to a patient's auto FCXM preferably using the same serum selected for allo-FCXM. Auto FCXM results can reveal that large channel shifts observed in the allo-FCXM are attributed to auto-reactivity [12]. Furthermore, as stated before when describing CDC-XM, Rituximab in the patient serum can additionally cause a strong false positive B cell crossmatch in FCXM as Rituximab is detected by the anti-human IgG secondary antibody bound to donor B cells. FCXM B cell channel shifts are elevated in this case as the assay is sensitive to high titer antibody and the ability to assess anti-HLA antibodies to class II antigens is uninterpretable. Given all the utility the physical crossmatch has to detect the binding of anti-HLA antibodies to donor cells and avoid hyper-acute and acute rejection episodes, there are fundamental situations as previously discussed of which the clinician needs to be aware when interpreting crossmatch results to ensure a patient is not denied a transplant due to an erroneous test result.

Virtual Crossmatch Assessment

The advancements in HLA typing have produced results which can be assessed quickly (under 4 hours) for a deceased donor typing; high resolution HLA typing is now used for confirmatory typing and living kidney donor transplants. These enhancements in speed and HLA allele resolution have allowed for a more accurate picture of antibody -antigen reactivity. Once a donor HLA type is available, a virtual crossmatch (VXM) can be performed assessing donor specific antibodies in a potential recipient's serum. However, the gold standard has always been a physical crossmatch (PXM). This assay gives a readout of recipient serum containing anti-HLA antibodies binding to HLA antigens expressed on the plasma membrane surface of either donor T cells or B cells. Through advancements in luminex technology the field has been able to place individual HLA antigens on the surface of luminex beads to detect anti-HLA antibodies binding their target antigen. Caveats to this method include denatured HLA antigens on beads, not a true representation of HLA expression on a plasma membrane cell surface; additionally, high background could lead to false positive s. Recipient serum requires treatment with either Ethylene Diamine Tetra acetic Acid (EDTA) or DTT to remove the inhibition effect of complement when high titers of anti-HLA antibodies are present. Even though there are drawbacks, this robust system has the ability to track anti-HLA antibody levels over time and predict the result of a physical crossmatch. This is an important point when considering deceased donor kidneys are shipped nationwide and the need to assess the histocompatibility of a donor-recipient pair when allocating an organ when no time exists for a physical crossmatch. With a virtual crossmatch, the HLA typing is performed by the donor typing center. This information is accessible to all centers with kidney patients on the waitlist and have serum evaluated for anti-HLA antibodies. By comparing the donor typing information with a waitlist candidate's anti-HLA antibody profile, a virtual crossmatch assessment can be performed and rules out any positives before physical crossmatches can be performed. This maximizes the use of donor cells, cuts down on the cold ischemia time, and decreases the time and effort to run multiple physical crossmatches.

When performing these assessments there are several guidelines which need to be considered to ensure the virtual crossmatch can most accurately reflect the physical crossmatch.

- The donor typing needs to be at single antigen bead resolution
- A plan for surrogate beads in case the donor's HLA antigen is not present in the HLA class I or II luminex panel used to assess a candidate's anti-HLA antibodies.
- An understanding of common HLA epitopes present which are targets for anti-HLA antibodies.
- Expression level of HLA molecules is different between the loci .

Next Generation sequencing has provided a cost -effective approach to sequence HLA molecules and therefore allows understanding of the amino acid sequence of each HLA locus. This knowledge translates into better understanding the target of what an anti-HLA antibody recognizes, which is called an epitope. Generation of epitope maps have been constructed to detail the positions of amino acid sequences which an anti-HLA antibody will recognize. Many of these epitopes are shared among various HLA antigens and is the reason why HLA antigens have groups called cross-reactive epitope groups (CREGs) [13]. Computer software has allowed mapping of epitopes to compare between donor and recipient level of epitope mismatch; it also allows assessment of an anti-HLA antibody profile from recipient serum. It is very important to recognize common epitopes such as Bw4 or Bw6 patterns in a recipient's serum. Common epitope sequences can be shared among multiple HLA alleles; the mean fluorescence intensity (MFI) of antibody binding this epitope can appear diluted as it is spread over multiple HLA antigens. A physical crossmatch where the donor cell surface may have either one or two copies of this epitope will yield a strong antibody binding response.

Epitope Mismatch Assessment

Having HLA mismatches has been proven to worsen kidney allograft survival. This was evident in the early days of kidney transplantation before immunosuppression was optimized. A cadaveric kidney donor that was a zero HLA A, B and DR mismatch had a one-year graft survival greater than 90%; however, this dropped significantly to 70% if HLA A, B and DR were all mismatched. But by the early 2000s, greater than 90% graft survival was observed at one year regardless of HLA mismatch [14]. There has been a paradigm shift in histocompatibility for renal transplantation; instead of matching donors and recipients for HLA antigens, we detect anti-HLA antibodies present in the patient sera that are donor specific and exclude only these antibodies as unacceptable. Over time, however, given the differences in HLA mismatches between a donor and recipient, the risk for developing antibody -mediated rejection increases. These changes in risk were not seen at the antigen or allele level differences in HLA but rather at the epitope level and predominately in HLA class II. An epitope refers to the sequence of amino acid residues which the antibody recognizes and to which it attaches. Until recently this area of study was challenging to explore. High resolution HLA typing combined with predictive computer algorithms now allows one to quantitate the number of HLA epitope mismatches. The resulting number of mismatches identified and how they can be applied as a clinical diagnostics has been reviewed [15]. HLA epitope matching provides an enhanced strategy to stratify recipients at risk of developing antibody-mediated rejection and is being considered for clinical use to help assess which patients need closer monitoring and whether immunosuppression can be tapered [16, 17]. Within these studies only the DR/DQ epitopes appear to have clinical relevance. The reasoning DR/DQ epitopes and not other HLA loci remains to be determined. Post kidney transplant, circulating de novo anti-HLA antibodies have also been predominantly anti-HLA DQ. Alloantibodies to HLA DQ can activate endothelial cells while reducing $FoxP3^+$ Treg proliferation [18]. HLA-DQ antigen expression is normally low; however, it can increase on the plasma membrane surface of endothelial cells when an inflammatory environment is present including IFN -γ and TNF -α cytokines.

Monitoring Patients for Donor Specific Antigens

Post-transplant monitoring for the development of DSA against donor HLA antigens is critical for the survival of the graft and to prevent continuous injury. Development of DSA for the first time after kidney transplant can vary between 10 and 40%. The development of de novo DSA has been shown consistently to be a predictor of allograft injury and reduced graft survival even more so than having a pre-existing DSA. It is crucial to identify de novo DSA early in the transplant course so treatments with plasmapheresis, IVIG, and/or Rituximab can be effective. If left unchecked or if there are issues with patient non-compliance, the diversity of potential injurious immune cells creating an inflammatory environment increases to a point where current immunosuppression methods may be unable to reverse. In order to ensure DSA monitoring is performed accurately, a few steps need to be taken into consideration.

- Confirmatory HLA type donor at the highest resolution possible with Next Generation Sequencing is preferable. In order to ensure accuracy of labeling a true DSA, HLA typing needs to be at the resolution of the HLA molecules conjugated to luminex beads. For each class I and II, there are 100 luminex beads each with a single HLA allele noted at the second field. HLA typing methods which only resolve HLA antigen to the first field constrain the DSA interpretation by either selecting the average of all the alleles with second field resolution or considering it an educated guess of the second field specific bead based on HLA haplotype frequencies.

- There are situations in which the donor HLA allele or HLA alpha-beta pair is not represented in a luminex bead panel. The best approach is to consider a surrogate bead that is within the panel which is most closely related in sequence to the allele or alpha-beta pair. Publicly available HLA alignment tools most notably from the IMGT (https://www.ebi.ac.uk/ipd/mhc/alignment/) provides a database of all known sequenced HLA alleles for comparison. Once the bead used to track a DSA is chosen, it is best to follow the same bead to track MFI levels over the course of transplantation.
- Lastly, anti-HLA antibodies are binding to epitopes, not just a single donor HLA specificity. The complete anti-HLA antibody profile needs to be assessed for specific donor specific epitopes and noted if they can be defined. Epitopes are commonly shared on multiple HLA molecules and DSA in the serum can bind to all HLA molecules sharing the sample epitope, which will lower the MFI signal. This is why MFI is not the sole metric that needs to be analyzed when assessing DSA development and tracking.

The characterization of DSA bound to C1q, the first member in the complement cascade, showed a significant increase in acute rejection, transplant glomerulopathy, and graft loss over a 10-year period [19, 20]. There were two populations at the high MFI range when comparing IgG DSA to IgG DSA that recruit complement. This would appear strange to have a group of antibodies at high MFI range using the IgG SAB test, yet unable to recruit complement. Further investigation would reveal IgG SAB MFI does directly correlate with C1q SAB MFI when various factors (prozone effect, denatured antigen beads) are removed and lead to false negative SAB results [21]. The prozone effect is related to the amount of complement within the serum. Various serum treatments with EDTA, DTT, or dilution are performed to eliminate the possibility of a false negative result.

Monitoring Patients for Non-HLA Antigens

In response to an allograft, B cells produce a polyclonal antibody to a variety of antigens. Although HLA is a common target for antibody production due to the high degree of polymorphism, other antigens have been found to elicit an alloantibody response. They may enhance the anti-HLA response by driving inflammation which in turn increases the expression of HLA molecules leading to a strengthening in the immune response. Biopsies with positive C4d staining confirm that an antibody has bound to cells in the graft, but in some cases this finding is not correlated with the presence of donor specific anti-HLA antibodies. In these cases, there is a search for the antibody responsible for this observation. Some antibodies have been consistently detected in the absence of anti-HLA antibodies and offer a better understanding of the humoral response to a renal allograft. Anti-angiotensin II type 1 receptor (AT1R) antibodies have been extensively studied and associated with allograft rejection. A clinical ELISA assay is able to detect the presence or absence of this antibody in patients' serum. Distinct from allorejection caused by anti-HLA antibodies, AT1R antibody was associated with renal patients having hypertension. On the biopsies of patients with AT1R antibodies, there is significantly more vascular rejection with arterial inflammation and higher levels of endothelial-associated transcripts which reflect an activation of the endothelium. Surprisingly, this pathology is also observed with no evidence of complement deposition in allograft capillaries [22]. Certain factors that significantly increase the likelihood that a patient will have anti-AT1R antibodies include young males, re-transplant patients, and those diagnosed with FSGS at the time of transplantation. These groups would potentially benefit from screening for non-HLA antibodies [23]. Many other non-HLA antigens have been described, but their association with renal transplant outcomes has not been conclusively demonstrated.

Immunology of Transplant Rejection

Cellular Arm of Transplant Rejection

Once a donor kidney is anastomosed and blood is perfused, there is an introduction of a foreign body to the host immune system. At this initial stage there is direct recognition in which the T cells of the host recognize foreign HLA molecules on the Antigen Presenting Cells (APC). Since these donor-derived APCs express HLA molecules with different epitopes, the recipient TCR receptor is able to identify these differences and bind to the foreign MHC peptides within the peptide binding groove, and start a signal transduction pathway. Further advancement of this signal requires costimulation with CD28 – B7 on the APC. These interactions lead to the release of interleukin 2 (IL-2) by the APC. This cytokine provides additional signal transduction through the IL-2 receptor. Emerging data provides further evidence that donor cells release extracellular vesicles (EV), which are taken up by recipient APC. The donor HLA molecules are stored within these vesicles [24]. The recipient APC will present these donor HLA molecules in similar fashion to their own HLA on the cell surface for recipient T cells to bind. This creates a micro-chimerism state. This process termed semi-direct or MHC cross-dressing allows recipient T cells to continue direct allorecognition even in the absence of donor APC. In murine models, cross-dressing of recipient APCs by small EV mediated delivery of donor MHC was the main pathway to directly stimulate allo-reactive T cells. Mastoridis et al. visually showed the presence of cross-dressed recipient cells expressing both recipient and donor HLA antigens using imaging flow cytometry after liver transplant and found their numbers significantly exceeding those of passenger leukocytes [25]. However, this process appears to decline rapidly post-transplant and is undetectable in as little as 30 days post-transplant. Given a patient's immunosuppression status and inflammatory environment, this process will remain dormant in the circulation active only in primary and secondary lymph node s. Host T cells that mediate allograft rejection interact with host dendritic cells (DCs) and differentiate into effector cells. DCs drive the rejection response mainly through displaying intact donor HLA on their surface in addition to processing of donor antigens into allopeptides, which are loading onto self-HLA molecules as a form of indirect presentation [26]. These processes are occurring in secondary lymphoid organs and can be challenging to assess as most blood or biopsy samples are either looking in the circulation or the graph itself. The kidney allograft is where the effector T cells migrate to and re-stimulate with host DCs to further their effector response. Release of chemokines and cytokines continue to drive the activation of the immune system by recruiting cells to the graft, adhere to the endothelium, and transmigrate with the end result to cause damage to essential renal allograft functions.

Antibody Arm of Transplant Rejection

Antibodies serve as a vital effector mechanism to target specific epitopes on proteins. A common target in the alloimmune response is for host B cells to make anti-HLA antibodies. Given HLA molecules are highly polymorphic in sequence, they can provide a diverse peptide repertoire for antigen presentation. Sensitization to HLA antigen occurs through a variety of mechanisms as follows:

- Blood transfusions: including platelets which express HLA class I antigens and can generate HLA class I antibodies
- Previous transplant /vein allograft
- Pregnancy in which anti-HLA antibodies are generated against the paternal HLA antigens
- Molecular mimicry in which sequence similarities between HLA and other peptides derived from other sources such as bacterial or viral exposure are cross-reactive

Before renal transplantation, alloantibodies to HLA molecules are tested. Antigens for which antibodies are found in high titers are avoided and listed as unacceptable. This ensures a patient will receive only a donor offer where the anti-HLA antibody levels are either negative or considered worth evaluating further. It was discovered early on that preformed cytotoxic antibodies were a contraindication to kidney transplantation [5]. Alloantibodies are required to be monitored and a crossmatch performed pre-transplant to avoid a hyper acute rejection. This occurs within minutes after a renal transplant is preformed due to high titers of antibodies specific to donor antigens. There have been three distinct pathways discovered in which antibodies harm their intended target. The most common method discussed involves the ability of the antibodies to recruit the complement cascade. Initially, IgG antibodies can fixate C1q and thereby activate the complement cascade, ultimately leading to the formation of the membrane attack complex, which structure creates pores within the target cell membrane lysing the cell. This process is done very efficiently by IgG1 and IgG3 subclasses while IgG2 and IgG4 exhibit no complement fixation due to their antibody structure hindering complement proteins from binding. Ironically, IgM is very good at recruiting complement, yet the presence of this antibody class does not lead to a hyperacute rejection response. Anti-HLA antibodies to IgM are routinely found in complement dependent cytotoxicity crossmatches (CDC -XM) and in the absence of IgG are not contraindicated for renal transplantation. A second method by which antibodies cause harm is through anti-HLA antibody binding through crosslinking of the HLA molecules at the cell surface which induces endothelial activation. Signal transduction pathways phosphorylate key proteins which leads to the upregulation of gene involved in cell proliferation, migration, and cell adhesion. Lastly, in association with the innate immune response, antibodies can induce lysis of target cells through a process of antibody-dependent cell mediated cytotoxicity [27, 28]. This occurs when the Fc portion of an anti-HLA antibody is bound to the donor kidney endothelium. The Fc portion will recruit a leucocyte, most commonly an NK cell, to induce apoptosis of the targeted endothelial cell which will in turn release cytokines to recruit additional inflammatory cells to the site of injury.

Innate Arm of Transplant Rejection

The innate immune response may provide the initial trigger that leads to activation of the adaptive immune response. Early after renal transplantation, innate immune transcripts for Toll-like receptors (TLR), specifically TLR-2 and TLR-4, allograft inflammatory factor-1 (AIF-1) and MyD88 were found to be elevated [29, 30]. Inflammatory signaling genes provide the initial stimulus to drive a dormant alloimmune response. Donor mitochondria released into the blood stream lead to increased endothelial cell activation and adhesion molecules in both EC and T cell s. These extracellular mitochondria are taken up by dendritic cells and endothelial cells increasing the expression of MHC class II molecules and eliciting a TH-1 cytokine response through increase in IFN -γ [31]. Cell free DNA has been shown to be increased in inflammatory processes. Detection of donor-derived cell-free DNA (dd-cfDNA) within a renal transplant patient's plasma has been shown to be predictive of histological rejection when the percentage of dd-cfDNA is above 1% [32, 33, 34.]

Natural Killer (NK) cells defined by the presence of CD56 on their cell surface have been found within the inflammation during active AMR. There is increased expression of

NK cell transcripts found within the biopsy which are not observed in the T cell -mediated rejection. Furthermore, quantitation of various cell types found in peritubular capillaries of biopsies classified as antibody -mediated rejection found a significant number of $CD56^+$ NK cells and $CD68^+$ macrophages. This recruitment is directly related to the antibody response as this infiltration is not seen in T cell-mediated rejection [35]. These results have been found in other studies which highlight that donor specific HLA antibodies induce innate immune response to areas of the graft [36]. Macrophage infiltration leads to enhanced antigen presentation in peritubular and perivascular compartment facilitating both T cell and antibody- mediated rejections [37]. In clinical practice, kidney transplant recipients who underwent biopsy for cause and had high scores of CD68(+) staining by immunohistochemistry were associated with increased risk of subsequent graft loss [38].

A detailed discussion of the pathology of acute and chronic rejection and Banff classification of rejection is presented elsewhere in this book.

Conclusion

This chapter describes the nomenclature, structure, and function of the HLA molecule and anti-HLA antibodies, which bind to specific epitopes found within the vast diversity of HLA antigens. The highly polymorphic nature of HLA requires a fundamental understanding of alleles, cross-reactive groups and epitopes which has been made possible through advancements in HLA typing methods, luminex technology, and computer -based software applications. Crossmatches, whether virtual or physical, will provide a pre-transplant immunologic readout that safeguards the recipients against any strong anti-donor response. Once the renal allograft is transplanted, the immune system provides an array of coordinated responses from both innate and adaptive sources within the context of an inflammatory milieu to recognize a donor allograft and response. Understanding these responses and how they can be identified with set criteria and modulated with immunosuppression can help ensure optimal kidney allograft survival.

References

[1] Wieczorek M, Abualrous ET, Sticht J, Alvaro-Benito M, Stolzenberg S, Noe F, et al. Major Histocompatibility Complex (MHC) Class I and MHC Class II Proteins: Conformational Plasticity in Antigen Presentation. *Front Immunol.* 2017;8:292.

[2] Apps R, Meng Z, Del Prete GQ, Lifson JD, Zhou M, Carrington M. Relative expression levels of the HLA class-I proteins in normal and HIV -infected cells. *J Immunol.* 2015;194(8):3594-600.

[3] Trolle T, McMurtrey CP, Sidney J, Bardet W, Osborn SC, Kaever T, et al. The Length Distribution of Class I-Restricted T Cell Epitopes Is Determined by Both Peptide Supply and MHC Allele-Specific Binding Preference. *J Immunol.* 2016;196(4):1480-7.

[4] Robson KJ, Ooi JD, Holdsworth SR, Rossjohn J, Kitching AR. HLA and kidney disease: from associations to mechanisms. *Nat Rev Nephrol.* 2018;14(10):636-55.

[5] Patel R, Terasaki PI. Significance of the positive crossmatch test in kidney transplantation. *N Engl J Med.* 1969;280(14):735-9.

[6] Kerman RH, Kimball PM, Van Buren CT, Lewis RM, DeVera V, Baghdahsarian V, et al. AHG and DTE/AHG procedure identification of crossmatch-appropriate donor-recipient pairings that result in improved graft survival. *Transplantation.* 1991;51(2):316-20.

[7] Desoutter J, Apithy MJ, Guillaume N. Unexpected Positive Prospective Crossmatches in Organ Transplant. *Exp Clin Transplant.* 2017;15(3):253-9.

[8] McCalmon RT, Jr., Tardif GN, Sheehan MA, Fitting K, Kortz W, Kam I. IgM antibodies in renal transplantation. *Clin Transplant.* 1997;11(6):558-64.

[9] Spees E, McCalmon R. Successful kidney transplantation with a positive IgM crossmatch. *Transplant Proc.* 1990;22(4):1887-8.

[10] Matsuda YH, T.; Li X; Watanabe, T. Characteristics of Immunoglobulin M Type Antibodies of Different Origins from the Immunologic and Clinical Viewpoints and Their Application in Controlling Antibody-Mediated Allograft Rejection. *Pathogens.* 2021;10(4).

[11] O'Rourke RW, Osorio RW, Freise CE, Lou CD, Garovoy MR, Bacchetti P, et al. Flow cytometry crossmatching as a predictor of acute rejection in sensitized recipients of cadaveric renal transplants. *Clin Transplant.* 2000;14(2):167-73.

[12] Hart JD, Lutz CT, Jennings CD, May JR, Nelson K, Jacobs S, et al. Falsely incompatible B-cell flow cytometry crossmatch after pronase treatment: a case report. *Transplant Proc.* 2015;47(3):831-3.

[13] El-Awar N, Jucaud V, Nguyen A. HLA Epitopes: The Targets of Monoclonal and Alloantibodies Defined. *J Immunol Res.* 2017;2017:3406230.

[14] D'Orsogna L, Fidler S, Irish A, Saker B, Moody H, Christiansen FT. HLA donor-specific antibody detected by solid phase assay identifies high-risk transplantation pairs irrespective of CDC crossmatch results: case reports and literature review. *Clin Transpl.* 2006:497-501.

[15] Cusick MF, Jindra PT. Human Leukocyte Antigen Epitope Matching in Solid Organ Transplantation. *Clin Lab Med.* 2018;38(4):595-605.

[16] Wiebe C, Kosmoliaptsis V, Pochinco D, Gibson IW, Ho J, Birk PE, et al. HLA - DR/DQ molecular mismatch: A prognostic biomarker for primary alloimmunity. *Am J Transplant.* 2019;19(6):1708-19.

[17] Davis S, Wiebe C, Campbell K, Anobile C, Aubrey M, Stites E, et al. Adequate tacrolimus exposure modulates the impact of HLA class II molecular mismatch: a validation study in an American cohort. *Am J Transplant.* 2021;21(1):322-8.

[18] Cross AR, Lion J, Poussin K, Assayag M, Taupin JL, Glotz D, et al. HLA -DQ alloantibodies directly activate the endothelium and compromise differentiation of FoxP3(high) regulatory T lymphocytes. *Kidney Int.* 2019;96(3):689-98.

[19] Yabu JM, Higgins JP, Chen G, Sequeira F, Busque S, Tyan DB. C1q-fixing human leukocyte antigen antibodies are specific for predicting transplant glomerulopathy and late graft failure after kidney transplantation. *Transplantation.* 2011;91(3):342-7.

[20] Loupy A, Lefaucheur C, Vernerey D, Prugger C, Duong van Huyen JP, Mooney N, et al. Complement-binding anti-HLA antibodies and kidney -allograft survival. *N Engl J Med.* 2013;369(13):1215-26.

[21] Taylor CJ, Kosmoliaptsis V, Martin J, Knighton G, Mallon D, Bradley JA, et al. Technical Limitations of the C1q Single-Antigen Bead Assay to Detect Complement Binding HLA -Specific Antibodies. *Transplantation.* 2017;101(6):1206-14.

[22] Lefaucheur C, Viglietti D, Bouatou Y, Philippe A, Pievani D, Aubert O, et al. Non-HLA agonistic anti-angiotensin II type 1 receptor antibodies induce a distinctive phenotype of antibody -mediated rejection in kidney transplant recipients. *Kidney Int.* 2019;96(1):189-201.

[23] Philogene MC, Zhou S, Lonze BE, Bagnasco S, Alasfar S, Montgomery RA, et al. Pre-transplant Screening for Non-HLA Antibodies: Who should be Tested? *Hum Immunol.* 2018;79(4):195-202.

[24] Gonzalez-Nolasco B, Wang M, Prunevieille A, Benichou G. Emerging role of exosomes in allorecognition and allograft rejection. *Curr Opin Organ Transplant.* 2018;23(1):22-7.

[25] Mastoridis S, Londono MC, Kurt A, Kodela E, Crespo E, Mason J, et al. Impact of donor extracellular vesicle release on recipient cell "cross-dressing" following clinical liver and kidney transplantation. *Am J Transplant.* 2020.

[26] Hughes AD, Zhao D, Dai H, Abou-Daya KI, Tieu R, Rammal R, et al. Cross-dressed dendritic cells sustain effector T cell responses in islet and kidney allografts. *J Clin Invest.* 2020;130(1):287-94.

[27] Valenzuela NM, Reed EF. Antibody-mediated rejection across solid organ transplants: manifestations, mechanisms, and therapies. *J Clin Invest.* 2017;127(7): 2492-504.

[28] Loupy A, Lefaucheur C. Antibody-Mediated Rejection of Solid-Organ Allografts. *N Engl J Med.* 2018;379(12):1150-60.

[29] McDaniel DO, Rigney DA, McDaniel KY, Windham WJ, Redmond P, Williams B, et al. Early expression profile of inflammatory markers and kidney allograft status. *Transplant Proc.* 2013;45(4):1520-3.

[30] Hosseinzadeh M, Ahmadpoor P, Yekaninejad MS, Pourrezagholi F, Foroughi F, Ghorbanpour M, et al. Expression patterns of Toll like receptor (TLR)-2, TLR-4 and myeloid differentiation primary response gene 88 (MYD88) in renal transplant patients developing allograft dysfunction; a cohort study. *Transpl Immunol.* 2018;48:26-31.

[31] Lin L, Xu H, Bishawi M, Feng F, Samy K, Truskey G, et al. Circulating mitochondria in organ donors promote allograft rejection. *Am J Transplant.* 2019;19(7):1917-29.

[32] Puliyanda DP, Swinford R, Pizzo H, Garrison J, De Golovine AM, Jordan SC. Donor-derived cell-free DNA (dd-cfDNA) for detection of allograft rejection in pediatric kidney transplants. *Pediatr Transplant.* 2020:e13850.

[33] Seeto RK, Fleming JN, Dholakia S, Dale BL. Understanding and using AlloSure donor derived cell-free DNA. *Biophys Rev.* 2020;12(4):917-24.

[34] Bloom RD, Bromberg JS, Poggio ED, Bunnapradist S, Langone AJ, Sood P, et al. Cell-Free DNA and Active Rejection in Kidney Allografts. *J Am Soc Nephrol.* 2017;28(7):2221-32.

[35] Hidalgo LG, Sis B, Sellares J, Campbell PM, Mengel M, Einecke G, et al. NK cell transcripts and NK cells in kidney biopsies from patients with donor-specific antibodies: evidence for NK cell involvement in antibody -mediated rejection. *Am J Transplant.* 2010;10(8):1812-22.

[36] Miyairi S, Baldwin WM, 3rd, Valujskikh A, Fairchild RL. Natural Killer Cells: Critical Effectors During Antibody-Mediated Rejection of Solid Organ Allografts. *Transplantation.* 2020.

[37] Bergler T, Jung B, Bourier F, Kuhne L, Banas MC, Rummele P, et al. Infiltration of Macrophages Correlates with Severity of Allograft Rejection and Outcome in Human Kidney Transplantation. *PLoS One.* 2016;11(6):e0156900.

[38] Paoletti E, Bussalino E, Bellino D, Tagliamacco A, Bruzzone M, Ravera M, et al. Early interstitial macrophage infiltration with mild dysfunction is associated with subsequent kidney graft loss. *Clin Transplant.* 2019;33(6):e13579.

In: Issues in Kidney Disease – Transplantation
Editors: B. V. R. Murthy and S. Z. Fadem ISBN: 978-1-53619-960-4

Chapter 5

Transplantation in the Highly Sensitized Recipient, and Living Donor Transplantation with Incompatible ABO Blood Group

Patricia West-Thielke**[*,1]**, PharmD, Pierpaolo Di Cocco**[1]**, MD, Enrico Benedetti**[1]**, MD and Bruce Kaplan**[2]**, MD

[1]Departments of Surgery and Pharmacy, University of Illinois at Chicago, Chicago, IL, USA

[2]Colorado Center for Transplant Care, Research and Education, University of Colorado, Aurora, CO, USA

Abstract

This chapter will review the management of highly sensitized kidney transplant recipients and recipients with incompatible donors. Transplant recipients who are highly sensitized or with an ABO-incompatible donor pose unique challenges in management. Desensitization for highly sensitized recipients can be performed in patients awaiting either living- or deceased-donor transplantation. Desensitization protocols are targeted on the prevention of early ABMR. There are many desensitization protocols combining different strategies which vary according to the immunological risk stratification. Crossing the ABO blood group barrier was historically considered to be a contraindication to transplantation because the formation of anti-blood group antibodies occurs when the recipient encounters foreign antigens. The protocols to accomplish ABOi living donor kidney transplantation are based plasmapheresis or immunoadsorption protocols to decrease the titer of anti-A and -B antibodies, B cell depletion, and immunosuppression. After the first two weeks post-transplant, ABOi recipients have similar graft outcomes to ABO compatible recipients.

[*] Corresponding Author's Email: .pmthielke@gmail.com.

Keywords: highly sensitized recipient, living donor transplantation, incompatible blood group

Introduction

Potential transplant recipients which are highly sensitized or with an ABO-incompatible donor pose unique challenges in management. The implementation of the new deceased donor Kidney Allocation System (KAS), which prioritizes highly sensitized candidates, improved desensitization protocols and the emergence of kidney paired donation programs (KPD) for incompatible living donor kidney transplantation have increased the likelihood of transplantation for these candidates [1]. Improving access to transplantation will translate in reduced waiting times and decreased waitlist mortality [2].

Approximately 30% of patients on the transplant waiting list have evidence of sensitization in the form of anti-Human Leukocyte Antigen (HLA) antibodies, generated from exposure to previous transplants, blood transfusion s, pregnancy, or other events. The presence of a panel-reactive antibody level of at least 80% (i.e., a high level of sensitization) creates difficulty in finding matched kidneys from compatible donors, leading to lower rates of transplantation in these patients compared to non-sensitized [3]. This chapter reviews the management of highly sensitized kidney transplant recipients and recipients with incompatible donors.

Highly Sensitized Recipients

History

In the late 1990s, the seminal work by Wolfe et al. brought to the attention of the medical community the fact that a successful kidney transplantation reduces mortality and improves quality of life compared to dialysis [4]. It soon became apparent that patients who remain on dialysis die at a high rate while waiting for an allograft [5-7]. As a consequence, at the same time, desensitization strategies emerged to address the immunologic barrier posed by sensitization to successful transplantation.

For the purposes of this chapter, desensitization is defined as the temporary removal or decreased production of antibodies. Sensitized individuals produce anti-HLA antibodies in response to exposure to the transplanted allograft [8]. This response is robust and involves plasma cells and memory B cells. True desensitization would require the elimination of memory cells which does not occur. Current desensitization protocols are impermanent, not enduring, as memory calls are still present.

In highly sensitized potential recipients, kidney transplantation with a negative standard crossmatch may not be easily attainable, therefore, lowering the levels of preformed antibodies may be the only feasible option. In summary, the rationale of desensitization has been twofold - increase the chance of successful kidney transplantation and prevent antibody -mediated rejection (ABMR). ABMR can be characterized as either early or late [9, 10]. Early ABMR is most commonly attributed to preexisting donor-specific antibodies (DSA) and occurs early after transplant, while late ABMR is associated with de novo DSA and generally occurs more than one-year post-transplant. Therefore, desensitization protocols are targeted on the prevention of early ABMR.

Desensitization can be performed in patients awaiting either living- or deceased-donor transplantation; however, the approach is slightly different considering the unpredictable timing of deceased-donor transplantation. Over the past 2 decades, several new therapeutic agents have been used in different protocols employing a combination of one of the following strategies:

1. Immunomodulation of the recipient immune system .
2. Removal of circulating anti-HLA antibodies .
3. Depletion of the B cell population responsible for anti-HLA antibody production.

Immunomodulation of the Recipient Immune System

Intravenous Immunoglobulin (IVIG)

IVIG is derived from human plasma pooled from thousands of donors and is primarily composed of IgG with trace amounts of IgA and IgM [11]. The new technology of chromatographic purification resulted in IgG products expressing higher concentrations and avidities [12]. In addition, IVIG in-vitro modification using tetra-Fc sialylation could enhance by 10-fold its immunomodulatory capacity [13]. Although their immunomodulatory effects were first recognized in studies from the early 1980s and subsequently found to have beneficial effects in autoimmune diseases and vasculitis, their mechanisms of immune modulation of innate and adaptive immune systems are several and still not fully characterized [11, 14]. The proposed mechanisms are complex and thought to involve most components of the immune system such as antibodies, complement, cytokines, most immune cells, including monocytes, macrophages, as well as both B and T cell s, and their receptors [11, 15-20].

Plasma-derived Immunoglobulin G (IgG) is now FDA approved for treatment of several primary and secondary immunodeficiency, and autoimmune inflammatory disease s, particularly those mediated by autoantibodies [11]. In addition, IVIG has multiple off-label use in prevention and treatment of ABMR of kidney allografts [21-23].

Efficacy in Desensitization

Jordan et al. in a multicenter prospective placebo -controlled trial conducted in the early 2000s highlighted the advantages of high dose IVIG (2 g/Kg) as a desensitizing agent, namely a reduction in PRA and improved transplantation rates among highly sensitized patients who received IVIG [17]. Subsequently, Montgomery et al., with a protocol of low dose IVIG (100 mg/kg) and plasma exchange (PLEX), demonstrated a significant survival benefit for patients with HLA sensitization who underwent living donor transplantation in comparison to patients who remained on dialysis or underwent HLA compatible transplantation [6].

Today, IVIG remains the cornerstone of all desensitization protocols. Most protocols use either high dose IVIG or low dose IVIG in combination with PLEX [6, 18]. The proposed mechanisms of IVIG desensitization include its inhibitory effect on B cells and T-cell proliferation, upregulation of anti-inflammatory Th2 cytokines and anti-idiotypic blockade of alloantibodies, and enhanced clearance of pathogenic IgG through blockade of FcR receptors [11, 18, 24].

However, several studies have shown that IVIG alone is not sufficient to sustain desensitization over the long term and is associated with antibody rebound post-transplant ation with ABMR [25-27].

In general, even high doses of IVIG are relatively safe with headache being the most common adverse event [17]. However, serious side effects have been reported, including acute renal dysfunction (likely related to high osmotic load), thrombotic events with rapid infusions, and aseptic meningitis [28].

Interleukin-6 (IL-6) Receptor Antagonist (Tocilizumab, Actemra®)

Tocilizumab is a humanized monoclonal antibody which binds to both soluble and membrane-bound forms of the interleukin-6 (IL-6) receptor [29, 30]. IL-6 is a key cytokine that regulates inflammation and the development, maturation, and activation of T cell s, B cells, and plasma cells [29]. Tocilizumab is now FDA approved for moderate to severe rheumatoid arthritis, systemic juvenile idiopathic arthritis (SJIA), and polyarticular juvenile idiopathic arthritis (PJIA) [31].

Efficacy in Desensitization

Animal models reveal that anti-IL-6 receptor therapy weakens alloantibody responses by increasing Treg and suppressing B-effector and plasma cells in bone marrow [30]. By targeting the IL-6/IL-6R pathway, reduction in antibody production and increases in Treg cells (CD4+, CD25+, FoxP3+) are likely [32]. This experimental evidence prompted Vo et al. to conduct a phase I/II trial of anti-IL-6R therapy on 10 highly sensitized patients who failed standard desensitization (IVIG + Rituximab ± PLEX) [33]. Patients received IVIG on days 0 and 30 at 2 g/kg and TCZ 8 mg/kg on day 15 and then monthly for 6 months. With this protocol, 7 of the 10 patients were transplanted and then received IVIG once and TCZ monthly for 6 months. Protocol biopsies (at 6 months) showed no evidence of ABMR or transplant glomerulopathy. The authors observed statistically significant reduction of donor specific antibody (DSA) strength and numbers at transplant and 12 months after transplantation. Although the results of this small trial are very encouraging, larger randomized controlled trials are needed to determine the overall efficacy of anti-IL6R drug therapy in desensitization. The infusions of Tocilizumab are overall well-tolerated, the most common side effects are hypertension, thrombocytopenia, and anemia .

Removal of Circulating Anti-HLA Antibodies

Plasmapheresis or Plasma Exchange and Immunoadsorption

Those are the two main strategies to remove antibodies and are regarded to be the fastest methods in doing so; in absence of randomized trials comparing their efficacy, their use remains center-dependent based on local expertise.

Plasmapheresis or Plasma Exchange (PLEX)

PLEX non-selectively removes immune complexes, protein bound toxins, circulating antibodies, complement components, and coagulation factors [34]. It is the most frequent modality applied in the United States and generally involves 1.0–1.5 volume exchange using albumin or plasma as replacement. PLEX is a reliable method of reducing antibodies and has been used in several desensitization protocols [35, 36]. However, antibody rebound is common if PLEX is used alone; it is therefore coupled with IVIG [6, 18]. PLEX is most commonly followed by low dose IVIG (100 mg/Kg), this strategy is considered by several authors more efficacious in preventing antibody rebound and antibody mediated rejection compared to high dose IVIG (2 g/Kg) [6, 37].

Commonly reported side effects (5-10%) include: allergic reactions that present as rigors and urticaria; symptoms of hypocalcemia such as paresthesia; and hypovolemia, which can manifest as muscle cramps and hypotension. Less frequent complications are related to the use of anticoagulants, the type of replacement fluid, and vascular access [34].

Immunoadsorption (IA)

IA is an extracorporeal hemofiltration technique based on affinity absorption [38, 39]. IA offers the advantage of no significant loss of clotting factors or albumin and therefore, requires no replacement of plasma [38, 40]. Disadvantages include higher cost, citrate reaction, hypotonia, reduced protective antibodies, and anaphylaxis. An obstacle of its use in United States is the fact that IA columns are not FDA approved. [36]. Several studies have reported the successful use of IA in highly sensitized patients alone or in combination with anti-CD20 therapy [41-43].

IgG Endopeptidase (Ides®)

IgG endopeptidase is a bacterial enzyme produced by *Streptococcus pyogenes* that cleaves all four human IgG subclasses at the lower hinge region of IgG heavy chains yielding $F(ab')_2$ and Fc fragments and can neutralize all IgG in the body within 4 hours of administration [44]. The rapid inactivation of IgG molecules inhibits both complement - dependent cytotoxicity (CDC) and antibody -dependent cytotoxicity (ADCC) [45]. There is a period of about 7 days during which both soluble IgG and the B cell receptor are not detectable, with a rebound and full reconstitution within 2 weeks [46].

Efficacy in Desensitization

Clinical trials in transplant patients have shown its ability to eliminate DSA; further, it has been used safely in highly sensitized individuals for desensitization [47, 48]. The main obstacle to its widespread use is the immunogenicity, anti-IdeS antibodies usually appear after only one or two doses [49]. An interesting area for future research would be for modulation of the immunogenicity of IdeS to allow for repeated dosing without production of anti-IdeS antibodies [50]. This drug will likely become part of desensitization protocols. Initial data are very promising showing complete removal of antibodies and may give hope to highly HLA sensitized patients who have received multiple rounds of desensitization without success.

Depletion of the B Cell Population Responsible for Anti-HLA Antibody Production

Rituximab (Rituxan®)

Rituximab is a chimeric monoclonal IgG antibody directed against the CD20 antigen expressed on the surface of both pre-B and mature B cells. Once bound to CD20, it causes B cell lysis via both complement -dependent cytotoxicity and antibody-dependent cell-mediated cytotoxicity. It is currently FDA approved for treatment of Non-Hodgkin's Lymphoma (NHL), Chronic Lymphocytic Leukemia (CLL), Rheumatoid Arthritis (RA), Granulomatosis with Polyangiitis (GPA) (Wegener's Granulomatosis) and Microscopic Polyangiitis (MPA).

Efficacy in Desensitization

Rituximab is an important adjunct for desensitization; according to some authors, B cell depletion prior to transplant would prevent post-transplant B cell activation, de novo DSA production, and transplant glomerulopathy [26, 27, 51, 52]. Vo et al. reported extensively on the efficacy of combination of high dose IVIG and rituximab in lowering anti-HLA antibodies and improving rates of transplantation in HLA sensitized patients [53]. A double-blinded, placebo -controlled trial of IVIG + placebo versus IVIG + rituximab for desensitization, conducted by the same group, was prematurely terminated due to serious adverse events (SAEs) and graft losses; the subsequent analysis showed that the SAEs were severe ABMRs and occurred in the IVIG + placebo group (26). Considering the limitations related to the small sample size, the IVIG + rituximab appeared more effective in preventing DSA rebound, ABMR, and development of transplant glomerulopathy determined by protocol biopsies after transplant. Since publication, other reports have demonstrated an important impact of rituximab on anamnestic responses to HLA antigens after transplant [51, 54, 55]. The most important impact of anti-CD20 therapy seems to be control and prevention of anamnestic responses, since rituximab has minimal effect in reducing antibody levels [54, 56].

Reported adverse effects include lung toxicity, hematologic toxicity, infectious and infusion related complications and, rarely, JC polyomavirus viremia [36, 57].

Bortezomib (Velcade®)

Bortezomib is a proteasome inhibitor which disrupts the normal intracellular protein degradation process and has been shown to induce plasma cell apoptosis and block anti-HLA antibody production [58]. It was FDA approved in 2008 for treatment of refractory multiple myeloma and has been used off label in the treatment of antibody mediated rejection with conflicting results [59, 60].

Efficacy in Desensitization

Woodle et al. with a proteasome inhibitor -based protocol achieved successful transplantation in 19 of 44 (43.2%) highly sensitized patients with low acute rejection rates (18.8%), with AMR rate of 12.5% and de novo DSA detected in 12.5% of transplanted patients [61]. Jeong et al. used a desensitization protocol of high dose IVIG, bortezomib, and rituximab and demonstrated an increased rate of deceased donor transplantation [62]. Limitations of the previous studies are related to the fact that they are open-labeled, nonrandomized trials, involving small numbers of patients; further multicenter, large-scale, randomized trials are needed to confirm these results.

Bortezomib is associated with significant side effects, mostly GI and hematologic toxicity, which limits enthusiasm for incorporation of this drug into most desensitization protocols [60].

Role of Complement

Emerging evidence over the past 15 years supports the concept that the complement cascade, traditionally considered a component of innate immunity, plays a major role as a mediator of graft injury [63].

C5 Inhibitor (Eculizumab ®, Soliris)

Eculizumab is a monoclonal antibody that binds protein C5 of the complement cascade, inhibiting its cleavage to C5a and C5b and formation of membrane attack complex C5b-9. It was approved by the FDA for use in the treatment of paroxysmal nocturnal hemoglobinuria and primary atypical hemolytic uremic syndrome. Eculizumab has been used off-label for antiphospholipid syndrome and the prevention and treatment of AMR in the kidney transplant population [64].

Efficacy in Desensitization

2 multicenter randomized Phase II trials have suggested a protective effect for administering eculizumab prior to clinical evidence of AMR in positive crossmatch HLA -incompatible living and deceased donor populations [65, 66]. However, studies with longer follow-up failed to show a statistically significant reduction in the incidence of chronic AMR, a finding likely related to the complexity of the mechanisms of antibody mediated injury besides complement activation [67, 68].

C1 Esterase Inhibitor (Berinert®, C1-INH)

C1 inhibitor (C1-INH) is a serine protease inhibitor that inactivates both C1r and C1s, thus regulating proteases in both the classical and lectin complement pathways and resulting in major downstream effects on regulation of the coagulation and inflammation cascade. Two C1-INH products, Berinert® (CSL Behring, Kankakee, IL, USA) and Cinryze® (Shire ViroPharma Inc., Lexington, MA, USA) are currently approved for use by the FDA in the treatment of hereditary angioedema. Proximal complement inhibition with C1-INH has also been studied as a therapeutic target in kidney transplant recipients with ABMR [69].

Efficacy in Desensitization

A recent blinded, placebo -controlled, phase I/II trial of C1-INH for prevention of ABMR in highly HLA sensitized patients was conducted by Vo et al. Twenty patients were enrolled in this phase I/II trial and results showed that no patient in the C1-INH group developed ABMR during the 1-month study period [70]. These preliminary results are encouraging and support the need for larger studies of C1-INH in this setting.

Protocols

There have been multiple iterations of desensitization protocols combining different available strategies. Most of the protocols applied vary according to the immunological risk stratification based on the result of the complement -dependent cytotoxicity (CDC) T and B cell crossmatch, and T and B cell flow cytometry crossmatch, the presence and intensity of DSAs, and the presence of living donor [71].

Table 1. Criteria and protocols for desensitization adopted by most transplant centers

Presence of potential living donor (Y/N)	Immunological status	Desensitization (Y/N)	Strategy/Protocols
Y	CDC positive	N Majority of Institutions	Consider different strategy (i.e., Kidney paired donation)
Y	CDC negative Positive flow	Y Majority of Institutions	PLEX (alternating day) plus low dose IVIG (100mg/kg post PLEX) OR PLEX (alternating day) plus low dose IVIG (100mg/kg post PLEX) plus rituximab 375 mg/m2 (approximately 4 weeks before transplant) OR Rituximab 375 mg/m2 on days 0 and 14 plus high-dose IVIG 2 g/kg on days 28 and 42*
Y	CDC negative Flow negative	N Majority of Institutions	The presence of DSAs may dictate close immunological monitoring post-transplant *
N		Y	Based on the likelihood to receive an offer (see text) Likely to receive an offer in the short term then: Rituximab 375 mg/m2 on days 0 and 14 plus high-dose IVIG 2 g/kg on days 28 and 42

*Some centers proceed with desensitization.

Use of alternating day plasmapheresis and low dose IVIG (100mg/kg post plasmapheresis session) has been shown to provide survival benefit for highly sensitized patients receiving renal transplants compared to remaining on dialysis [6]. Protocols that have expanded on this strategy have added a single dose of rituximab 4 weeks prior to transplant for depletion of B-cell populations. This is followed by removal of circulating anti-HLA antibodies via PLEX or IA approximately a week prior to transplant [72]. The timing of surgery and the length of the desensitization is driven by the level of the antibody titers which would allow a successful transplantation. Another strategy of desensitization involves using high-dose IVIG (2g/kg) combined with rituximab; however, multiple trials have demonstrated high rates of ABMR and allograft loss [26, 73]. Lastly, small scale studies using protocols with the proteasome inhibitor Bortezomib for plasma cell apoptosis combined with rituximab and plasmapheresis demonstrated suppression of anti-HLA antibody levels for several weeks after treatment [61]. In highly sensitized patients without living donor options, a strategy applied to some centers is to offer pretransplant desensitization if the patient is likely to receive a deceased donor offer in the short term, based upon the number of years of waiting time and the points allotted by the kidney allocation system for his/her degree of allosensitization [71].

Outcomes

Better immunological risk stratification with sensitive DSA screening assays, avoidance techniques, and the implementation of KAS has led to improved transplantation rates. Highly sensitized patients with a potential live donor, even if incompatible, have more options; however, still, only approximately 6.5% of highly sensitized patients receive a transplant each year [74]. Transplantation across a complement -dependent cytotoxicity crossmatch historically has shown poor outcomes and the goal of desensitization is to reduce the antibody level in order to obtain a negative flow crossmatch or lower than a predetermined cutoff [75]. With this goal in mind, several different protocols have been used with varying success; the combination of IVIG + rituximab ± plasma exchange, especially for patients with DSAs of low to moderate intensity, has consistently shown acceptable short- and long-term outcomes and improvement in long-term patient survival compared to remaining on dialysis [6, 73, 76]. From the studies present in the literature, it is evident that transplanting highly sensitized patients carries an increased risk of ABMR; 25%–50% of transplants will have an early ABMR [37, 53, 77, 78]. Most of these rejections can be successfully treated, but a high rate of transplant glomerulopathy and chronic ABMR leading to accelerated allograft failure is common [79]. The evidence that after prolonged blockage of the complement system with eculizumab chronic damage to the allograft still occurs raises the suspicion that complement-independent pathways play a role [64, 67]. Thus, the optimal desensitization protocol before transplant and the best maintenance immunosuppression remains to be determined.

Incompatible Donors

Incompatible ABO Blood Group

Patients with blood type O or B can spend beyond 5 years on the waiting list before receiving a transplant translating to a 50% mortality rate [80]. ABO-incompatible (ABOi) transplantation has been shown to increase this survival rate from 50% to roughly 90% at 5 years. However, Scientific Registry of Transplant Recipients (SRTR) data still shows that even with current desensitization protocols, there remains a significantly lower graft survival rate amongst ABOi renal transplants when compared to their compatible counterparts, driven mostly by graft loss in the first 14 days. In fact, after the first two weeks post-transplant, ABOi recipients have similar graft outcomes to ABO compatible recipients.

History

The first attempt at crossing the ABO barrier was made in 1955 by Hume et al. [81, 82]. In that series, 8 of 10 ABOi renal allografts were lost within the first few postoperative days because of hyperacute rejection. Although in 1964 Starzl et al. reported 3 successful kidney transplants across the ABO barrier, over the next 2 decades several case reports of unsuccessful attempts at kidney transplant across ABO antigens were published. A large case series was published in 1987, revealed a graft survival rate of 4% at 1 year in 25 ABOi kidney transplants. Therefore, ABO incompatibility generally was considered an absolute contraindication to kidney transplantation .

One promising area identified quite early was the potential use of A2 donors for O and B recipients [81, 83]. It was shown that the expression of A antigens on erythrocytes from A2 individuals was much weaker than the expression in A1 individuals. In whites, the A2 subtype constitutes approximately 20% of blood group A individuals. Based on this premise and previous experiments using skin grafts from both A1 and A2 donors, trials began to transplant blood group A2 donors into O recipients. In 1987, Rydberg et al. reported that in 20 transplants performed under this protocol, 8 were lost within a month, whereas 12 maintained long- term function [83]. With improvements in immune-suppression medications and intensive immunologic monitoring, results of A2 donors into O or B recipients have now reached outcomes equal to that of compatible donors [84]. These findings have been able to help a minority of kidney transplant candidates with available ABOi living donors.

The modern era of effective and reliable desensitization in ABOi living donor kidney transplant was introduced by Alexandre et al. between 1982 and 1987 [85]. The Belgian group was the first to introduce plasmapheresis as a strategy to reduce the titers of anti-A or -B antibodies. Furthermore, after 3 transplants failed secondary to hyperacute rejection, they introduced recipient splenectomy at the time of the kidney transplant to minimize the risk of ABMR. Immunosuppression included cyclosporine, steroids, and azathioprine, with induction based on antilymphocyte globulin. In the original series of 26 patients, the investigators reported a 75% 1-year graft survival rate. Further development in the field has come from centers in Japan [86]. Living donor transplantation is virtually the only chance at life without dialysis since cadaver kidney transplants are rarely performed in Japan for primarily cultural reasons. The next significant development was the replacement of splenectomy with rituximab, a humanized monoclonal antibody that binds to CD20 on the B cell membrane.

Immunologic Considerations

Crossing the ABO blood group barrier was historically considered to be a contraindication to transplantation because the formation of anti-blood group antibodies occurs when the recipient encounters foreign antigens [87]. Isoagglutinins are antibodies produced due to an ABO incompatibility between the recipient and donor and the subsequent reaction results in complement activation. Blood group O is known to express higher antibody titers to both A and B antigens which results in a higher incidence of ABMR. In addition, as described above, the expression of A antigens on erythrocytes from A2 individuals is much weaker than the expression in A1 individuals.

Accommodation is the lack of an antigen -antibody reaction despite the presence of donor specific antibodies in the recipient [88]. The end result in ABOi transplant recipients is no significant allograft injury despite activation of complement by antibodies in the recipient. One of the hallmarks of accommodation is C4d deposition, with reports of detection in up to 90-95% of ABOi kidney transplant recipients. No clear mechanism for this has been fully elucidated, but it may be due to decreased ABO antigen expression, up-regulation of complement inhibiting molecules, and endothelial chimerism.

Measurement of ABO titers pre-transplant is considered standard of care [80, 88, 89]. Most protocols are developed with the intent of achieving a minimum anti-donor blood group titer of ≤1:8 at the time of transplant, but this varies per center. The role of ABO titers post-transplant is controversial. There is no consensus of the positive predictive value of post-transplant elevated ABO titers for the occurrence of ABMR in the presence of elevated ABO titer [90, 91].

Strategies

The protocols to accomplish ABOi living donor kidney transplantation are based on 3 main strategies: (1) plasmapheresis or immunoadsorption protocols to decrease the titer of anti-A and -B antibodies; (2) B cell depletion, which was historically accomplished with splenectomy, but rituximab is currently used, and (3) immunosuppression with use of polyclonal antibodies for induction.

Removal of Anti-A/B Antibodies

Plasmapheresis or plasma exchange (PLEX) with or without intravenous immune globulin has been the mainstay of all protocols aimed at reducing the titers of anti-A/B antibody levels in preparation for an ABOi kidney transplant. PLEX non-selectively removes immune complexes, protein bound toxins, circulating antibodies, complement components, and coagulation factors [34]. This modality is still the standard in the United States and involves 1.0–1.5 volume exchange using albumin or plasma as replacement. This method reduces anti-A/B antibodies by approximately 20% per session but also removes protective immunoglobulins and coagulation factors [88]. Another method developed in Japan is double-filtration plasmapheresis which involves a second plasma filter which permits some of the smaller molecules to be returned back to the patient, thereby avoiding some of the safety concerns associated with removal of coagulation factors [92].

Several European centers have implemented the use of immunoadsorption (IA) to selectively remove anti-A and -B antibodies, stating that it is as efficient as plasmapheresis and has the distinct advantage to avoid an indiscriminate depletion of serum proteins, including clotting factors and albumin, with excellent results. Selective immune absorption seems to be a more logical way to specifically remove preformed anti-A and -B antibodies [39, 72, 93-95]. There are different types of columns for IA. IA columns can utilize immobilized antibodies (Therasorb), immobilized staphylococcal protein A (Immunosorba), and immobilized antigens (Glycosorb-ABO). The specificity of each type for IgG antibodies varies. The Glycosorb-ABO system is not FDA approved; however, it is the most commonly utilized modality for removal of anti-A/B antibodies outside of the United States .

B Cell Depletion

Historically, splenectomy was utilized for B cell depletion; however, this came with several risks, including surgical and infectious complications. Sawada et al. first published the use of rituximab in a single ABOi case in 2002 but had also included splenectomy [96]. Rituximab is a chimeric monoclonal IgG antibody directed against the CD20 antigen expressed on the surface of both pre-B and mature B cells. Once bound to CD20, it causes B cell lysis via both complement -dependent cytotoxicity and antibody-dependent cell-mediated cytotoxicity. Subsequently, many investigators have investigated protocols without splenectomy utilizing rituximab at varying doses and time points.

Gloor et al. in 2005 published a comparison of splenectomy versus a protocol including rituximab with more intensive post-transplant plasmapheresis and concluded that splenectomy is not essential for successful ABOi kidney transplantation [97]. This was a retrospective review of 2 protocols, one with splenectomy and one without. The protocol without splenectomy included rituximab administered just prior to starting pre-transplant plasmapheresis, pre-transplant plasmapheresis with IVIG to achieve a titer of $\leq$ 1:8, aggressive immunosuppression with polyclonal antibody induction, tacrolimus, mycophenolate and prednisone, and post-transplant plasmapheresis with IVIG to maintain the IgG titer to $\leq$1:8 in the first week and $\leq$1:16 in the second week.

The protocol developed at the Karolinska University Hospital in Sweden has been widely adopted across Europe. This was first published by Tyden et al. in 2003 and was subsequently adjusted and published as a 3-year follow-up in 2008 concluding that their protocol achieves similar results in ABOi compared to ABOc [72, 98]. The protocol utilized one dose of rituximab (375 mg/m2) given 2–4 weeks before IA, followed by a conventional triple-drug immunosuppressive protocol consisting of tacrolimus with a targeted trough level of 15–20 ng/mL, mycophenolate mofetil (2–3 g) and prednisolone (30 mg), starting 1 week before IA. Induction therapy was not used. Postoperatively, tacrolimus trough level of 15 ng/mL during the first month, 10 ng/mL during the second month and 5 ng/mL thereafter, and mycophenolate mofetil of 2 g during the first 3 months and thereafter, of 1 g. The prednisolone dose was increased to 100 mg on the first postoperative day, and then decreased every day by 10 mg until 20 mg, which was maintained for the first month. The dose was 15 mg during the second month and 10 mg thereafter. Preoperatively, the anti-A or anti-B antibodies were removed using antigen - specific immunoadsorption (Glycosorb ABO, Glycorex Transplantation, Lund, Sweden). Four preoperative apheresis sessions were used to achieve a preoperative antibody titer of IgG <1:8. If this was not achieved after four sessions, the transplantation was postponed for 1 week and four more sessions were performed. Postoperatively, three more apheresis sessions were given every third day over the total period of 9 days. If there was a significant increase in the antibody titers, extra sessions were considered.

Montgomery et al. 2009 published a retrospective review of 60 consecutive ABOi transplant performed between 1999 and 2007 [99]. The treatment protocol developed over this time frame from one that included to splenectomy, to replacement of splenectomy with rituximab, to removal of both methods of B cell depletion. The protocol always included pre-transplant plasmapheresis with CMVIg and the number of treatments ranged from 2-6 based on the isoagglutinin AHG titer. Tacrolimus and mycophenolate mofetil were started at the onset of pre-transplant PP/CMVIg. A minimum of 2 post-transplant PP/CMVIg were performed but this was increased in cases of antibody rebound, high starting titers and antibody mediated rejection. The immunosuppression regimen consisted of daclizumab (IL2), dexamethasone 100 mg intraoperatively and 25 mg every 6 hour for six doses postoperatively, followed by prednisone 30 mg/day decreased to 5-10mg/day once tacrolimus therapeutic. The outcomes demonstrated that this regimen, without B-cell depleting therapy, allowed for successful ABOi transplantation with low rate of ABMR.

Immunosuppression

Due to the immunologic risk with ABOi kidney transplantation, aggressive immunosuppressive protocols have been used since the 1980s to reduce the risk of immunologic graft loss. Most centers in the US and Japan have used quadruple therapy with polyclonal or monoclonal (anti-CD25) antibodies as induction and chronic immunosuppression based on tacrolimus, mycophenolate mofetil, and corticosteroids [80, 92, 97]. The introduction of a commercially available anti-CD20 antibody that specifically targets B cells has led to several trials in which this molecule was implemented into ABOi protocols. The timing of administration has been either 2-4 weeks before the transplant or at the time of transplant and the dose varies from 100-500 mg/m^2; however, a single dose 4 weeks before transplant is the most common. The intended goal was to decrease the chance of humoral rejection and eliminate the need for splenectomy. As discussed previously, those trials have been extremely successful, although the combination of multiple innovations in the treatment make it difficult to dissect the real value of each single component of the protocol. As already mentioned, ABOi kidney transplants have already been performed successfully without anti-CD20 induction. The role of anti-CD20 therapy in this setting deserves further investigation. Eculizumab, a monoclonal antibody against C5, has been investigated in the setting of ABOi with some success [100-102].

Table 2. ABOi protocols [72, 80, 92, 94, 97, 99]

	Pretxp tx	Rituximab	Posttxp tx	Pre-Immunosuppression	Post-Immunosuppression
Gloor 2005; Mayo Clinic	PP/IVIG to achieve IgG < 1:8	375 mg/m2 just prior to PP/IVIG regimen	PP/IVIG to achieve IgG < 1:8 during week 1 and < 1:16 during week 2	Mycophenolate 1g twice daily starting 1-5 days pre-transplant,	Thymoglobulin 1.5mg/kg, 5-7 doses; tacrolimus (12-15 ng/ml 1st month, 10-12 to 3 months, 6-8 after), mycophenolate, Methylprednisolone 500mg intra-operatively, prednisone tapered to 30mg/day by end of week1 and to 5mg.day by month 3
Genberg 2008/Tyden 2005; Karolinska	IA x 4-8 sessions to achieve IgG < 1:8	375 mg/m2 at 2-4 weeks pre-IA	IA x3 sessions more if needed	Tacrolimus (15-20 ng/ml), mycophenolate (2-3g), prednisolone (30mg) starting 1 week pre-IA	Tacrolimus (15ng/ml 1st month, 10ng.ml 2nd month and 5ng/ml after), mycophenolate (2g for 3 months then 1g), prednisolone (100mg on POD1, then decreased by 10mg/day till dose of 20mg, 15 mg 2nd month and 10mg after)
Okumi 2019; Japan	1-3 sessions of double filtration plasmapheresis	200g/body (equivalent to 125 mg/m^2)5 days before transplant		Tacrolimus, mycophenolate, and prednisone started 7 days before transplant	Basiliximab (20mg days 1 and 4)
Montgomery 2009; Johns Hopkins	PP/ CMVIg to achieve IgG < 1:16	None in most recent protocol	PP/IVIG – minimum of 2	Tacrolimus and mycophenolate mofetil beginning on the first day of their pretransplant PP/ IVIG	Daclizumab (2 mg/kg initial dose and 1 mg/kg every 2 weeks for 5 total doses; dexamethasone 100 mg intraoperatively and 25 mg every 6 hr for six doses postoperatively, followed by prednisone 30 mg/day decreased to 5-10mg/day once tacrolimus therapeutic

Protocols

Okumi et al. published a review of ABOi protocols used in Japan since their first ABOi transplant in 1989 [92]. The current protocol includes 1-3 sessions of double filtration plasmapheresis, tacrolimus, mycophenolate, and prednisone started 7 days before transplant, induction with basiliximab (20mg days 1 and 4), and rituximab 200g/body (equivalent to 125 mg/m^2) 5 days before transplant which has achieved similar rates of patient and graft survival (99.1% and 05.9% versus 90.2% and 88.3%, respectively). The table below summarizes the protocols that have been discussed above and are commonly seen in the literature.

Conclusion

Significant advances have been made in the management of highly sensitized kidney transplant recipients awaiting either living- or deceased-donor transplantation. Desensitization can be performed either using immunomodulation of the recipient immune system, removal of circulating anti-HLA antibodies, or depletion of the B cell population responsible for anti-HLA antibody production. Most commonly, a combination of these are used. Transplantation of these highly sensitized patients carries an increased risk of ABMR, most of them early after transplantation. While most of these rejections can be successfully treated, a high rate of transplant glomerulopathy and chronic ABMR leading to accelerated allograft failure is common. The optimal desensitization protocol before transplant and the best maintenance immunosuppression remains to be determined.

ABOi transplantation among living donors is being performed increasingly with excellent outcomes. These protocols include plasmapheresis or immunoadsorption, B cell depletion, and immunosuppression with polyclonal antibodies for induction. The use of these protocols significantly improves access to transplantation in these complex populations.

References

[1] Israni AK, Salkowski N, Gustafson S, et al. New national allocation policy for deceased donor kidneys in the United States and possible effect on patient outcomes. *J Am Soc Nephrol.* 2014; 25: 1842–48.

[2] Sapir-Pichhadze R, Tinckam KJ, Laupacis A, Logan AG, Beyene J, Kim SJ. Immune Sensitization and Mortality in Wait-Listed Kidney Transplant Candidates. *J Am Soc Nephrol.* 2016; 27: 570–78.

[3] Cecka JM, Kucheryavaya AY, Reinsmoen NL, Leffell MS. Calculated PRA: initial results show benefits for sensitized patients and a reduction in positive crossmatches. *Am J Transplant.* 2011; 11: 719–24.

[4] Wolfe RA, Ashby VB, Milford EL, et al. Comparison of mortality in all patients on dialysis, patients on dialysis awaiting transplantation, and recipients of a first cadaveric transplant. *N Engl J Med.* 1999; 341: 1725–30.

[5] Gill JS, Tonelli M, Johnson N, Kiberd B, Landsberg D, Pereira BJ. The impact of waiting time and comorbid conditions on the survival benefit of kidney transplantation. *Kidney Int.* 2005; 68: 2345–51.

[6] Montgomery RA, Lonze BE, King KE, et al. Desensitization in HLA-incompatible kidney recipients and survival. *N Engl J Med.* 2011; 365: 318–26.

[7] Kahwaji J, Jordan SC, Najjar R, et al. Six-year outcomes in broadly HLA-sensitized living donor transplant recipients desensitized with intravenous immunoglobulin and rituximab. *Transpl Int.* 2016; 29: 1276–85.

[8] Aubert O, Loupy A, Hidalgo L, et al. Antibody-Mediated Rejection Due to Preexisting versus *De Novo* Donor-Specific Antibodies in Kidney Allograft Recipients. *J Am Soc Nephrol.* 2017; 28: 1912–23.

[9] Haas M, Loupy A, Lefaucheur C, et al. The Banff 2017 Kidney Meeting Report: Revised diagnostic criteria for chronic active T cell-mediated rejection, antibody-mediated rejection, and prospects for integrative endpoints for next-generation clinical trials. *Am J Transplant.* 2018; 18: 293–307.

[10] Haas M, Mirocha J, Reinsmoen NL, et al. Differences in pathologic features and graft outcomes in antibody-mediated rejection of renal allografts due to persistent/recurrent versus de novo donor-specific antibodies. *Kidney Int.* 2017; 91: 729–37.

[11] Jordan SC, Toyoda M, Vo AA. Intravenous immunoglobulin a natural regulator of immunity and inflammation. *Transplantation.* 2009; 88: 1–6.

[12] Zuercher AW, Spirig R, Baz Morelli A, KäsermannF. IVIG in autoimmune disease - Potential next generation biologics. *Autoimmun Rev.* 2016; 15: 781–85.

[13] Washburn N, Schwab I, Ortiz D, et al. Controlled tetra-Fc sialylation of IVIg results in a drug candidate with consistent enhanced anti-inflammatory activity. *Proc Natl Acad Sci. 2USA.* 2015; 112: E1297–306.

[14] Gilardin L, Bayry J, Kaveri SV. Intravenous immunoglobulin as clinical immune-modulating therapy. *CMAJ.* 2015; 187: 257–64.

[15] Basta M. Ambivalent effect of immunoglobulins on the complement system: activation versus inhibition. *Mol Immunol.* 2008; 45: 4073–79.

[16] Toyoda M, Pao A, Petrosian A, Jordan SC. Pooled human gammaglobulin modulates surface molecule expression and induces apoptosis in human B cells. *Am J Transplant.* 2003; 3: 156–66.

[17] Jordan SC, Tyan D, Stablein D, et al. Evaluation of intravenous immunoglobulin as an agent to lower allosensitization and improve transplantation in highly sensitized adult patients with end-stage renal disease: report of the NIH IG02 trial. *J Am Soc Nephrol.* 2004; 15: 3256–62.

[18] Glotz D, Antoine C, Julia P, et al. Desensitization and subsequent kidney transplantation of patients using intravenous immunoglobulins (IVIg). *Am J Transplant.* 2002; 2: 758–60.

[19] Tyan DB, Li VA, Czer L, Trento A, Jordan SC. Intravenous immunoglobulin suppression of HLA alloantibody in highly sensitized transplant candidates and transplantation with a histoincompatible organ. *Transplantation.* 1994; 57: 553–62.

[20] Glotz D, Haymann JP, Sansonetti N, et al. Suppression of HLA-specific alloantibodies by high-dose intravenous immunoglobulins (IVIg). A potential tool for transplantation of immunized patients. *Transplantation* 1993; 56: 335–37.

[21] Levine MH, Abt PL. Treatment options and strategies for antibody mediated rejection after renal transplantation. *Semin Immunol.* 2012; 24: 136–42.

[22] Montgomery RA, Loupy A, Segev DL. Antibody-mediated rejection: New approaches in prevention and management. *Am J Transplant.* 2018; 18 (suppl 3): 3–17.

[23] Schinstock CA, Mannon RB, Budde K, et al. Recommended Treatment for Antibody-mediated Rejection After Kidney Transplantation: The 2019 Expert Consensus From the Transplantion Society Working Group. *Transplantation.* 2020; 104: 911–22.

[24] Jordan SC, Toyoda M, Vo AA. Regulation of immunity and inflammation by intravenous immunoglobulin: relevance to solid organ transplantation. *Expert Rev Clin Immunol.* 2011; 7: 341–48.

[25] Vo AA, Lukovsky M, Toyoda M, et al. Rituximab and intravenous immune globulin for desensitization during renal transplantation. *N Engl J Med.* 2008; 359: 242–51.

[26] Vo AA, Choi J, Cisneros K, et al. Benefits of rituximab combined with intravenous immunoglobulin for desensitization in kidney transplant recipients. *Transplantation.* 2014; 98: 312–19.

[27] Loupy A, Suberbielle-Boissel C, Zuber J, et al. Combined posttransplant prophylactic IVIg/anti-CD 20/plasmapheresis in kidney recipients with preformed donor-specific antibodies: a pilot study. *Transplantation.* 2010; 89: 1403–10.

[28] Rault R, Piraino B, Johnston JR, Oral A. Pulmonary and renal toxicity of intravenous immunoglobulin. *Clin Nephrol.* 1991; 36: 83–86.

[29] Tanaka T, Kishimoto T. The biology and medical implications of interleukin-6. *Cancer Immunol Res.* 2014; 2: 288–94.

[30] Kim I, Wu G, Chai NN, Klein AS, Jordan S. Anti-interleukin 6 receptor antibodies attenuate antibody recall responses in a mouse model of allosensitization. *Transplantation.* 2014; 98: 1262–70.

[31] Rossi JF, Lu ZY, Jourdan M, Klein B. Interleukin-6 as a therapeutic target. *Clin Cancer Res.* 2015; 21: 1248–57.

[32] Fogal B, Yi T, Wang C, et al. Neutralizing IL-6 reduces human arterial allograft rejection by allowing emergence of CD161+ CD4+ regulatory T cells. *J Immunol.* 2011; 187: 6268–80.

[33] Vo AA, Choi J, Kim I, et al. A Phase I/II Trial of the Interleukin-6 Receptor-Specific Humanized Monoclonal (Tocilizumab) + Intravenous Immunoglobulin in Difficult to Desensitize Patients. *Transplantation.* 2015; 99: 2356–63.

[34] Okafor C, Ward DM, Mokrzycki MH, Weinstein R, Clark P, Balogun RA. Introduction and overview of therapeutic apheresis. *J Clin Apher.* 2010; 25: 240–49.

[35] Zachary AA, Montgomery RA, Ratner LE, et al. Specific and durable elimination of antibody to donor HLA antigens in renal-transplant patients. *Transplantation.* 2003; 76: 1519–25.

[36] Abu Jawdeh BG, Cuffy MC, Alloway RR, Shields AR, Woodle ES. Desensitization in kidney Transplantation: review and future perspectives. *Clin Transplant.* 2014; 28: 494–507.

[37] Stegall MD, Gloor J, Winters JL, Moore SB, Degoey S. A comparison of plasmapheresis versus high-dose IVIG desensitization in renal allograft recipients with high levels of donor specific alloantibody. *Am J Transplant.* 2006; 6: 346–51.

[38] Schwenger V, Morath C. Immunoadsorption in nephrology and kidney transplantation. *Nephrol. Dial Transplant.* 2010; 25: 2407–13.

[39] Speer C, Kälble F, Nusshag C, et al. Outcomes and complications following ABO-incompatible kidney transplantation performed after desensitization by semi-selective immunoadsorption - a retrospective study. *Transpl Int.* 2019; 32: 1286–96.

[40] Belàk M, Borberg H, Jimenez C, Oette K. Technical and clinical experience with protein A immunoadsorption columns. *Transfus Sci. 2* 1994; 15: 419–22.

[41] Lorenz M, Regele H, Schillinger M, et al. Peritransplant immunoadsorption: a strategy enabling transplantation in highly sensitized crossmatch-positive cadaveric kidney allograft recipients. *Transplantation.* 2005; 79: 696–701.

[42] Bartel G, Wahrmann M, Regele H, et al. Peritransplant immunoadsorption for positive crossmatch deceased donor kidney Transplantation. *Am J Transplant.* 2010; 10: 2033–42.

[43] Morath C, Beimler J, Opelz G, et al. Living donor kidney transplantation in crossmatch-positive patients enabled by peritransplant immunoadsorption and anti-CD20 therapy. *Transpl Int.* 2012; 25: 506–17.

[44] von Pawel-Rammingen U, Björck L. IdeS and SpeB: immunoglobulin-degrading cysteine proteinases of Streptococcus pyogenes. *Curr Opin Microbiol.* 2003; 6: 50–55.

[45] Johansson BP, Shannon O, Björck L. IdeS: a bacterial proteolytic enzyme with therapeutic potential. *PLoS One.* 2008; 3: e1692.

[46] Järnum S, Bockermann R, Runström A, Winstedt L, Kjellman C. The Bacterial Enzyme IdeS Cleaves the IgG-Type of B Cell Receptor (BCR), Abolishes BCR-

Mediated Cell Signaling, and Inhibits Memory B Cell Activation. *J Immunol.* 2015; 195: 5592–601.

[47] Jordan SC, Lorant T, Choi J, et al. IgG Endopeptidase in Highly Sensitized Patients Undergoing Transplantation. *N Engl J Med.* 2017; 377: 442–53.

[48] Lonze BE, Tatapudi VS, Weldon EP, et al. IdeS(Imlifidase): A Novel Agent That Cleaves Human IgG and Permits Successful Kidney Transplantation Across High-strength Donor-specific Antibody. *Ann Surg.* 2018; 268: 488–96.

[49] Winstedt L, Järnum S, Nordahl EA, et al. Complete Removal of Extracellular IgG Antibodies in a Randomized Dose-Escalation Phase I Study with the Bacterial Enzyme IdeS--A Novel Therapeutic Opportunity. *PLoS One.* 2015; 10: e0132011.

[50] Lorant T, Bengtsson M, Eich T, et al. Safety, immunogenicity, pharmacokinetics, and efficacy of degradation of anti-HLA antibodies by IdeS(imlifidase) in chronic kidney disease patients. *Am J Transplant.* 2018; 18: 2752–62.

[51] Kohei N, Hirai T, Omoto K, Ishida H, Tanabe K. Chronic antibody-mediated rejection is reduced by targeting B-cell immunity during an introductory period. *Am J Transplant.* 2012; 12: 469–76.

[52] van den Hoogen MW, Kamburova EG, Baas MC, et al. Rituximab as induction therapy after renal transplantation: a randomized, double-blind, placebo-controlled study of efficacy and safety. *Am J Transplant*. 2015; 15: 407–16.

[53] Vo AA, Peng A, Toyoda M, et al. Use of intravenous immune globulin and rituximab for desensitization of highly HLA-sensitized patients awaiting kidney transplantation. *Transplantation.* 2010; 89: 1095–102.

[54] Zachary AA, Lucas DP, Montgomery RA, LeffellMS. Rituximab prevents an anamnestic response in patients with cryptic sensitization to HLA. *Transplantation.* 2013; 95: 701–04.

[55] Jackson AM, Kraus ES, Orandi BJ, Segev DL, Montgomery RA, Zachary AA. A closer look at rituximab induction on HLA antibody rebound following HLA-incompatible kidney transplantation. *Kidney Int.* 2015; 87: 409–16.

[56] Vieira CA, Agarwal A, Book BK, et al. Rituximab for reduction of anti-HLA antibodies in patients awaiting renal transplantation: 1. Safety, pharmacodynamics, and pharmacokinetics. *Transplantation.* 2004; 77: 542–48.

[57] Toyoda M, Thomas D, Ahn G, et al. JC polyomavirus viremia and progressive multifocal leukoencephalopathy in human leukocyte antigen-sensitized kidney transplant recipients desensitized with intravenous immunoglobulin and rituximab. *Transpl Infect Dis.* 2015; 17: 838–47.

[58] Perry DK, Burns JM, Pollinger HS, et al. Proteasome inhibition causes apoptosis of normal human plasma cells preventing alloantibody production. *Am J Transplant.* 2009; 9: 201–09.

[59] Everly MJ, Everly JJ, Susskind B, et al. Bortezomib provides effective therapy for antibody- and cell-mediated acute rejection. *Transplantation.* 2008; 86: 1754–61.

[60] Eskandary F, Regele H, Baumann L, et al. A Randomized Trial of Bortezomib in Late Antibody-Mediated Kidney Transplant Rejection. *J Am Soc Nephrol.* 2018; 29: 591–605.

[61] Woodle ES, Shields AR, Ejaz NS, et al. Prospective iterative trial of proteasome inhibitor-based desensitization. *Am J Transplant.* 2015; 15: 101–18.

[62] Jeong JC, Jambaldorj E, Kwon HY, et al. Desensitization Using Bortezomib and High-dose Immunoglobulin Increases Rate of Deceased Donor Kidney Transplantation. *Medicine (Baltimore).* 2016; 95: e2635. (Baltimore).

[63] Cravedi P, Heeger PS. Complement as a multifaceted modulator of kidney transplant injury. *J Clin Invest.* 2014; 124: 2348–54.

[64] Stegall MD, Diwan T, Raghavaiah S, et al. Terminal complement inhibition decreases antibody-mediated rejection in sensitized renal transplant recipients. *Am J Transplant.* 2011; 11: 2405–13.

[65] Marks WH, Mamode N, Montgomery RA, et al. Safety and efficacy of eculizumab in the prevention of antibody-mediated rejection in living-donor kidney transplant recipients requiring desensitization therapy: A randomized trial. *Am J Transplant.* 2019; 19: 2876–88.

[66] Glotz D, Russ G, Rostaing L, et al. Safety and efficacy of eculizumab for the prevention of antibody-mediated rejection after deceased-donor kidney transplantation in patients with preformed donor-specific antibodies. *Am J Transplant*. 2019; 19: 2865–75.

[67] Cornell LD, Schinstock CA, Gandhi MJ, KremersWK, Stegall MD. Positive crossmatch kidney transplant recipients treated with eculizumab: outcomes beyond 1 year. *Am J Transplant*. 2015; 15: 1293–302.

[68] Schinstock CA, Bentall AJ, Smith BH, et al. Long-term outcomes of eculizumab-treated positive crossmatch recipients: Allograft survival, histologic findings, and natural history of the donor-specific antibodies. *Am J Transplant.* 2019; 19: 1671–83.

[69] Montgomery RA, Orandi BJ, Racusen L, et al. Plasma-Derived C1 Esterase Inhibitor for Acute Antibody-Mediated Rejection Following Kidney Transplantation: Results of a Randomized Double-Blind Placebo-Controlled Pilot Study. *Am J Transplant.* 2016; 16: 3468–78.

[70] Vo AA, Zeevi A, Choi J, et al. A phase I/II placebo-controlled trial of C1-inhibitor for prevention of antibody-mediated rejection in HLA sensitized patients. *Transplantation.* 2015; 99: 299–308.

[71] Sethi S, Choi J, Toyoda M, Vo A, Peng A, Jordan SC. Desensitization: Overcoming the Immunologic Barriers to Transplantation. *J Immunol Res.* 2017; 2017: 6804678.

[72] Genberg H, Kumlien G, Wennberg L, Berg U, Tydén G. ABO-incompatible kidney transplantation using antigen-specific immunoadsorption and rituximab: a 3-year follow-up. *Transplantation.* 2008; 85: 1745–54.

[73] Vo AA, Petrozzino J, Yeung K, et al. Efficacy, outcomes, and cost-effectiveness of desensitization using IVIG and rituximab. *Transplantation.* 2013; 95: 852–58.

[74] Jackson KR, Covarrubias K, Holscher CM, et al. The national landscape of deceased donor kidney transplantation for the highly sensitized: Transplant rates, waitlist mortality, and posttransplant survival under KAS. *Am J Transplant.* 2019; 19: 1129–38.

[75] Orandi BJ, Alachkar N, Kraus ES, et al. Presentation and Outcomes of C4d-Negative Antibody-Mediated Rejection After Kidney Transplantation. *Am J Transplant* .2016; 16: 213–20.

[76] Orandi BJ, Luo X, Massie AB, et al. Survival Benefit with Kidney Transplants from HLA-Incompatible Live Donors. *N Engl J Med.* 2016; 374: 940–50.

[77] Thielke JJ, West-Thielke PM, Herren HL, et al. Living donor kidney transplantation across positive crossmatch: the University of Illinois at Chicago experience. *Transplantation.* 2009; 87: 268–73.

[78] Gloor JM, DeGoey SR, Pineda AA, et al. Overcoming a positive crossmatch in living-donor kidney transplantation. *Am J Transplant.* 2003; 3: 1017–23.

[79] Bentall A, Cornell LD, Gloor JM, et al. Five-year outcomes in living donor kidney transplants with a positive crossmatch. *Am J Transplant.* 2013; 13: 76–85.

[80] Montgomery JR, Berger JC, Warren DS, James NT, Montgomery RA, Segev DL. Outcomes of ABO-incompatible kidney transplantation in the United States. *Transplantation.* 2012; 93: 603–09.

[81] Thielke J, Kaplan B, Benedetti E. The role of ABO-incompatible living donors in kidney transplantation: state of the art. *Semin Nephrol.* 2007; 27: 408–13.

[82] Cook DJ, Graver B, Terasaki PI. ABO incompatibility in cadaver donor kidney allografts. *Transplant Proc.* 1987; 19: 4549–52.

[83] Rydberg L, Breimer ME, Samuelsson BE, BryngerH. Blood group ABO-incompatible (A2 to O) kidney transplantation in human subjects: a clinical, serologic, and biochemical approach. *Transplant Proc.* 1987; 19: 4528–37.

[84] Gloor JM, Lager DJ, Moore SB, et al. ABO-incompatible kidney transplantation using both A2 and non-A2 living donors. *Transplantation.* 2003; 75: 971–77.

[85] Alexandre GP, Squifflet JP, De Bruyère M, et al. Present experiences in a series of 26 ABO-incompatible living donor renal allografts. *Transplant Proc.* 1987; 19: 4538–42.

[86] Takahashi K, Saito K, Takahara S, et al. Excellent long-term outcome of ABO-incompatible living donor kidney transplantation in Japan. *Am J Transplant.* 2004; 4: 1089–96.

[87] Cen M, Wang R, Kong W, Deng H, Lei W, Chen J. ABO-incompatible living kidney transplantation. *Clin Transplant.* 2020; 34: e14050.

[88] Salvadori M, Tsalouchos A. Current protocols and outcomes of ABO-incompatible kidney transplantation. *World J Transplant.* 2020; 10: 191–205.

[89] Zschiedrich S, Kramer-Zucker A, Jänigen B, et al. An update on ABO-incompatible kidney transplantation. *Transpl Int.* 2015; 28: 387–97.

[90] Tobian AA, Shirey RS, Montgomery RA, et al. ABO antibody titer and risk of antibody-mediated rejection in ABO-incompatible renal transplantation. *Am J Transplant.* 2010; 10: 1247–53.

[91] Ishida H, Kondo T, Shimizu T, Nozaki T, Tanabe K. Postoperative rebound of antiblood type antibodies and antibody-mediated rejection after ABO-incompatible living-related kidney transplantation. *Transpl Int.* 2015; 28: 286–96.

[92] Okumi M, Kakuta Y, Unagami K, et al. Current protocols and outcomes of ABO-incompatible kidney transplantation based on a single-center experience. *Transl Androl Urol.* 2019; 8: 126–33.

[93] Becker LE, Siebert D, Süsal C, et al. Outcomes Following ABO-Incompatible Kidney Transplantation Performed After Desensitization by Nonantigen-Specific Immunoadsorption. *Transplantation.* 2015; 99: 2364–71.

[94] Tydén G, Kumlien G, Genberg H, Sandberg J, Lundgren T, Fehrman I. ABO incompatible kidney transplantations without splenectomy, using antigen-specific immunoadsorption and rituximab. *Am J Transplant.* 2005; 5: 145–48.

[95] Genberg H, Kumlien G, Wennberg L, Tydén G. Isoagglutinin adsorption in ABO-incompatible transplantation. *Transfus Apheresis Sci. 2* 2010; 43: 231–35.

[96] Sawada T, Fuchinoue S, Teraoka S. Successful A1-to-O ABO-incompatible kidney transplantation after a preconditioning regimen consisting of anti-CD20 monoclonal antibody infusions, splenectomy, and double-filtration plasmapheresis. *Transplantation.* 2002; 74: 1207–10.

[97] Gloor JM, Lager DJ, Fidler ME, et al. A Comparison of splenectomy versus intensive posttransplant antidonor blood group antibody monitoring without splenectomy in ABO-incompatible kidney transplantation. *Transplantation.* 2005; 80: 1572–77.

[98] Tydén G, Kumlien G, Fehrman I. Successful ABO-incompatible kidney transplantations without splenectomy using antigen-specific immunoadsorption and rituximab. *Transplantation.* 2003; 76: 730–31.

[99] Montgomery RA, Locke JE, King KE, et al. ABO incompatible renal transplantation: a paradigm ready for broad implementation. *Transplantation.* 2009; 87: 1246–55.

[100] West-Thielke P, Progar K, Campara M, et al. Eculizumab for Prevention of Antibody-Mediated Rejection in Blood Group-Incompatible Renal Transplantation. *Transplant Proc.* 2018; 50: 66–69.

[101] Locke JE, Magro CM, Singer AL, et al. The use of antibody to complement protein C5 for salvage treatment of severe antibody-mediated rejection. *Am J Transplant.* 2009; 9: 231–35.

[102] Biglarnia AR, Nilsson B, Nilsson T, et al. Prompt reversal of a severe complement activation by eculizumab in a patient undergoing intentional ABO-incompatible pancreas and kidney transplantation. *Transpl Int.* 2011; 24: e61–66.

In: Issues in Kidney Disease – Transplantation
Editors: B. V. R. Murthy and S. Z. Fadem
ISBN: 978-1-53619-960-4

Chapter 6

IMMUNOSUPPRESSION IN TRANSPLANTATION

Vishnu Parvathareddy[1], MD and Nidhi Aggarwal[2,*], MD
[1]Selzman Institute for Kidney Health, Section of Nephrology,
Baylor College of Medicine, Houston, TX, USA
[2]Selzman Institute for Kidney Health, Section of Nephrology,
and Michael E. DeBakey Veterans Affairs Medical Center,
Baylor College of Medicine, Houston, TX, USA

ABSTRACT

Kidney transplantation is considered the best choice for renal replacement therapy for most patients with chronic kidney disease. Pharmacologic immunosuppression has played a major role in the success of kidney transplantation. High levels of immunosuppression (induction immunosuppression) are required in the early post-transplant period due to the highest risk of acute rejection. Later post-transplant period is managed with lower level of immunosuppression (maintenance immunosuppression). Drug protocols vary among different transplant centers, and anywhere from two to four drugs in different combinations are used. While the main goal of these agents is to prevent rejection and maintain long-term allograft function, toxic side effects may necessitate modification of drug regimens from time to time.

Keywords: immunosuppression, rejection, tacrolimus, antithymocyte globulin, mycophenolate mofetil, azathioprine, alemtuzumab, basiliximab, sirolimus, everolimus, cyclosporine, belatacept, steroid sparing strategy

[*] Corresponding Author's Email: Nidhi.Aggarwal@bcm.edu.

Introduction

A fundamental knowledge of the immune system and its various signaling pathways has played a critical role in the ability to prolong life by successfully transplanting organs. Kidney transplantation provides the best possible outcomes for a patient with end-stage kidney disease. Immunosuppressive medications, vital to the success of a transplant, involve many classes of drugs. In this chapter, basic immunology, immunological risk stratification, induction, and maintenance immunosuppression are discussed. Side effects of these agents as well as certain special situations where modification of immunosuppression may be required are also discussed.

Brief History of Kidney Transplantation

Early attempts at kidney transplantation with the use of total body irradiation were futile. Later, steroids alone were used, also without much success. In the early 1960s, development of 6-mercaptopurine followed by azathioprine, ushered in a new era of pharmacological immunosuppression. Though not without significant adverse effects, the combination of steroids and azathioprine became the standard of care over the next several years. With increasing understanding of the role of the immune system in rejection of the transplanted organ, therapies targeted to specific immunoregulatory sites became possible. The first polyclonal antilymphocyte globulin was used in 1967, followed by development of other polyclonal and monoclonal antibodies.

Introduced in 1983, cyclosporine, a calcineurin inhibitor, when used in combination with azathioprine and steroids, reduced the incidence of acute rejection and dramatically improved graft survival. The next advance came in 1994 with the introduction of mycophenolate mofetil followed by tacrolimus and sirolimus in 1999. Use of these medications has led to significant improvement in short-term outcomes.

Basic Immunology

The process of organ rejection involves multiple steps of T-cell activation and proliferation, and can be described by the 3-signal model [1]. *Signal 1* is *alloantigen recognition,* in which a foreign antigen, bound to the host major histocompatibility complex (MHC) on the antigen-presenting cell (APC), binds to the T-cell receptor (TCR) on the surface of T cells (Figure 1). *Signal 2 (costimulation)* is essential for complete T-cell activation, and involves binding of several ligands (CD80, CD86) on the surface of APC to different TCRs (e.g., CD28). This leads to internalization of the TCR complex which binds to immunophilin and stimulates calcineurin, a calcium and calmodulin-dependent phosphatase. Calcineurin dephosphorylates and activates nuclear factor of activated T cells (NFAT), which then translocates to the nucleus where it leads to expression of interleukin -2 (IL-2). Then IL-2 binds to IL-2 receptors (IL-2R) on the T cell surface in an autocrine fashion. This stimulates T-cell proliferation through the mammalian target of rapamycin (mTOR) and phosphoinositide-3-kinase pathway (*clonal expansion, Signal 3*). This leads to secretion of a large number of cytokines, chemokines, and adhesion molecules, leading to cell-mediated cytotoxicity, delayed type hypersensitivity response, and antibody production by B cells.

Suppression of immune response can be achieved by depletion of lymphocytes, preventing lymphocytes from infiltrating the graft, downregulation and inhibition of T-cell surface receptors, or by blocking various lymphocyte response signal pathways. No single agent is perfect as an immunosuppressant on its own. Multiple agents targeting various steps of this process (Figure 1), and drugs in various combinations, are used to achieve the optimal immunosuppressive regimen while minimizing toxicity. Different drug combinations are used during different phases in the post-transplant period. Immediately post-transplant, intense immunosuppression (induction therapy) is needed to prevent acute rejection. Long term prevention of acute and chronic rejection is done with maintenance immunosuppression. Treatment of episodes of rejection is based on the type and severity of rejection and is discussed elsewhere in this book.

INDUCTION IMMUNOSUPPRESSION

Induction therapy is high-intensity immunosuppression administered at the time of kidney transplantation when the risk of allograft rejection is highest. It involves the use of higher doses of drugs than are used for maintenance, with or without additional use of antibody therapy. Use of induction therapy in combination with maintenance therapy is superior in reducing allograft rejection and graft failure when compared to maintenance therapy alone [2, 3]. Antibody therapy includes T-cell-depleting agents and nondepleting agents. The depleting antibodies can be polyclonal or monoclonal agents. Polyclonal antibodies are antilymphocyte or antithymocyte globulin. Alemtuzumab is a humanized monoclonal antibody. Basiliximab is a nondepleting monoclonal antibody.

Polyclonal Antibody

Polyclonal antithymocyte globulins (ATG) are immunoglobin G (IgG) derived from horses or rabbits that are immunized with human thymocytes or T-cell line s. ATG binds to TCR and causes T-cell depletion in blood and peripheral lymphoid tissues through complement -dependent lysis and T-cell activation-induced apoptosis. In addition,

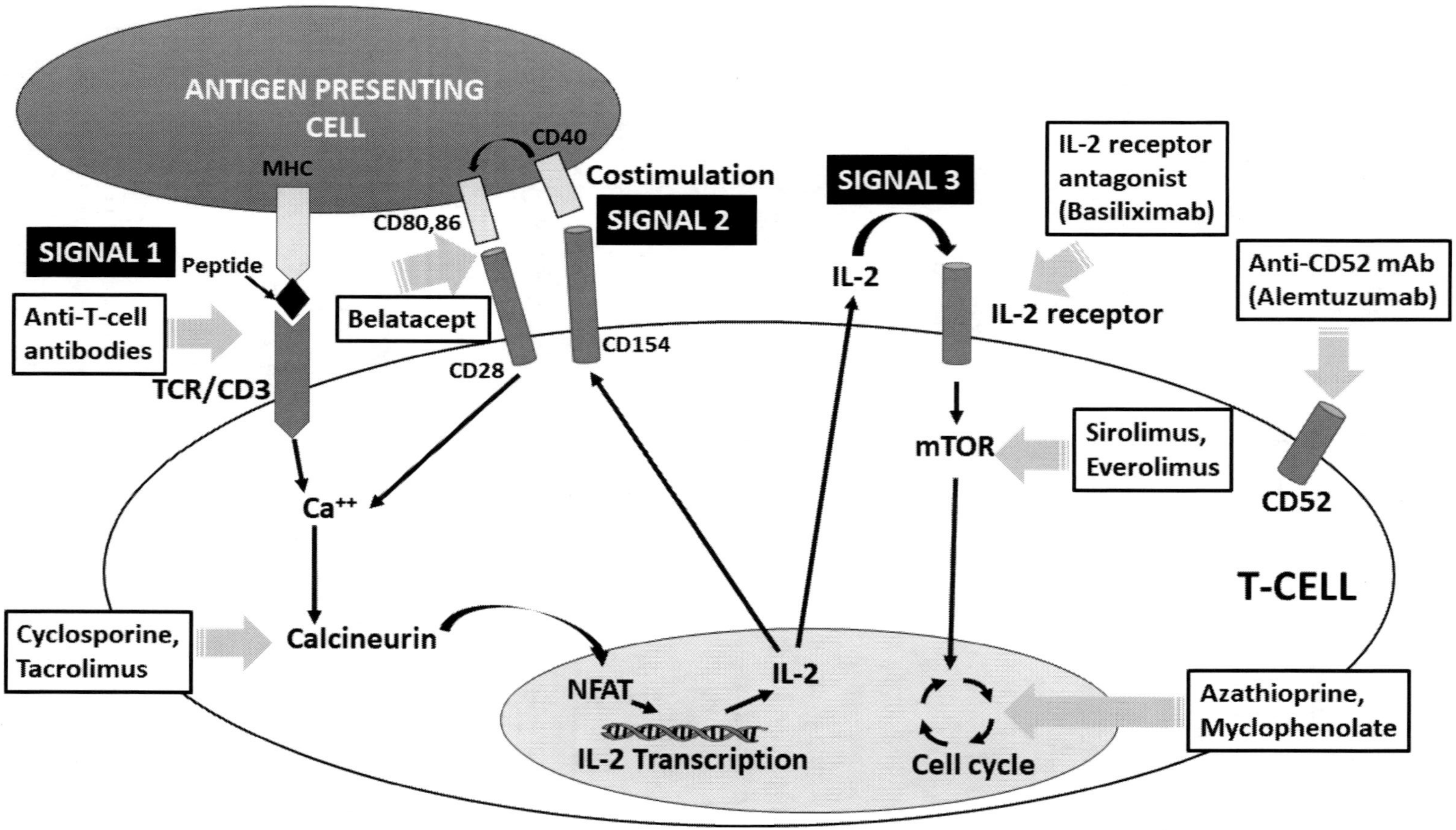

Figure 1. Mechanisms of action and targets of immunosuppressive drugs used in renal transplantation. (TCR, T-cell receptor; Ca^{++}, Calcium; NFAT, nuclear factor of activated T-cells; IL-2, Interleukin-2; mTOR, mammalian target of rapamycin).

it induces B-cell apoptosis, modulates key cell surface adhesion molecules and chemokine receptor s, and interferes with dendritic cell maturation and migration. ATG can be used as an induction agent as well as for treatment in cases of severe acute rejection. Most widely used preparations are horse ATG (hATG) and rabbit ATG (rATG). Due to better tolerability, fewer acute rejection episodes and higher allograft survival than hATG, rATG is the preferred agent [4].

As an induction therapy, rATG is generally administered at a dose of 1.5 mg/kg/day via high flow vein for 3 to 10 days for a cumulative dose of 4.5 to 10.5 mg/kg. Dosing varies depending upon patient-related factors and transplant center protocols. Close monitoring of vital signs should be performed during administration of ATG. Cytokine-release syndrome (CRS), most pronounced with the first dose, is a potentially life-threatening, systemic inflammatory response which can occur during or after administration of this drug. Symptoms can be mild such as fever, chills, myalgia and fatigue, to severe, including cardio-respiratory compromise resulting in severe hypotension, tachycardia, pulmonary edema with respiratory failure, and even renal failure. Premedication with acetaminophen, antihistamine and corticosteroids, along with reduction in rate of infusion can help to minimize reactions. Other adverse effects associated with this drug are leukopenia, anemia and thrombocytopenia, and may necessitate medication dose adjustments. Serum sickness is an immune complex-mediated illness, and presents with fever, rash, arthritis, lymph adenopathy and/or glomerulonephritis, usually 1-4 weeks after initiation of ATG. It is usually a self-limited disease, which can be treated with a course of corticosteroids, with or without plasmapheresis. Increased incidence of opportunistic infections and malignancy, particularly lymphoproliferative disorders, are long-term side effects of polyclonal antibodies.

Alemtuzumab

Alemtuzumab is a humanized monoclonal antibody directed against the CD52 cell surface antigen present on all peripheral blood lymphocytes, and depletes T cells and B cells through antibody - and complement -dependent cytotoxicity, leading to profound and long-lasting lymphopenia. This in turn helps prevent acute rejection and allows for lower calcineurin inhibitor doses in the early post-transplant period.

Alemtuzumab is usually given as a single dose of 30 mg intraoperatively, with premedication with acetaminophen, antihistamines, and corticosteroids. It has shown similar efficacy in terms of prevention of early acute rejection episodes, including graft and patient survival when compared to ATG, with fewer infusion related symptoms. However, rates of late (>12 months post-transplant) rejection episodes are found to be higher with alemtuzumab [5]. Adverse effects of alemtuzumab include first-dose reactions, infections, leukopenia, anemia, and (rarely) pancytopenia and autoimmunity (e.g., hemlytic anemia, thrombocytopenia, and hyperthyroidism).

Basiliximab

Basiliximab is a non-depleting, chimeric (human /murine) monoclonal antibody that binds with high affinity to the α subunit of the IL-2R on the surface of activated T lymphocytes. Thus, it acts as an IL-2R antagonist and inhibits IL-2-mediated T cell proliferation and differentiation, without causing T cell depletion. The efficacy of basiliximab is similar to rATG in patients at lower immunological risk for rejection, but less in higher risk patients [5, 6]. Two doses of 20 mg each are administered intravenously for induction therapy, one each on the day of transplant and then on post-transplant day 4. It is generally well tolerated and has a more favorable side effect profile when compared to ATG. There is less incidence of fever, leukopenia, infections and malignancies associated with basiliximab.

Choice of induction immunosuppression varies at different transplant centers and is generally guided by the baseline immunologic risk for rejection of an organ recipient. Certain factors are associated with an increased risk of rejection (*higher immunologic risk*) – history of prior sensitization with high panel reactive antibodies, prior history of rejection or graft loss, higher number of human leukocyte antigen (HLA) mismatches, positive B-cell crossmatch, presence of preformed donor-specific antibodies, ABO-incompatible transplant, advanced age of donor, younger recipient, deceased donor transplant, delayed graft function, and cold ischemia time >24 hours. Unless otherwise contraindicated, ATG or alemtuzumab is used as an induction agent for higher risk patients. For patients at lower immunological risk, basiliximab is considered a safer option, which provides similar efficacy.

MAINTENANCE IMMUNOSUPPRESSION

The purpose of maintenance immunosuppression is to prevent acute and chronic rejection, and to preserve long-term allograft function. Initiated at the time of surgery, a single agent or a combination of multiple agents are maintained for the life of the allograft. The most frequently used maintenance immunosuppressants include calcineurin inhibitors, antimetabolites, mammalian target of rapamycin inhibitors, corticosteroids, and T-cell costimulation blockers. Like induction therapy, maintenance immunosuppressive regimens also vary between transplant centers. According to the Scientific Registry of Transplant Recipients (SRTR), annual data report of 2018, the triple drug combination of tacrolimus (Tac), mycophenolate mofetil (MMF), and prednisone (PDN) is the most common initial maintenance immunosuppression regimen used for kidney transplants in the United States [7]. Some centers use dual agent maintenance with tacrolimus and mycophenolate after rapid corticosteroid withdrawal within the first week post-transplant. Table 1 lists some of the maintenance immunosuppressive agent s, their doses, and common adverse effects.

Table 1. Doses and adverse effects of commonly used immunosuppressant drugs for kidney transplantation

Drug	Dose	Adverse effects
Anti-thymocyte globulin (rabbit)	1.5 mg/kg/day IV x 3-10 d	Leukopenia, thrombocytopenia, rash, fever, cytokine release syndrome, serum sickness
Alemtuzumab	30 mg IV x 1 dose on POD 0	First-dose reactions, leukopenia, anemia, thrombocytopenia, autoimmunity (hemolytic anemia, thrombocytopenia, hyperthyroidism) .
Basiliximab	20 mg IV x 2 doses (POD 0 and POD 4)	Hypersensitivity reactions
Cyclosporine	4 to 8 mg/kg/day PO (2 divided doses)	Nephrotoxicity, gingival hyperplasia, hirsutism, gynecomastia, hyperuricemia, hypertension, hyperlipidemia, glucose intolerance, neurotoxicity, hypomagnesemia, hyperkalemia
Tacrolimus	1.1 to 0.2 mg/kg/day PO (2 divided doses)	Nephrotoxicity, neurotoxicity, alopecia, hypertension, hyperlipidemia, glucose intolerance, nephrotoxicity, hyperkalemia, hypomagnesemia
Mycophenolate mofetil	500-1000 mg twice daily	Leukopenia, thrombocytopenia, gastrointestinal disturbances, teratogenicity
Mycophenolic acid	360-720 mg twice daily	
Sirolimus	2-10 mg/day PO daily	Anemia, leukopenia, thrombocytopenia, oral ulcers, delayed wound healing, hyperlipidemia, gastrointestinal disturbances, edema, interstitial pneumonitis, proteinuria, teratogenicity
Everolimus	0.75 mg PO twice daily	
Belatacept	10 mg/kg POD 0, POD 5, and at end of 2, 4, 8, and 12 weeks, and then, 5 mg/kg every 4 weeks	Post-transplant lymphoproliferative disorder, progressive multifocal leukoencephalopathy
Corticosteroids	Induction: 250-500 mg IV (Variable) Maintenance: 5-10 mg/day PO	Weight gain, acne, skin- thinning, bruising, osteoporosis, Cushingoid appearance, hyperglycemia, hyperlipidemia, cataracts, psychologic effects, gastrointestinal bleeding

IV: Intravenous; POD: Post-operative day; PO: Per oral.

Calcineurin Inhibitors

The calcineurin inhibitors (CNI) are a major class of immunosuppressive drugs, and are used in combination with other classes of immunosuppressants. The two commonly used CNIs are cyclosporine and tacrolimus, both of which bind with high affinity to T-cell cytoplasmic proteins (immunophilins), cyclophilin and FK506-binding protein 12 (FKBP12), respectively. This drug-receptor complex then binds to and inhibits calcineurin [8]. This prevents activation and migration of NFAT to the nucleus, and impairs transcription of IL-2 and several other critical cytokine genes that promote T-cell activation and proliferation. CNIs are usually started immediately after transplantation, but their initiation can be delayed up to 1-2 weeks post-transplant ation such as in cases of delayed graft function (where antibody induction therapy has been used).

Cyclosporine is a hydrophobic cyclic polypeptide produced as a metabolite by the fungus species *Tolypocladium inflatum,* and is available as a capsule, solution, or injection. Cyclosporine dosing depends on multiple factors, including type of transplant (kidney alone or multi-organ), timing from transplantation, concomitant medications, and patient factors. Usual dose ranges from 4 to 8 mg/kg/day orally divided into 2 equal doses. Drug levels, either C2 (peak level 2 hours after intake) or C0 (trough level 12 hours after intake), should be monitored due to narrow therapeutic index. C2 levels (goal 600 to 2000 ng/ml), though more reliable, are difficult to obtain. Goal trough concentrations range from 150 to 300 ng/ml in the first 3 months, and 50-150 ng/ml in the subsequent months. The oral dose of cyclosporine is approximately 3 times the IV dose.

Table 2. Common drug interactions of calcineurin inhibitors and mTOR inhibitors

Mechanism	Interacting medications	Drug levels of CNI and mTORi
CYP3A4 inhibitors	Erythromycin Clarithromycin Diltiazem Verapamil Azole antifungals Protease inhibitors Fluoxetine Fluvoxamine Grapefruit juice	Increase
CYP3A4 inducers	Carbamazepine Phenobarbital Phenytoin INH Rifampin Rifabutin St. John's Wort	Decrease

CYP3A4: Cytochrome P-450 3A4; CNI: Calcineurin inhibitor; mTORi: mammalian Target of Rapamycin inhibitor.

Tacrolimus is a macrolide antibiotic derived from a soil bacterium, *Streptomyces tsukubaensis.* It inhibits calcineurin with greater potency than cyclosporine. The 2009

KDIGO (Kidney Disease: Improving Global Outcomes) Clinical Practice Guidelines suggest using tacrolimus as the first line CNI for renal transplant patients (Level of recommendation 2A) [9]. When compared with cyclosporine, tacrolimus is associated with reduced incidence of biopsy -proven acute rejection and steroid-resistant acute rejection, with better graft survival [10, 11]. Longer follow-up data has shown similar patient survival with both these agents.

Tacrolimus is available as capsules or intravenous formulations. Initial dosing is 0.1 to 0.2 mg/kg/day orally divided into 2 doses. Single dose formulations are also available. Tacrolimus absorption is best when taken on an empty stomach, since food decreases its bioavailability. Like cyclosporine (CYA), dosing of tacrolimus is variable, depending on multiple factors, and needs careful monitoring by measuring trough drug concentrations. Goal trough concentrations range from 8-12 ng/ml in the early, and 4-8 ng/ml in the late post-transplant period. The oral dose of tacrolimus is approximately 3 to 5 times the IV dose. It can be administered sublingually at half the oral dose.

Both CYA and tacrolimus are metabolized by the p-glycoprotein and cytochrome - P450 (CYP) 3A4 enzyme system in the gut and the liver. Concomitant administration of agents inducing the CYP3A4 system can reduce CNI levels, therefore, decreasing the overall level of immunosuppression, which can lead to allograft rejection. On the other hand, drugs inhibiting this enzyme system can increase the levels of CNI and lead to potential toxicity. These various drug and food interactions are shown in Table 2.

Calcineurin inhibitors can cause acute and chronic nephrotoxicity through dose-related, reversible renal vasoconstriction, thrombotic microangiopathy, and chronic interstitial fibrosis. Common electrolyte abnormalities associated with CNI use include hypomagnesemia and hyperkalemia. Neurotoxicity, more marked with tacrolimus, can range from coarse tremors and headaches to seizures, delirium, and coma. Few patients can develop posterior reversible encephalopathy syndrome (PRES), which may occur with or without supratherapeutic levels of CNI. PRES, confirmed by radiological imaging, can present clinically with mental status change s, visual disturbances, headache and/or focal neurological deficits [12]. Post-transplant diabetes or hyperglycemia caused by CNI may be reversible or require treatment with insulin. Several adverse effects are common to tacrolimus and cyclosporine. However, tacrolimus has a lower incidence of hyperlipidemia, hypertension, hyperuricemia, and cosmetic problems such as hirsutism, gingival hyperplasia, and gynecomastia, but is more likely than cyclosporine to cause GI side-effects, alopecia, post-transplant diabetes, and neurotoxicity.

Antiproliferative Agents

The antiproliferative agents, also known as antimetabolites, include azathioprine and mycophenolate mofetil (MMF) or its enteric-coated form, mycophenolic acid (MPA).

These drugs work by inhibiting purine base synthesis required for T- and B-cell proliferation. Azathioprine is a prodrug that releases 6-mercaptopurine (6-MP). It antagonizes purine metabolism and inhibits DNA, RNA and protein synthesis [13]. MMF is a prodrug, derived as a fermentation product of several Penicillium species. It is metabolized in the liver to its active moiety, mycophenolic acid. It is a selective, non-competitive, and reversible inhibitor of inosine monophosphate dehydrogenase (IMPDH), causing inhibition of guanine nucleotide synthesis. Azathioprine blocks all purine synthesis (both de novo and salvage), while MMF/MPA blocks only de novo purine synthesis. Since all cells except for lymphocytes have a "salvage pathway " for purine synthesis, MMF/MPA specifically targets proliferation of lymphocytes. Most transplant centers use MMF as the first-line antimetabolite as it is shown to be superior to azathioprine in preventing acute rejections with fewer side effects [14].

Azathioprine is available as an oral formulation and is used as a maintenance immunosuppressive agent at a dose of 1 to 3 mg/kg/day. Major adverse effects are hematologic and gastrointestinal. Dose-dependent myelosuppression, leading to leukopenia and thrombocytopenia can occur, necessitating dose reduction or drug interruption. Other purine analogues, such as allopurinol, inhibit xanthine oxidase, the enzyme which breaks down azathioprine, thus increasing the toxicity of azathioprine when administered concomitantly.

MMF is available in capsule, tablet, suspension, and injectable forms, and the usual starting dose post-kidney transplantation is 1000 mg twice daily, given orally or intravenously. MPA, the delayed-release formulation of mycophenolate, has better gastrointestinal tolerability than MMF, and is also approved for renal allograft rejection prophylaxis with usual starting dose of 720 mg twice daily. Given variable blood concentration due to enterohepatic circulation, MPA levels are not routinely measured. Combination of MMF and tacrolimus is more immunosuppressive than MMF and cyclosporine, as cyclosporine interrupts enterohepatic circulation of MMF, thus decreasing MMF levels. Drug doses are adjusted based on complete blood count.

Besides opportunistic infections and increased risk of malignancies, major adverse effects of MMF/MPA include gastrointestinal (nausea, vomiting, diarrhea and abdominal pain) and hematologic (anemia, leukopenia, and thrombocytopenia). Dose reduction or interruption is usually done for severe leukopenia, anemia, thrombocytopenia, or in cases of severe infections or malignancies. Rare cases of progressive multifocal leukoencephalopathy (PML) have also been described. Due to risk of first trimester pregnancy loss and congenital malformations, women of childbearing age should be counseled on pregnancy prevention and planning with the use of mycophenolate. Dual mode of contraception is recommended in women of childbearing age when using MMF/MPA. During pregnancy, immunosuppression can be switched to alternate agents (e.g., azathioprine).

Mammalian Target of Rapamycin Inhibitors

The mammalian target of rapamycin inhibitors (mTORi) are sirolimus and everolimus. Sirolimus is a macrolide antibiotic compound, produced by the bacterium *Streptomyces hygroscopicus.* Everolimus is a derivative of sirolimus with a shorter half-life. The mTORi binds to FKBP12, and this drug-protein complex then binds to proteins called mTOR, causing inhibition of a multi-functional serine -threonine kinase, preventing both DNA and protein synthesis, resulting in cell-cycle arrest and thereby, preventing IL-2 driven cell-proliferation (Figure 1, Signal 3).

Sirolimus is available as a tablet and solution, and everolimus is available in tablet form. Sirolimus has a half-life of 62 hours and is given once daily, while everolimus has a half-life of 30 hours and is given twice daily. Trough drug levels are measured for adequate dosing, and goal trough levels depend on the timing from transplant, presence of infections, patient factors, and whether used as primary agent or as adjunct to CNI. Like CNIs, these drugs are extensively metabolized in the liver by CYP3A4 and p-glycoprotein, and therefore, have similar drug interactions with CYP3A4 inducers and inhibitors (Table 2).

The major early adverse effects of mTORi are wound dehiscence, lymphocele formation , and prolongation of delayed graft function. Most transplant centers delay initiating these drugs until wound healing is complete. The main nonimmune toxic effects include hyperlipidemia, hyperglycemia, oral ulcers, gastrointestinal side-effects, and bone marrow suppression resulting in anemia, leukopenia, and thrombocytopenia. Tubular toxicity may produce hypokalemia and hypomagnesemia, while podocyte toxicity can cause proteinuria and even nephrotic syndrome. Other reported complications are a non-infectious interstitial pneumonitis (bronchiolitis obliterans organizing pneumonia), delayed recovery from acute tubular necrosis, thrombotic microangiopathy, limb edema and angioedema. These agents are fetotoxic, and their use is contraindicated in pregnancy. Contraception is recommended when giving these drugs to women of childbearing age .

These drugs have been used as part of initial maintenance immunosuppression regimen, either with a CNI in place of an anti-metabolite, or with an anti-metabolite as a replacement for CNI. Meta-analysis of studies has shown that use of mTORi with an antimetabolite (when compared with CNI use with antimetabolite), is associated with an increased risk of graft loss and biopsy -proven acute rejection [15]. mTORi can be potentially used with CNIs as an alternative to antimetabolites, given similar rates of graft loss and acute rejection but reduced risk of cytomegalovirus (CMV) infections [15]. However, use of mTORi is associated with more complications related to wound healing, and increased need to change immunosuppression related to adverse effects .

Costimulation Blocker: Belatacept

Belatacept is a fusion protein composed of the Fc fragment of human IgG1 linked to the extracellular domain of cytotoxic T lymphocyte-associated protein 4 (CTLA 4). It binds to the CD 80/86 on the APC, and prevents them from interacting with CD 28 on T-cells *(costimulation blockade)*, which selectively inhibits T-cell activation and proliferation. In studies comparing it with cyclosporine, belatacept has shown similar graft survival and better preservation of renal function [16-18]. It was approved in 2011 for prevention of graft rejection in adult kidney transplant recipients as a substitute for CNIs.

Belatacept is available as a reconstituted solution which is administered intravenously over 30 minutes. Its dosing is divided into 2 phases. First dose of 10 mg/kg is given on the day of transplantation, with subsequent doses 96 hours later and at the end of weeks 2, 4, 8, and 12. Maintenance dose is 5mg/kg every 4 weeks starting at week 16. Its use is associated with higher risk of post-transplant lymphoproliferative disorders and PML. Its use, however, is contraindicated in patients who are seronegative for Ebstein-Barr virus (EBV) or whose serostatus is unknown.

Corticosteroids

Corticosteroids exert immunosuppressive and anti-inflammatory effect through various mechanisms. They inhibit dendritic cell s, and inhibit nuclear factor kappa B (NFκB), a transcription factor needed for the expression of various cytokines that are integral for T-cell activation [19]. In addition, they induce lymphopenia as a result of lymphocyte migration from the vascular compartment to the lymphoid tissue.

Corticosteroids are available in several formulations including tablets, liquid, and injectable. All patients receive steroids as induction therapy, usually in the form of high dose intravenous doses for 3-7 days. Maintenance therapy is usually tapered to 5-10 mg daily oral dose. Major side effects include glucose intolerance, growth impairment, cosmetic changes (weight gain, central adiposity, moon facies and buffalo hump), peptic ulcer, hypertension, dyslipidemia, osteonecrosis, osteoporosis, impaired wound healing, glaucoma, cataracts, and psychological effects. Most dangerous side effect of chronic steroid administration is development of secondary adrenal insufficiency, in case steroids are withdrawn suddenly after long-term maintenance.

Steroid Sparing Strategies and Outcomes

Due to significant morbidity associated with long-term use of high-dose corticosteroids, several steroid-sparing strategies have been attempted by various transplant centers. Most centers continue steroids at a low maintenance dose for their patients. However, about one-third patients have the steroids withdrawn within a few days of transplant *(steroid avoidance)*, and some later *(steroid-withdrawal)*. Various studies have looked at short-term and long-term outcomes of these steroid-sparing protocols. When compared to steroid maintenance, a recent meta-analysis failed to demonstrate any significant beneficial effect of steroid-avoidance or steroid-withdrawal on mortality or new-onset diabetes within five years [20]. There was no significant difference in graft loss or CMV infection, but the risk of acute rejection increased significantly in both steroid-withdrawal and avoidance groups. Regardless, the kidney function was similar in all the groups at five years post-transplant.

IMMUNOSUPPRESSION MODIFICATION IN SPECIAL SITUATIONS

Modifications of the maintenance immunosuppressive regimen, either temporary or permanent, may be required in certain conditions. Some of these situations are discussed below. Management of acute and chronic rejection will be discussed elsewhere in the book.

BK Virus Nephropathy

BK virus nephropathy is a serious complication occurring in kidney transplant patients and bears a special mention. Almost 80% of the general adult population is seropositive for BK virus antibodies [21]. Primary infection with BK virus occurs during early childhood and usually manifests as a non-specific upper respiratory tract infection. Thereafter, the virus becomes latent and persists in the cells of different organs including the kidneys, ureters, brain, and peripheral blood leukocytes. In immunocompetent patients, BK virus can undergo asymptomatic reactivation, and be transiently shed in the urine (*BK viruria*). However, in immunocompromised kidney transplant patients, BK virus reactivation can present as viruria in up to 30-40%, and as *BK viremia* in almost 10-20% of the patients. It can invade the renal allograft tissue and cause tubulointerstitial nephritis, the BK virus nephropathy (*BKVN*). It is characterized by inclusions of viral bodies in the nuclei of tubular epithelial cells as well as signs of inflammation and tubular damage. Widespread tubular necrosis or death can lead to graft loss.

Polyoma BK virus is a small, non-enveloped DNA virus, first discovered in 1971 in the urine of a kidney transplant patient [22]. Its clinical significance was only realized in the mid-1990s, when increasing use of more potent immunosuppressive agents lead to increased prevalence of BKVN [23]. Since then, it has emerged as an important cause of graft dysfunction, affecting 1-10% of the kidney transplants, with most cases occurring during the first year. If left unchecked, this infection leads to allograft loss in almost half of these patients, and the rest go on to develop chronic allograft dysfunction. BKVN may occur concurrently with acute rejection, and the two processes are sometimes difficult to differentiate, and a challenge to treat.

The risk factors for the development of BKVN are not consistent among different studies. Some of the risk factors that are implicated include donor factors such as seropositivity for BKV antibodies, deceased donor with mechanical or ischemic reperfusion injury, female gender, and African American ethnicity. Recipient factors include extremes of age, male gender, non-black race, HLA or ABO mismatching, ureteral stents, use of lymphocyte depleting agents, tacrolimus or MMF based regimens, delayed graft function, and treatment of acute rejection. Of all the implicated risk factors, it is the 'net degree of immunosuppression ' that is considered as the strongest risk factor for BK virus reactivation in transplant recipients. Use of highly potent immunosuppressants has coincided with the dramatic rise in the incidence of BKVN [23]. Reduction of maintenance immunosuppression, with or without the use of adjuvant antiviral agents, is the mainstay of therapy. Despite this, a significant proportion of patients with BKVN develop progressive allograft dysfunction. As such, there has been an increasing emphasis on early diagnosis and preemptive reduction of immunosuppression.

The gold standard for diagnosis of BKVN is the demonstration of viral cytopathic changes in renal allograft biopsy. Majority of cases of BKVN are preceded by a period of persistent and significant viruria without any changes noted in the renal function [24]. Viruria can be detected either by demonstration of 'decoy cells' on urine cytology, or by polymerase chain reaction (PCR) based studies. Sustained *BK viruria* is often followed within weeks by the development of *BK viremia.* Persistent *BK viremia* can lead to the development of BKVN, which in most cases eventually leads to deterioration of allograft function. *BK viremia* is almost inevitably preceded by *BK viruria*, and BKVN almost never occurs in the absence of *BK viremia.* Current practice guidelines recommend measurement of BK virus load in the plasma, and reduction of immunosuppression if the level of BK virus in the plasma is high (usually $>10^4$ copies/ml but may vary at different laboratories) [9]. Figure 2 shows the suggested algorithm for post-transplant monitoring and management of BK virus infection.

Immunosuppression in Patients Undergoing Elective Surgery

Careful attention to drug regimens should be paid in patients prior to undergoing elective surgery. Immunosuppression may need modification if patients are on an mTORi-based regimen. Since mTORi are associated with an increased risk of wound healing complications, these drugs should be switched over to an alternative regimen several days before the surgery is planned. Once the wound is healed, the mTORi can be reinitiated.

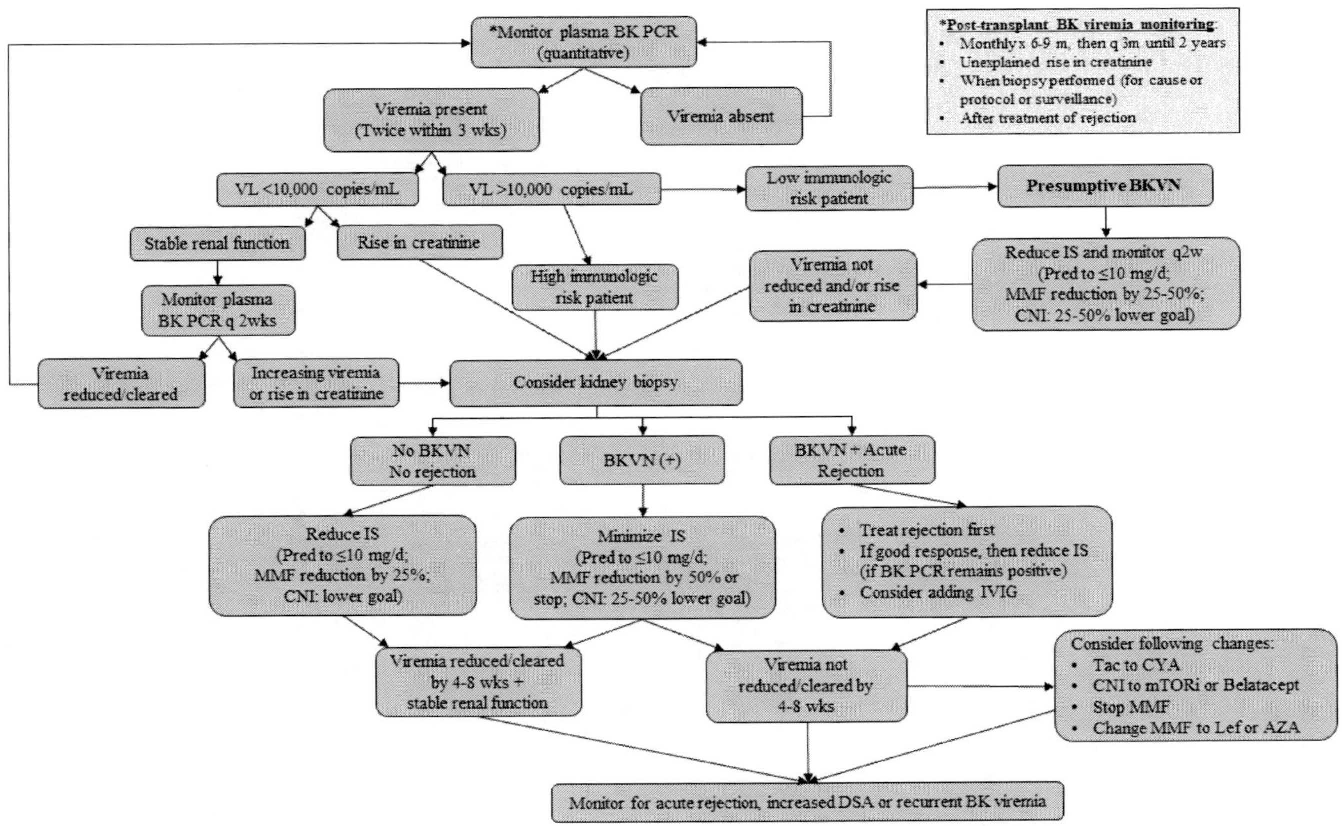

Figure 2. Algorithm for post-transplant monitoring and management of BK virus infection in kidney transplant recipients. The immunosuppression dose changes are suggestions and may vary from one transplant center to another. (AZA, Azathioprine; CNI, Calcineurin inhibitor; CYA, Cyclosporine; DSA, Donor-specific antibody; IS, Immunosuppression; IVIG, Intravenous immunoglobulin; Lef, Leflunomide; MMF, Mycophenolate; mTORi, mammalian target of rapamycin inhibitor; Pred, Prednisone; Tac, Tacrolimus; VL, Viral load).

Patients on maintenance corticosteroids may develop secondary adrenal insufficiency, which may manifest in situations of increased stress to the body, such as high-risk surgeries. For most minor to moderate intensity surgeries, no additional steroids are required. For patients undergoing major surgery, short course of stress dose steroids, usually hydrocortisone IV 50-100 mg, can be given in the perioperative period. This can be rapidly changed to baseline steroid dose within 24-72 hours of the surgery.

Adjunctive Therapies

Use of potent immunosuppression increases the risk of opportunistic infections in a predictable pattern in the post-transplant period [25]. Antimicrobial prophylaxis against certain bacterial, fungal and viral pathogens is given for a variable period of time after transplant, ranging from weeks to months. Sulfamethoxazole/trimethoprim is used for prophylaxis against *Pneumocystis jirovecii* pneumonia, and provides additional coverage for *Toxoplasma gondii*, Nocardia and certain urinary tract infection s. For patients with sulfa allergy, alternative agents such as dapsone, pentamidine or atovaquone can be used. Nystatin suspension or clotrimazole troches are used for prevention of oral candidiasis. Oral fluconazole can be given to patients living in endemic areas of coccidioides. Oral valganciclovir or IV ganciclovir is used for prophylaxis against viral infections like cytomegalovirus (CMV), herpes simplex virus, human herpes virus 6 and 7, EBV and varicella-zoster virus. Acyclovir or valacyclovir do not provide adequate coverage for CMV but can be used for prophylaxis against herpes viruses in patients who are at low risk for developing CMV infection.

Electrolyte replacements, such as magnesium and phosphorus supplements are often required for patients who develop hypomagnesemia or hypophosphatemia. Other agents are individualized to patient needs and co-morbid conditions, and may include anti-hypertensive medications, vitamin D supplements, anti-hyperglycemic drugs, statins, or anti-platelet agents. Initiation of any new medications requires careful review of drug interactions and effect on the transplanted organ.

CONCLUSION

The goals of a successful immunosuppressive regimen are to prevent graft rejection, improve graft and patient survival, reduce complications, minimize adverse effects, and improve overall quality of life. In the absence of an ideal agent, the current approach to immunosuppression is to combine various drugs to achieve the best possible outcomes while minimizing toxicity. An understanding of these medications allows careful monitoring for adverse effects, drug interaction s, and cautious modification of regimen when clinical situation changes.

References

[1] Halloran PF. Immunosuppressive drugs for kidney transplantation. *N Engl J Med.* 2004;351(26):2715-29.

[2] Cai J, Terasaki PI. Induction immunosuppression improves long-term graft and patient outcome in organ transplantation: an analysis of United Network for Organ Sharing registry data. *Transplantation*. 2010;90(12):1511-5.

[3] Hill P, Cross NB, Barnett ANR, Palmer SC, Webster AC. Polyclonal and monoclonal antibodies for induction therapy in kidney transplant recipients. *Cochrane Database of Systematic Reviews*. 2017(1).

[4] Gaber AO, First MR, Tesi RJ, Gaston RS, Mendez R, Mulloy LL, et al. Results of the double-blind, randomized, multicenter, phase III clinical trial of Thymoglobulin versus Atgam in the treatment of acute graft rejection episodes after renal transplantation. *Transplantation*. 1998;66(1):29-37.

[5] Hanaway MJ, Woodle ES, Mulgaonkar S, Peddi VR, Kaufman DB, First MR, et al. Alemtuzumab induction in renal transplantation. *N Engl J Med.* 2011;364(20): 1909-19.

[6] Killen JP, Chadban S. Antithymocyte globulin versus basiliximab in renal transplantation. *N Engl J Med*. 2007;356(6):634; author reply -5.

[7] Hart A, Smith JM, Skeans MA, Gustafson SK, Wilk AR, Castro S, et al. OPTN/SRTR 2018 Annual Data Report: Kidney. *American Journal of Transplantation*. 2020;20(s1):20-130.

[8] Clipstone NA, Crabtree GR. Identification of calcineurin as a key signalling enzyme in T-lymphocyte activation. *Nature*. 1992;357(6380):695-7.

[9] KDIGO clinical practice guideline for the care of kidney transplant recipients. *Am J Transplant.* 2009;9 Suppl 3:S1-155.

[10] Ekberg H, Tedesco-Silva H, Demirbas A, Vítko S, Nashan B, Gürkan A, et al. Reduced exposure to calcineurin inhibitors in renal transplantation. *N Engl J Med*. 2007;357(25):2562-75.

[11] Webster AC, Woodroffe RC, Taylor RS, Chapman JR, Craig JC. Tacrolimus versus ciclosporin as primary immunosuppression for kidney transplant recipients: meta-analysis and meta-regression of randomised trial data. *BMJ*. 2005;331(7520):810.

[12] Hinchey J, Chaves C, Appignani B, Breen J, Pao L, Wang A, et al. A Reversible Posterior Leukoencephalopathy Syndrome. New England Journal of Medicine. 1996;334(8):494-500.

[13] Elion GB. The George Hitchings and Gertrude Elion Lecture. The pharmacology of azathioprine. *Ann N Y Acad Sci.* 1993;685:400-7.

[14] Wagner M, Earley AK, Webster AC, Schmid CH, Balk EM, Uhlig K. Mycophenolic acid versus azathioprine as primary immunosuppression for kidney transplant recipients. *Cochrane Database Syst Rev*. 2015(12):Cd007746.

[15] Hahn D, Hodson EM, Hamiwka LA, Lee VW, Chapman JR, Craig JC, et al. Target of rapamycin inhibitors (TOR-I; sirolimus and everolimus) for primary immunosuppression in kidney transplant recipients. *Cochrane Database Syst Rev*. 2019;12(12):Cd004290.

[16] Vincenti F, Larsen C, Durrbach A, Wekerle T, Nashan B, Blancho G, et al. Costimulation blockade with belatacept in renal transplantation. *N Engl J Med.* 2005;353(8):770-81.

[17] Vincenti F, Charpentier B, Vanrenterghem Y, Rostaing L, Bresnahan B, Darji P, et al. A phase III study of belatacept-based immunosuppression regimens versus cyclosporine in renal transplant recipients (BENEFIT study). *Am J Transplant.* 2010;10(3):535-46.

[18] Durrbach A, Pestana JM, Pearson T, Vincenti F, Garcia VD, Campistol J, et al. A phase III study of belatacept versus cyclosporine in kidney transplants from extended criteria donors (BENEFIT-EXT study). *Am J Transplant*. 2010;10(3):547-57.

[19] Karin M. New twists in gene regulation by glucocorticoid receptor: is DNA binding dispensable? *Cell*. 1998;93(4):487-90.

[20] Haller MC, Royuela A, Nagler EV, Pascual J, Webster AC. Steroid avoidance or withdrawal for kidney transplant recipients. *Cochrane Database of Systematic Reviews*. 2016(8).

[21] Egli A, Infanti L, Dumoulin A, Buser A, Samaridis J, Stebler C, et al. Prevalence of polyomavirus BK and JC infection and replication in 400 healthy blood donors. *J Infect Dis.* 2009;199(6):837-46.

[22] Gardner SD, Field AM, Coleman DV, Hulme B. New human papovavirus (B.K.) isolated from urine after renal transplantation. *Lancet*. 1971;1(7712):1253-7.

[23] Ramos E, Drachenberg CB, Portocarrero M, Wali R, Klassen DK, Fink JC, et al. BK virus nephropathy diagnosis and treatment: experience at the University of Maryland Renal Transplant Program. *Clin Transpl*. 2002:143-53.

[24] Hirsch HH, Knowles W, Dickenmann M, Passweg J, Klimkait T, Mihatsch MJ, et al. Prospective study of polyomavirus type BK replication and nephropathy in renal-transplant recipients. *N Engl J Med*. 2002;347(7):488-96.

[25] Fishman JA. Infection in solid-organ transplant recipients. *N Engl J Med.* 2007;357(25):2601-14.

In: Issues in Kidney Disease – Transplantation
Editors: B. V. R. Murthy and S. Z. Fadem

ISBN: 978-1-53619-960-4

Chapter 7

THE BANFF CLASSIFICATION OF KIDNEY TRANSPLANT REJECTION

Sadhna Dhingra[1], MD and Luan D. Truong[2,*], MD

[1]Department of Pathology and Immunology, Baylor St. Luke's Medical Center, Baylor College of Medicine, Houston, TX, USA

[2]Department of Pathology and Genomic Medicine, Houston Methodist Hospital, Houston, TX, USA

ABSTRACT

Renal allograft biopsy evaluation is essential to determine etiology of renal allograft dysfunction. The Banff classification is a consensus classification that provides histologic criteria for standardized reporting of renal allograft rejection and other transplant related diseases. The classification was first introduced in the year 1991, and since then the classification had multiple updates based on the evolution of pathogenetic understanding of disease. The foundation of Banff classification is pathogenesis related tissue changes and their scoring. The chapter focusses on pathology and pathogenesis of renal allograft rejection and describe the diagnostic criteria from the most recent version, the Banff classification 2017. We describe the pathology of all phases (acute, chronic active and chronic) of antibody -mediated rejection and T cell -mediated rejection. Updated criteria for suspicious/borderline for acute rejection are described. Evolving role of molecular diagnostics in determining renal allograft rejection is discussed. Last but not the least, the strengths and weakness of Banff classification are outlined.

Keywords: Banff classification, kidney transplant rejection, pathology

* Corresponding Author's Email: ltruong@houstonmethodist.org.

INTRODUCTION

The Banff classification of kidney transplant pathology is a comprehensive classification of diseases causing human renal allograft dysfunction, with an emphasis on transplant rejection. The classification is developed by renal pathologists with input from renal transplant physicians and scientists focused on transplant related research [1]. Renal biopsy evaluation is essential to determine etiology of graft dysfunction. The classification provides histologic criteria for diagnosis of rejection and other transplant-related diseases. The histologic changes in the renal allograft biopsies are disease-specific and reflect the current pathogenetic understanding, especially of rejection. The classification is used by the pathologists to diagnose disease and assess its severity in renal allograft biopsies; it is reproducible. Moreover, it is used by the transplant physicians to treat and prognosticate patients.

Table 1. Banff meetings and major modifications

Meeting Years	Report Year (Ref.)	Major Modifications
1991	1993 [2]	Fundamental classification frame work; TCMR recognized with tubulitis and arteritis; ABMR barely mentioned
1995	1996 [3]	Recognition of chronic allograft injury and its scoring
1997	1999 [4]	*First comprehensive classification: All major histologic types of rejection recognized; Comprehensive scoring systems defined; Biopsy tissue adequacy established*
2001	2002 [5]	Focus on "IFTA" (interstitial fibrosis and tubular atrophy)
2003	2004 [6]	Introduction of molecular diagnosis; C4 d as a marker for ABMR, scoring of peritubular capillaritis
2005	2007 [7]	Focus on ABMR; Acute vs chronic/active ABMR; Tissue markers for ABMR (C4d tissue staining, peritubular capillaritis; glomerulitis, transplant glomerulopathy Variants of ABMR (C4d staining without tissue changes, isolated vasculitis) Recognition of chronic active TCMR Chronic injury not related to rejection
2007	2008 [8]	*Comprehensive update Banff classification, new scoring system (peritubular capillaritis, total inflammation, hyalin arteriolar thickening, C4d) Variants of ABMR (C4d staining without tissue changes, isolated vasculitis), recognition of chronic TCMR Recognition of interstitial fibrosis and tubular atrophy*
2009	2010 [9]	Creation of topic-focused working groups
2011	2012 [10]	Refinement of diagnostic criteria for ABMR including recognition of C4d-negative ABMR
2013	2016 [11], 2014 [15]	Revision and updated diagnostic criteria for ABMR; C4d-positive vs negative ABMR; Scoring for glomerulitis and transplant glomerulopathy
2015	2017 [12]	Interstitial inflammation in both scarred and non-scarred areas for diagnosis Arteritis/arteriopathy in both TCMR and ABMR; Adoption of molecular pathology to diagnosis
2017	2018 [13]	*Comprehensive updated classification scheme; Adopting interstitial inflammation in scarred areas for the diagnosis/grading of chronic active TCMR; Addition of molecular classifiers for diagnosis*
2019	2020 [14]	Comprehensive report on molecular diagnosis

Abbreviations: ABMR = antibody -mediated rejection; IFTA = interstitial fibrosis /tubular atrophy; TCMR = T cell -mediated rejection.

Table 2. Banff 2017 classification of renal allograft rejection

Category 1	Normal biopsy or nonspecific changes
Category 2	Antibody mediated changes
	Active ABMR; all 3 criteria must be met for diagnosis
	1. Histologic evidence of acute tissue injury, including 1 or more of the following:
	Microvascular inflammation (g>0 and/or ptc >0), in the absence of recurrent or de novo glomerulonephritis, although in the presence of acute TCMR, borderline infiltrate, or infection, ptc ≥ 1 alone is not sufficient and g must be ≥ 1.
	Intimal or transmural arteritis (v > 0).
	Acute thrombotic microangiopathy, in the absence of any other cause.
	Acute tubular injury, in the absence of any other apparent cause.
	2. Evidence of current/recent antibody interaction with vascular endothelium, *including 1 or more of the following*:
	Linear C4d staining in peritubular capillaries (C4d2 or C4d3 by IF on frozen sections, or C4d > 0 by IHC on paraffin sections).
	At least moderate microvascular inflammation ([g + ptc] ≥2) in the absence of recurrent or de novo glomerulonephritis, although in the presence of acute TCMR, borderline infiltrate, or infection, ptc ≥ 2 alone is not sufficient and g must be ≥1.
	Increased expression of gene transcripts/ classifiers in the biopsy tissue strongly associated with ABMR, *if thoroughly validated*
	3. Serologic evidence of donor-specific antibodies (DSA to HLA or other antigens)
	C4d staining or expression of validated transcripts/ classifiers as noted above in criterion 2 may substitute for DSA; However thorough DSA testing, including testing for non-HLA antibodies if HLA antibody testing is negative, is strongly advised whenever criteria 1 and 2 are met.
	Chronic active ABMR; all 3 criteria must be met for diagnosis
	1. Morphologic evidence of chronic tissue injury, including 1 or more of the following:
	Transplant glomerulopathy (cg >0) if no evidence of chronic TMA or chronic recurrent/ de novo glomerulonephritis; includes changes evident by electron microscopy (EM) alone (cg1a).
	Severe peritubular capillary basement membrane multilayering (requires EM).
	Arterial intimal fibrosis of new onset, excluding other causes; leukocytes within the sclerotic intima favor chronic ABMR if there is no prior history of TCMR, but are not required.
	2. Identical to criterion 2 for active ABMR, above
	3. Identical to criterion 3 for active ABMR, above, including strong recommendation for DSA testing whenever criteria 1 and 2 are met
	C4d Staining without Evidence of Rejection; all 4 features must be present for diagnosis
	1. Linear C4d staining in peritubular capillaries (C4d2 or C4d3 by IF on frozen sections, or C4d>0 by IHC on paraffin sections)
	2. Criterion 1 for active or chronic, active ABMR not met
	3. No molecular evidence for ABMR as in criterion 2 for active and chronic, active ABMR
	4. No acute or chronic active TCMR, or borderline changes
Category 3	Borderline changes
	Suspicious (Borderline) for acute TCMR
	Foci of tubulitis (t > 0) with minor interstitial inflammation (i0 or i1), or moderate-severe interstitial inflammation (i2 or i3) with mild (t1) tubulitis; retaining the i1 threshold for borderline with t > 0 is permitted although this must be made transparent in reports and publications.
	No intimal or transmural arteritis (v = 0)
Category 4	T Cell Mediated Rejection
	Acute T Cell Mediated Rejection
	Grade IA Interstitial inflammation involving >25% of nonsclerotic cortical parenchyma (i2 or i3) with moderate tubulitis (t2) involving 1 or more tubules, not including tubules that are severely atrophic.
	Grade IB Interstitial inflammation involving >25% of nonsclerotic cortical parenchyma (i2 or i3) with severe tubulitis (t3) involving 1 or more tubules, not including tubules that are severely atrophic.

Table 2. (Continued)

Category 4	T Cell Mediated Rejection
	Grade IIA Mild to moderate intimal arteritis (v1), with or without interstitial inflammation and/or tubulitis
	Grade IIB Severe intimal arteritis (v2), with or without interstitial inflammation and/or tubulitis
.	Grade III Transmural arteritis and/or arterial fibrinoid necrosis of medial smooth muscle with accompanying mononuclear cell intimal arteritis (v3), with or without interstitial inflammation and/or tubulitis.
	Chronic T cell Mediated Rejection
	Grade 1A. Interstitial inflammation involving >25% of the total cortex (ti score 2 or 3) and >25% of the sclerotic cortical parenchyma (i-IFTA score 2 or 3) with moderate tubulitis (t2) involving 1 or more tubules, not including tubules; severely atrophic other known causes of i-IFTA should be ruled out.
	Grade1B. Interstitial inflammation involving >25% of total cortex (ti score 2 or 3) and >25% of the sclerotic cortical parenchyma (i-IFTA score 2 or 3) with severe tubulitis (t3) involving 1 or more tubules, not including severely atrophic tubules; other known causes of i-IFTA should be ruled out.
	Grade II. Chronic allograft arteriopathy (arterial intimal fibrosis with mononuclear cell inflammation in fibrosis and formation of neo-intima.

The origin of classification dates back to the first meeting held in the town of Banff located in, Alberta, Canada on August 2-4, 1991. The meeting was organized by Kim Solez and Lorraine C. Racusen; it included US-based and international renal transplant experts of that era. The intent was to develop a consensus classification of renal allograft diseases for standardized reporting in order to guide therapy in transplant recipients, and to help establish an objective rejection end point in clinical trials [1]. The proceedings of the meeting were published as Banff working class ification of kidney transplant pathology in 1993 [2]. Thereafter, the Banff group has organized a meeting every two years and the classification has evolved based on new literature and experience of experts. Impact of changes to the diagnostic criteria for causes of transplant dysfunction are reviewed at each meeting and modifications implemented in new recommendations. So far, there has been a total of 15 Banff meetings with proceedings published in 13 articles, which report comprehensive updated classification or focus only on specific topics (such as C4d staining or molecular methods) as interim reports [2-15]. Meetings with major progresses/ modifications are summarized in Table 1.

This chapter will focus on the pathology of renal allograft rejection and describe the diagnostic criteria from the most recent version, the Banff classification 2017 (Table 2).

Foundation of the Banff Classification: Pathogenesis-Related Tissue Changes and Their Scoring

The pathogenesis of rejection is complex and remains under investigation. However, some fundamental pathogenetic considerations are described below to facilitate the understanding of how, why, and what morphologic changes are used to achieve the diagnosis.

Table 3. Morphologic changes of rejection and their scoring

Lesion	Abbreviation	Quantified Criteria	Score 0	Score 1	Score 2	Score 3
Interstitial inflammation	*i*	Percentage of interstitial areas with inflammation	<10%	10-25%	26-50%	>50%
Tubulitis (inflammatory cells within tubular epithelium)	*t*	Number of inflammatory cells/ tubular cross section	None	1-4	5-10	>10
Arteritis	*v*	Percentage of vascular lumen reduction due to inflammatory cell infiltration of vascular wall	0%	<25%	>25%	Transmural inflammation/ fibrinoid necrosis
Glomerulitis (inflammatory cells within glomerular capillary lumens)	*g*	Percentage of affected glomeruli	0%	< 25%	26-50%	>50%
Peritubular capillaritis (inflammatory cells within PCT lumen)	*ptc*	Percentage of affected PTCs and number of inflammatory cells/ per PTC lumen	<10%	>10% + maximum 3-4 cells/lumen	>10% + maximum 5-10 cells/lumen	>10% + maximum > 10 cells/lumen
C4d staining of PTCs	*C4d*	Percentage of positive PTCs	0%	< 10%	10-50%	>50%
Interstitial fibrosis	*ci*	Percentage of affected cortical area	<5%	6-25%	26-50%	>50%
Tubular atrophy	*ct*	Percentage of affected cortical area	0%	<25%	26-50%	>50%
Arterial intimal fibrosis	*cv*	Percentage of vascular lumen reduction due to intimal fibrous expansion	0%	< 25%	26-50%	>50%
Transplant glomerulopathy	*cg*	Percentage of capillaries with double contour of the GBM in the most severely affected glomerulus	0%	<25% or only by EM	26-50%	>50%
Total inflammation	*ti*	Percentage of tissue area with interstitial inflammation including both scarred and non-scarred areas	<10%	10-25%	26-50%	>50%
Inflammation in areas with IFTA	*i-IFTA*	Percentage of tissue area with interstitial inflammation including only areas with IFTA	<10%	10-25%	26-50%	>50%

Abbreviations: EM = electron microscopy; GBM = glomerular basement membrane; IFTA = interstitial fibrosis /tubular atrophy; PCT = peritubular capillaries.

Rejection is a complex immune mediated process in which the transplanted organ is recognized as foreign by the recipient's immune system. The adaptive immune response that attacks allograft is either T cell -mediated, antibody -mediated, or a combination of both. Antibody-mediated rejection often co-exists with T cell-mediated rejection. These pathogenetic pathways result in a vast array of tissue changes of variable severity, some of which are specific for rejection, whereas most others represent nonspecific tissue injury frequently seen in rejection but can also be encountered in unrelated conditions. These considerations are central in the scoring of tissue changes as a cornerstone for the Banff classification. Scoring is needed since the mere presence of some lesions indicates rejection (e.g., tubulitis or arteritis), whereas, both the presence and severity (scores) of other lesions are needed for diagnosis (e.g., glomerulitis, peritubular capillaritis). In addition, scoring reflects the severity of parenchymal injury, has prognostic value, and guides treatment. The scoring system has evolved as our mechanistic understanding of the rejection evolved; this is reflected in the Banff updates. Major rejection-related Banff morphologic changes and associated scores are summarized in Table 3.

Antibody-Mediated Rejection

Donor-specific antibodies (DSA) play a pivotal role in graft rejection. The rejection sequentially involves the development of circulating DSAs, their binding to the target antigens within the graft and, through both complement activation and complement-independent pathways causes tissue injury. This mechanism is reflected in the requirement in the Banff classification of the simultaneous presence of each of these three steps for a definitive diagnosis of antibody -mediated rejection (ABMR) (Table 2). However, not infrequently, fewer than three criteria could be documented (mostly for technical reasons, see below) in an otherwise convincing episode of ABMR, for which a "suspicious for/suggestive of" diagnosis is offered.

ABMR can be hyperacute, acute or chronic. The DSAs may be present before transplantation in hyperacute ABMR, develop at variable interval post-transplant and cause temporal acute tissue injury in acute ABMR, or persist and cause progressive ongoing graft injury in chronic active ABMR. The targets of these antibodies include mostly the major histocompatibility complex (MHC /HLA) class I and class II antigens, or less frequently other antigens including major histocompatibility complex class I related chain A (MICA), angiotensin type 1 receptor, vimentin and perlecan [16, 17]. Routine testing is limited to DSAs against HLA, perhaps partly explaining the observation that in about a third of episodes of ABMR, DSA is not detected. These antigens are localized mostly to vascular endothelial cells, making renal vasculature a major target of antibody -mediated tissue injury manifesting as thrombotic microangiopathy, microvascular inflammation involving glomerular capillaries *(glomerulitis*), peritubular capillaries (*peritubular capillaritis*), or inflammation of arteries (*arteritis)* (Table 2). The presence and the scored severity of many of these changes (*g, ptc*, and *v* scores) (Table 3) carry diagnostic and prognostic significance for ABMR.

Once the circulating antibodies ligate their targeted antigens, injury to the targeted tissue can be mediated by *in situ* activation of the complement system. Traditionally, this is manifested as tissue deposition of immunoglobulins and complement components. However, in the context of rejection, these molecules, for poorly understood reasons, are not seen in tissue, leaving C4d, a component of C4 formed during C4 activation and bound to the target tissue, the most sensitive and specific footprint of complement activation. These observations lead to the recognition of the presence of *C4d staining along the peritubular capillary* (PTC) wall and its scored extent (C4d score, Table 3) as a diagnostic requirement for ABMR.

Tissue injury may be complement -independent, including direct target injury by DSA, or recruitment of cytotoxic natural killer cells through binding the Fc fragment of DSAs. This mechanism accounts for the Banff diagnostic category of *C4d-negative ABMR*, in which the evidence of DSA-mediated microvascular injury is provided by findings other than C4d stain, including severe microvascular inflammation or molecular markers of endothelial injury.

DSAs may persist and actively cause progressive ongoing graft injury in chronic active ABMR. The tissue manifestation of this injury may be non-specific including interstitial fibrosis /tubular atrophy (IFTA), or may be DSA-specific, including transplant glomerulopathy and multilayering of basement membrane of PTCs. Transplant glomerulopathy is a morphologic complex lesion, but one of the most reliable change is double contour of the glomerular basement membrane by light microscopy, which is also amenable to scoring (cg score), although this score has not been incorporated in the diagnostic scheme. Multilayering of basement membrane of PTCs can only be reliably identified by electron microscopy (EM), and its scoring has not been developed since perhaps the mere presence vs absence of this lesion is of diagnostic significance.

DSAs may bind to target antigens and activate complement; however, this activation may not be completed. This is a process in which C4 activation is achieved resulting in the tissue deposition of C4d, but subsequent progression is blocked, preventing the formation of tissue-damaging complement components such as C5a or C5-9. The tissue manifestation of this pathway is the expression of C4d in PTC but without the tissue injury traditionally observed in rejection. This is the foundation for the category of “C4d only” in the Banff classification.

T Cell-Mediated Rejection

T cell -mediated rejection (TCMR) is mediated by either CD8+ cytotoxic T lymphocytes or CD4+ helper T lymphocytes. The major antigenic difference between donor and recipient is in the highly polymorphic major histocompatibility complex (MHC) molecules, class I and class II. The dendritic cells in the allograft are the antigen presenting cells (APCs) that express class I and class II MHC molecules. They travel to secondary lymphoid tissue and stimulate both direct and indirect pathways of allorecognition by recipient T cells. In the direct pathway, CD8+ T cells recognize class I MHC/HLA molecules on exposure to APCs and differentiate into active cytotoxic T lymphocytes that migrate to the graft, undergo transendothelial migration and kill graft cells. The direct pathways is predominantly responsible for acute T cell-mediated rejection. In the indirect pathway, recipient T lymphocytes recognize donor MHC/HLA antigens when presented by recipient APCs. This stimulates CD4+ helper T cells to proliferate and differentiate, produce cytokines like gamma-interferon and trigger a delayed hypersensitivity reaction resulting in graft infiltration by lymphocytes and macrophages. The CD4+ T cells also stimulate B lymphocytes to produce antibodies.

Both pathways result in T cell infiltration of various renal compartments including interstitium (*interstitial inflammation),* tubules *(tubulitis),* and arteries *(arteritis).* The severity of the infiltration, which portends both diagnostic and prognostic significance, is reflected in the *i (interstitial), t (tubulitis), and v (vasculitis)* scores (Table 3). Although both CD4 and CD8 T cells and other types of inflammatory participate in cell-mediated rejection, only T cell infiltration is keyed in the Banff classification. This limitation mainly reflects the limited technical capability to differentially phenotype the different types of renal tissue infiltrating inflammatory cells in routine diagnostic settings.

Acute TCMR often responds well to immunosuppression with often complete resolution of the rejection changes. However, TCMR may persist with inflammation cell infiltrate in tubules, interstitium, and arteries, and at the same time cause progressive chronic graft injury including tubular atrophy, interstitial fibrosis and arterial intimal fibrous thickening. These changes indicate the presence of chronic active TCMR, the diagnosis of which depends not only on the presence of the chronic changes but also their scored severity, i.e., *ci, ct, and cv* scores (Table 3). In the early Banff classification, only interstitial inflammation in areas without significant interstitial fibrosis and tubular atrophy IFTA is keyed in as diagnostic changes. However, inflammation of the entire renal tissue areas and also that in areas of significant IFTA and their severity (*ti* and *i-IFTA* scores, Table 3) are recognized in the diagnosis of chronic active TCMR.

Interstitial inflammation and tubulitis can be seen in rejection and other conditions. Therefore, not only their presence but also their severity reaching a minimal threshold is required for the definite diagnosis of TCMR. However, there are instances in which these thresholds are not met, leading to the diagnostic category "suspicious for T-cell mediated rejection. "

Common Final Pathway

Most grafts finally fail. The common change of the failed graft is severe IFTA, with or without other changes that may reveal the cause of graft failure. Many conditions can cause graft failure including infection, immunosuppressive drug toxicity, hypertension, *de novo* or recurrent renal diseases, or chronic rejection of either cell- or antibody -mediated type. These considerations are reflected in the diagnosis of "IFTA." This diagnostic category is recognized in the 2007 Banff classification but not listed in the most recent 2017 Banff classification, perhaps recognizing that the causes of IFTA are often multifactorial and cannot be clearly attributed to rejection in most cases.

Pathology and Diagnostic Criteria

Antibody-Mediated Rejection (ABMR)

ABMR includes 3 subgroups: active ABMR, chronic active ABMR, and C4d staining without evidence of rejection. A category of chronic ABMR might have been considered but is not officially recognized, perhaps reflecting the fact that the causes of the advanced chronic changes is probably multifactorial and may not be readily attributable to antibody -mediated injury in most cases.

Active Antibody-Mediated Rejection

The diagnosis requires a *simultaneous* presence of (1) Histologic evidence of acute tissue injury thought to be mediated by antibodies; (2) Evidence of current/recent antibody interaction with vascular endothelium; (3) Serologic evidence of circulating donor-specific antibodies (Table 2).

Criteria 1: Acute Tissue Injury

There are four histologic changes indicative of active ABMR: (a) microvascular inflammation (Figure 1A, 1B); (b) intimal or transmural arteritis (Figure 2A-2C); (c) acute thrombotic microangiopathy (Figure 2D); (d) acute tubular injury (Figure 2E). One or more of these changes can be seen in each episode of acute AMR.

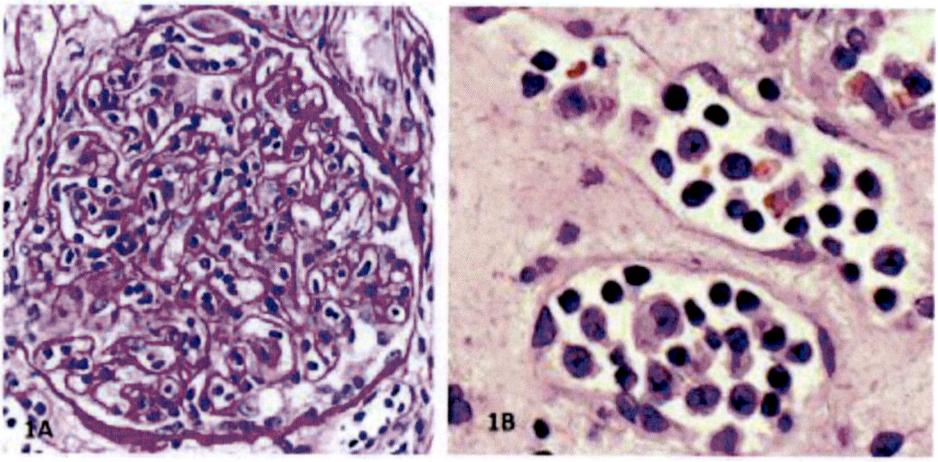

Figure 1. Microvascular inflammation. A. Glomerulitis (PAS x400); B. Peritubular capillaritis (HE x600).

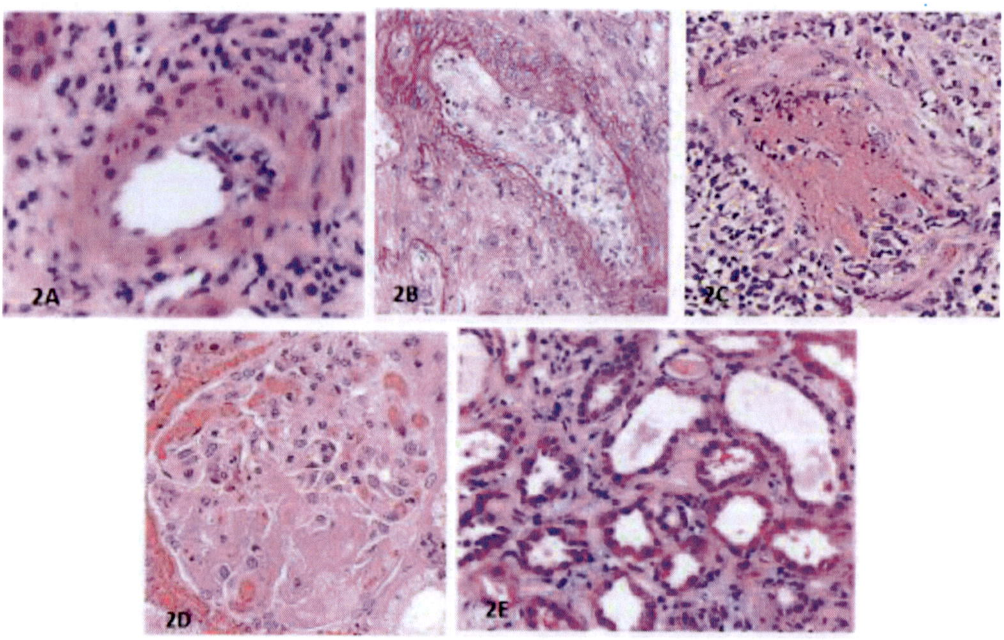

Figure 2. A. Intimal arteritis, mild v1 (HE x400); B. Intimal arteritis, moderate v2 (PAS x400); C. Transmural arteritis with fibrinoid necrosis, v3 (HE x400); D. Fibrin thrombi in glomerular capillaries (HE x400); E. Acute tubular injury (HE x200).

Microvascular Inflammation (Figure 1A, 1B): Microvascular inflammation is manifested by glomerulitis and peritubular capillaritis that reflects complement activation due to antibody interaction with endothelial antigens, leading to local recruitment of inflammatory cells. These histologic lesions are nonspecific by themselves and can be seen in active TCMR and other causes of renal injury. *Glomerulitis (lesion "g")* is characterized leucocytic infiltration of glomerular capillaries with endothelial cell swelling, causing complete or partial occlusion of capillary lumina. The diagnosis requires at least one glomerular capillary lumen showing this change. The leukocytes are mononuclear inflammatory cells, T lymphocytes or macrophages, with or without neutrophils. Electron microscopic evaluation shows discreet, floating leucocytes in the capillary lumina with endothelial cell swelling. Glomerulitis is scored (g1-g3, Table 2). *Peritubular capillaritis* (lesion *"ptc"*) is defined as dilated peritubular capillaries containing 3 to 4 or more inflammatory cells per cross-section in more than 10% of PTCs in non-atrophic cortex. The inflammatory cells are monocytes/macrophages, lymphocytes or less often neutrophils. Neutrophils are more frequent in ABMR in early post-transplant period. Peritubular capillaritis is assessed in the cortex and not in the medulla. This occurs because vasa recta of medulla can contain inflammatory cells as a normal component and peritubular capillaritis is often seen in acute tubular necrosis. Peritubular capillaritis is scored (*ptc 1-3*, Table 2).

Microvascular inflammation as a marker for the diagnosis of acute AMR is utilized in different contexts. Its presence regardless of severity ($g> 0$ and/or $pct>0$) can be a diagnostic criteria (Criteria 1, Table 2). Furthermore when they are severe, they can be used as a surrogate marker for the DSA-endothelium interaction $g+pct \geq 2$.

Arteritis (lesion *"v"*) includes intimal arteritis and transmural arteritis (Figure 2A-2C). The most common form is intimal arteritis characterized by presence of subendothelial T lymphocytes or macrophages within the intima. The overlying endothelium shows features of activation characterized by endothelial cell enlargement and nuclear hyperchromasia. These changes lead to intimal edema and thickening causing variable degree of narrowing of the lumina. Much less frequent is severe transmural arteritis characterized by transmural inflammation and myoid fibrinoid necrosis with or without thrombosis. These arteritic lesions can involve interlobular arteries of all caliber and can even be appreciated in arterioles. It can be focal thus seen in only a few levels in serial sections of the biopsy. Arteritis is virtually specific to active rejection and can be seen in both ABMR and TCMR. It is not known to occur in other conditions affecting the renal allograft. Arteritis is scored as *v0-v3*, with *v0-2* reflecting the extent of vascular lumen narrowing, whereas *v3* is assigned to the transmural vasculitis, regardless of luminal changes (Table 3).

Acute Thrombotic Microangiopathy (TMA) (Figure 2D) is characterized by endothelial cell swelling, mesangiolysis and fibrin thrombi in glomerular capillaries, with or without involvement of arterioles or small arteries. Electron microscopy shows subendothelial rarefaction and fragmented red blood cells (RBCs) in the subendothelium and mesangium. TMA can be seen in ABMR and several other conditions including hemolytic uremic syndrome, calcineurin inhibitor toxicity or antiphospholipid syndrome, thus the qualifying statement "Acute thrombotic microangiopathy, in the absence of any other cause" for the use of TMA as a diagnostic criteria since its presence, regardless of severity, has diagnostic value. TMA is not scored.

Acute Tubular Necrosis (ATN) (Figure 2E) or acute tubular epithelial injury with minimal inflammation can be multifactorial in renal allografts. However, it can rarely be the only tissue injury mediated by DSA

Aside from these "DSA-specific" lesions, other nonspecific changes are often seen including interstitial edema and hemorrhage, as a result of microvascular injury. Minor interstitial inflammation is often seen with mature plasma cells, but significant interstitial inflammation is not a manifestation of active ABMR, and its presence often indicates a concurrent TCMR.

Criteria 2: Current/Recent Antibody Interaction with Vascular Endothelium

Any of these three findings would fulfil this requirement: C4d staining of PTC, moderate microvascular inflammation, or gene expression of endothelial injury .

C4d Staining (Figure 3): C4d staining of PTC is a sensitive and specific marker for complement activation due to DSA-endothelium interaction. C4d staining is recommended for diagnostic work-up of all renal allograft biopsies. C4d staining can be seen not only in PTC, but also less frequently in other renal structures. However, only C4d staining of PTC is diagnostic for active ABMR. C4d expression was originally determined by immunofluorescent staining on frozen tissue, and now can also be evaluated by immunohistochemical staining on formalin-fixed paraffin-embedded tissue. Since the mere presence of C4d staining of PTC is nonspecific, the staining extent must reach the minimal threshold for diagnostic use (this threshold is denoted as "*positive for C4d*" in the Banff classification). For this goal C4d staining is scored (*c4d 0-3*, Table 3), and a minimum score is required for a "*c4d positivity.*" Since the immunofluorescence (IF) technique is more sensitive than immunohistochemical, this minimal threshold is different between these two methods. Strong, linear and circumferential C4d staining involving ≥10% of PTC (C4d 2), on immunofluorescence is considered "positive" (Figure 3A). In contrast, any positive immunohistochemical staining performed on paraffin embedded tissue (C4d1) is considered "positive" (Figure 3B).

Moderate Microvascular Inflammation: Microvascular inflammation, at least of moderate severity (score *g+pct* ≥2) may serve as the surrogate marker for DSA-endothelium interaction. This reflects the knowledge that DSA-endothelium interaction may initiate tissue injury by a mechanism independent of complement, thus an absence of C4d in PTC, but still resulting in significant microvascular inflammation.

Gene Expression of Endothelial Injury: The same consideration as above leads this "aspirational" criteria. It, however, has not reached clinical use, reflecting technical and interpretational drawback.

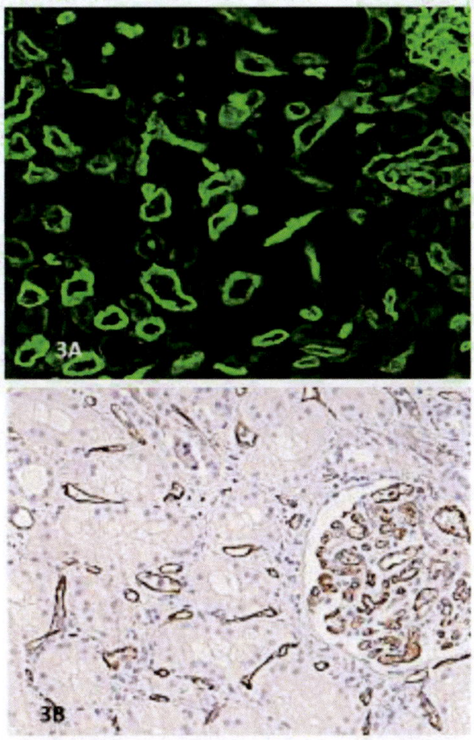

Figure 3. A. Diffuse and strong C4d staining in peritubular capillaries by immunofluorescence; B. Diffuse staining in peritubular capillaries and glomerular capillary loops with immunohistochemical stain for C4d.

Criteria 3: Serologic Evidence of Circulating Donor-Specific Antibodies

Laboratory detection of DSAs is complex and is not discussed in detail here. However, some observations are pertinent to the Banff classification. Current laboratory setting allows for routine testing for DSAs against donor HLA antigens, but not other antigens that can potentially induce rejection. Thus, this criterion may not be fulfilled in up to about 30% of episodes with features otherwise typical for acute ABMR. There is a high correlation (about 90%) of positive C4d staining of PTC and circulating DSAs. Thus, a positive C4d stain of PTC is permitted to serve as a surrogate marker for the presence of circulating DSAs.

Chronic Active Antibody-Mediated Rejection

This diagnosis requires a *simultaneous* presence of: (1) Histologic evidence of *chronic* tissue injury thought to be mediated by antibodies; (2) Evidence of current/recent antibody interaction with vascular endothelium; and (3) Serologic evidence of circulating donor-specific antibodies

Criteria 1: Chronic Tissue Injury

Morphologic hallmarks of chronic tissue injury mediated by antibodies include transplant glomerulopathy, multilayering of PTC basement membrane, and arterial intimal fibrosis. In addition, concomitant acute antibody -mediated changes are also often seen, justifying the term chronic "*active.*"

Transplant glomerulopathy (TG, lesion *"cg"*) (Figure 4) is a constellation of glomerular changes occurring as a result of chronic repetitive DSA-mediated endothelial injury and activation, resulting in glomerular basement membrane (GBM) remodeling, characterized ultrastructurally by subendothelial electron lucent and subendothelial neo-densa glomerular basement membrane [18]. On light microscopy, this is visualized as double contours of GBM, best appreciated by PAS and Jones silver stains (Figure 4A, 4B). Other changes can be seen including mild mesangial sclerosis /hypercellularity, mesangiolysis, focal segmental or global glomerulosclerosis or glomerulitis. However, these changes are not defining features of TG. Of note, glomerulitis often accompanies TG, and may even be a precursor lesion. Indirect immunofluorescence for IgA, IgG, C1q, kappa light chains and lambda light chains is negative, whereas IgM and C3 can be positive in the mesangium and along capillary wall and represent nonspecific entrapment. Staining for C4d is only seen in one-fourth of cases and when present it is positive in the capillary walls [19]. Negative C4d staining in TG could be due to clearance of previous C4d deposition over time, or other mechanism including non-complement binding DSA, or mechanism unrelated to DSA. Electron microscopic evaluation shows endothelial cell injury including cytoplasmic swelling, plasmalemmal disruption, disorganization of organelles, loss of fenestrations, subendothelial widening by electron lucent or electron variegated material, and formation of circumferential or discontinuous, single or layered new lamina densa distinct from the original GBM (Figure 4C) [20]. Immune complex type electron dense deposits are not typically seen in TG but, occasionally, few small scattered nonspecific electron dense deposits are seen.

TG is scored (*cg*, Table 3) based on the presence and extent of GBM double contours. The score is not incorporated in the diagnostic scheme but does carry significance in its correlation with the severity of the disease including renal function and protein excretion

TG detected by light microscopy is rare in the first year post-transplant, therefore, it is considered a feature of chronic rejection [19]. However, ultrastructural changes of early TG can be seen within 1-3 months post-transplant [18, 21]. In most cases, TG is mediated by anti-HLA antibodies (class II predominantly) leading to complement activation and complement mediated endothelial injury. Other causes of endothelial injury causing TG include non-HLA alloantibodies, autoantibodies, cell-mediated rejection, hepatitis C viral infection and thrombotic microangiopathy.

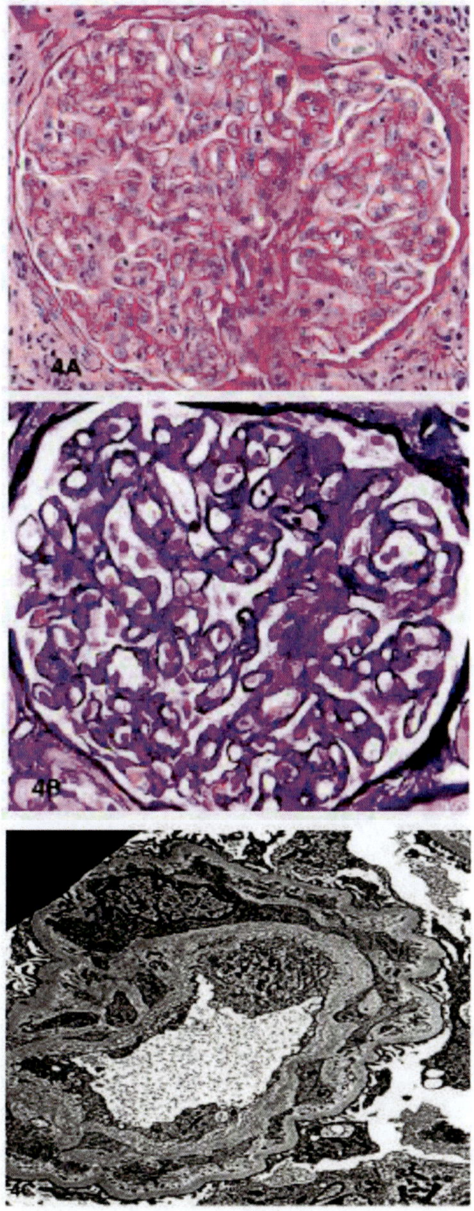

Figure 4. Transplant glomerulopathy. A and B. Glomerulus with double contours of basement membranes (PAS and Jones stain x400); C. Electron photomicrograph showing glomerular basement membrane with endothelial injury and two layers of lamina densa.

Severe Peritubular Capillary Basement Membrane Multilayering (Figure 5): This is a specific histologic feature of chronic antibody -mediated injury caused by persistent and repetitive immunologic endothelial damage. This change is not scored; however, a diagnostic threshold is needed for diagnostic criteria. Normally, the PTC basement membrane has 1-3 layers. Mild increase in basement membrane layers (up to 3-5 layers) can be multifactorial. Severe multilayering characterized by 7 or more layers of basement membrane in one capillary, or 5 or more layers in two capillaries is specific for chronic ABMR (Figure 5A,5B). Concurrent presence of intraluminal inflammatory cells is frequent and may indicate an active component of ABMR.

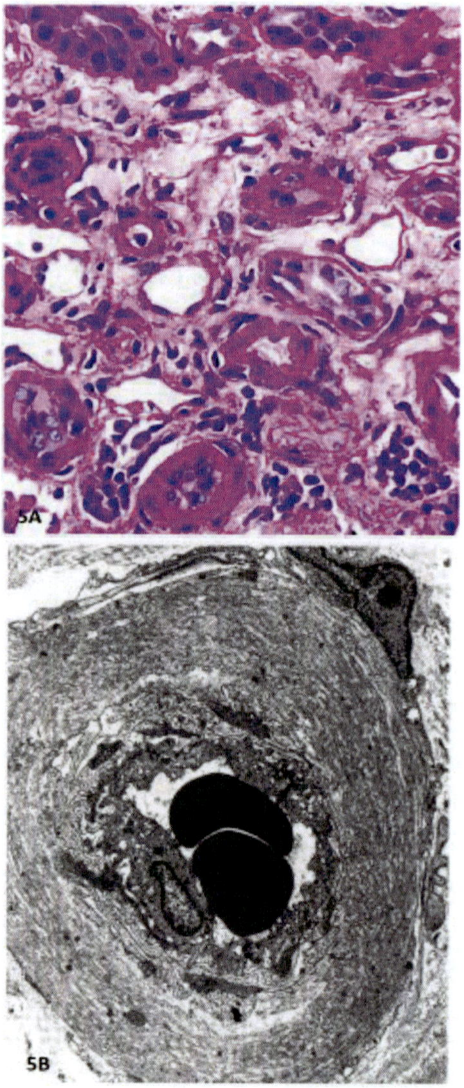

Figure 5. A. Thickened peritubular capillaries on light microscopy (PAS stain x400); B. Electron photomicrograph showing multiple lamellations of peritubular capillary basement membrane s.

Arterial Intimal Fibrosis (lesion *"cv,"* Figure 6A-6C, Table 3) is composed of concentric myofibroblastic proliferation involving the tunica intima and leading to intimal fibrous or fibromyxoid thickening. There is variable degree of cellularity. Neointima may occasionally be seen. This is referred to as "transplant arteriopathy" and can occur secondary to ABMR or TCMR. The presence of intimal lymphocytes, foamy macrophages, or transmural inflammation with thrombosis is indicative of a concurrent component of active rejection.

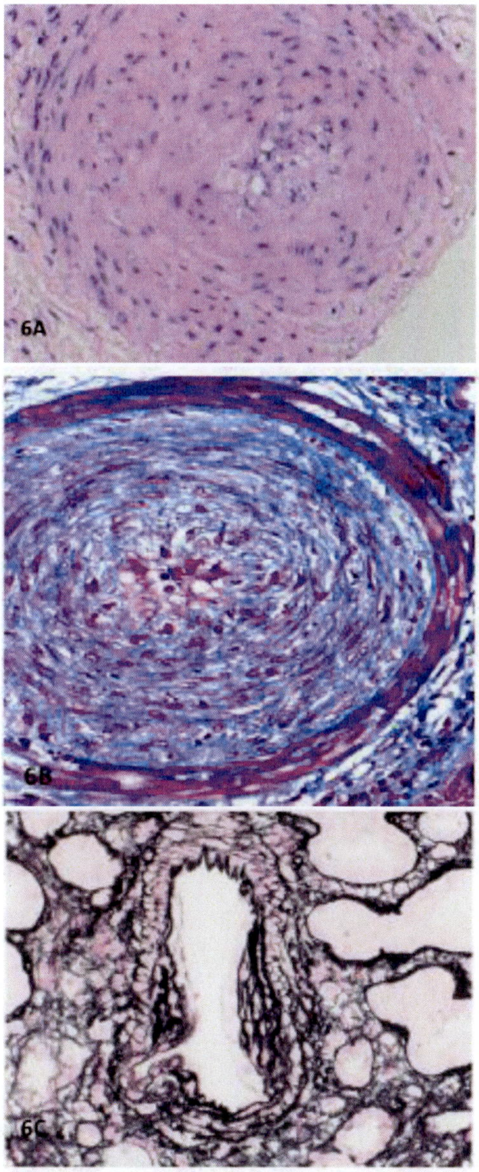

Figure 6. A and B. Arterial intimal fibrosis with myofibroblastic proliferation (HE stain and trichrome stain x200); C. Arterial profile with neointima (Jones stain).

Criteria 2 and 3: Evidence of Current/Recent Antibody Interaction with Vascular Endothelium and Serologic Evidence of Circulating Donor-Specific Antibodies

These criteria are the same as the corresponding criteria for active ABMR and denote an ‘active" component of the rejection

Chronic Antibody-Mediated Rejection

As previously mentioned, this category is not listed in the current Banff classification, but should represent a diagnostic possibility. Chronic (inactive) ABMR is characterized by morphologic evidence of antibody -mediated chronic tissue injury, and *prior* documented diagnosis of active or chronic active ABMR, and/or documented prior evidence of DSA. Evidence of current/recent antibody interaction with endothelium is not required.

C4d Staining without Evidence of Rejection

This requires the presence of linear C4d staining in PTC, concomitant with the absence of features of active or chronic active antibody - or cell-mediated rejection or borderline changes. In addition, molecular evidence of DSA-endothelium interaction should also be absent (Table 2). As mentioned previously, this reflects incomplete complement activation leading to C4d in PTC but not graft injury .

T Cell-Mediated Rejection

Three subcategories include: (1) acute T cell -mediated rejection (TCMR); (2) chronic active T-cell mediated rejection, and 3) suspicious (borderline) for acute T cell-mediated rejection.

Acute T Cell-Mediated Rejection

The morphologic features of T cell -mediated rejection (TCMR) are tubulitis, interstitial inflammation and arteritis (Figure 7A-7C). Depending on the extent and severity of these changes implied in their scores, acute TCMR is subdivided in grade 1A, IB, II A, IIB, and III, reflecting increasing severity.

Interstitial Inflammation (lesion *"i"*) as a component of acute TCMR is defined as mononuclear interstitial inflammation occurring in the nonsclerotic cortex. Nodular infiltrates, if occurring in unscarred cortex are also included in the score. Interstitial inflammation involving scarred cortex, immediate subcapsular cortex and in adventitia around large veins and lymphatics is excluded [22]. The traditional inflammatory cells of rejection are mononuclear cells, primarily lymphocytes and macrophages. Plasma cells or eosinophils form a minor component of the inflammatory infiltrate in a classical form of acute TCMR but may be more pronounced (>5-10% of total cell density and may signify an aggressive course. Scant neutrophils can be present but are not a specific component of acute TCMR. However, significant neutrophil infiltration implies a concomitant acute ABMR.

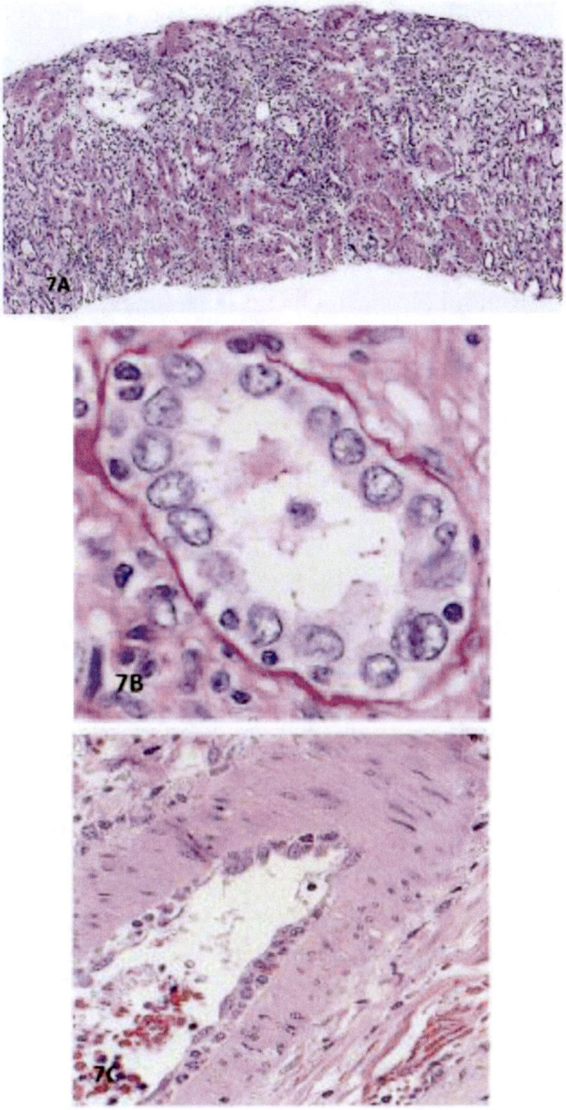

Figure 7. Acute T cell mediated rejection. A. Interstitial inflammation. (HE stain x100); B. Tubulitis (HE stain x400); C. Intimal arteritis (HE stain x400).

Tubulitis (lesion *"t"*) is characterized by penetration of lymphocytes and macrophages through tubular basement membrane to infiltrate into tubular epithelial cells. Acute tubuloepithelial injury is often associated with changes. Although tubulitis can develop in tubules regardless of the level of preexisting injury, only tubulitis in tubules without severe atrophy is of diagnostic value. Severely atrophic tubules are defined by a diameter of less than 25% of that of unaffected or minimally affected tubules with thickened irregular basement membrane and lined by cuboidal or flattened epithelium. Very small endocrine - like tubules with very narrow lumens also comprise atrophic tubules even though the basement membranes are not thickened. This limitation reflects the observation that tubulitis in severely atrophic tubules can developed in chronic kidney injury regardless of cause. Tubulitis predominantly affects distal tubules but depending on the severity it can also involve proximal tubules and renal medulla too. Tubulitis is scored as *t0 - t3* (Table 3).

Arteritis: This lesion is identical to the arteritic lesion in acute ABMR and was previously described in detail.

Although these changes define acute T cell mediated rejection, each of them displays a wide range of severity in an episode of acute T cell rejection. These observations lead to the subdivision of TCMR in subtypes with increasing clinical severity. These subtypes and their diagnostic threshold reflecting the *i, t*, and *v* scores are summarized in Table 2.

Chronic Active T Cell-Mediated Rejection

This diagnostic category a cknowledges the concept that TCMR can be ongoing and cause progressive chronic graft injury. The diagnostic criteria thus retain the inflammation of interstitium, tubules, and arteries, like in acute TCMR, and, in addition, associated with chronic tissue changes as additional criteria. The morphologic changes of chronic active TCMR include chronic allograft arteriopathy, total inflammation, and inflammation in IFTA areas.

*Chronic Allograft Arteriopathy (*lesion *"cv")* is defined by arterial intimal fibrosis with mononuclear inflammation infiltrating in intimal fibrosis, and formation of neointima. This lesion can also be seen in chronic active ABMR, as described previously.

Total inflammation (lesion *"ti")* includes "total" cortical inflammation. In contrast to the *"i"* score which includes only inflammation in intact cortical area, The *"ti"* score includes all cortical parenchyma including intact areas, areas of IFTA, subcapsular cortex and perivascular cortex along with nodular infiltrates. This lesion is scored as *ti 0-3* (Table 3).

Inflammation in areas of IFTA (lesion *"i-IFTA"*) evaluates inflammation limited to cortical areas with tubular atrophy and interstitial fibrosis (Figure 8). This lesion is scored as *i-IFTA 0-3* (Table 3).

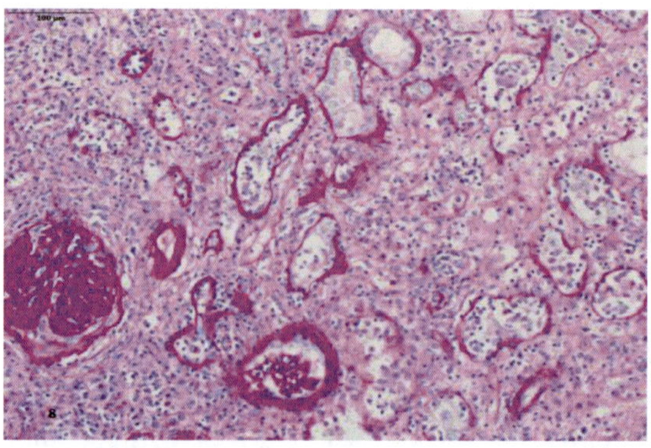

Figure 8. Chronic active T cell mediated rejection. Interstitial fibrosis and tubular atrophy in a background of moderate interstitial inflammation and presence of tubulitis in atrophic tubules, i-IFTA (PAS stain x200).

Up until the Banff 2015 update, the only lesion that qualified as chronic active TCMR was chronic allograft arteriopathy. The Banff 2015 introduced the concept that chronic active TCMR may also manifest in the tubulointerstitial compartment as interstitial inflammation in areas of IFTA (*i-IFTA*), based on well-documented association of *i-IFTA* with poor graft survival [12, 23, 24]. These concepts were fully adopted in the Banff 2017 classification in which the diagnosis of chronic active TCMR is again recognized, but with an expanded diagnostic criterion and a subtyping reflecting the severity of both acute and chronic changes. The severity of total inflammation (lesion *ti* scores), or inflammation in areas of IFTA (lesion *i-IFTA* scores) is summarized in Table 3. The subtypes of chronic active TCMR and their diagnostic thresholds are summarized in Table 2.

Borderline (Suspicious) for Acute T Cell-Mediated Rejection

A definitive diagnosis of acute TCMR requires at least moderate interstitial inflammation (26% to 50% of cortex, i2) and moderate tubulitis (5-10 lymphocytes /tubule, t2). The category "borderline for acute T cell mediated rejection " is used when the morphologic changes are below the minimal diagnostic threshold for acute TCMR. The concept of "suspicious" for acute rejection was introduced in 1993, because of the negative impact of subclinical inflammation on allograft outcome. Since then the diagnostic criteria have undergone multiple mild modifications, reflecting uncertainty on the level at which the changes, although below the diagnostic threshold for a definite diagnosis for acute TCMR, signify weak or pending rejection or merely represent an innocent by-stander.

The current Banff 2017 update defines borderline (suspicious) for acute TCMR as 1) foci of tubulitis of any severity *t1-t3*) with mild interstitial inflammation (Banff *i1*); or 2) mild tubulitis (Banff *t1*) with moderate to marked interstitial inflammation (*i2, i3*)

MOLECULAR DIAGNOSIS OF TRANSPLANT REJECTION

During rejection, several genes belonging to various pathogenetic pathways would be activated resulting in the expression of their corresponding mRNAs in tissue, blood or urine. It is conceivable that the pathogenic mRNA profiles would enable a specific diagnosis including rejection. This is the cornerstone for the molecular approach to the diagnosis of transplant rejection and its different diagnosis. This concept was first introduced in the 2003 Banff classification and has been emphasized as an "aspirational" goal in every updated Banff classification. In addition to a goal for a comprehensive approach, molecular changes have also been formally incorporated as a surrogate for specific morphologic lesion. Thus, gene expression of endothelial injury is accepted as evidence of DSA-endothelium interaction, in parallel with C4d staining of PTC [25]. These approaches, collectively termed "Molecular Diagnostics" in the 2019 Banff Meeting interim report, however, have not reached routine clinical application. This drawback reflects several challenges including reported studies focusing on different gene sets subjected to different platforms of detection, a lack of diagnostic gold standard and clinical validation, cost concern, slow turn-around time, and the requirement for fresh frozen tissue. Although a few molecular diagnostic tests are currently commercially available, these limitations prevent popular utilization [14]. The Banff 2019 molecular diagnostics is proposing a unified platform aiming at overcoming these drawbacks with the final goal of clinical implementation of molecular diagnosis for transplantation rejection [14]. This platform includes evaluation of mRNA of a set of 770 genes representing all known pathogenetic pathways leading to rejection or transplant injury, subjected to detection by a reliable platform known to work well for archival paraffin embedded tissue (NanoString platform). This however is still an ongoing preliminary study, with no clinical utilization. In spite of these drawbacks, molecular diagnostics has been recommended in a few instances in which the Banff criteria are equivocal or not amenable to a specific diagnosis [26].

Clinical Implication

The Banff classification has a profound implication in the diagnosis, treatment, and prognosis of renal transplant. It also serves as a foundation for further research advancement in this area (Table 4). In spite of its strength, the Banff classification is limited by an array of weaknesses, partially inherent to any morphologic scheme of classification (Table 4). Yet, not only the strengths, but even more so the weaknesses that have inspired a constant refinement of this scheme. As the transplant science matures, the Banff classification has and will well serve the transplant community of patients and physicians.

Table 4. Strength and weaknesses

Strength
Based on the current understanding of mechanism of rejection
Morphologic markers specific for rejection
Comprehensive and applicable to tissue; which is still the diagnostic "gold standard"
Carries prognostic/therapeutic significance, down to subgroup categories
Dynamic/self-updating, not be outdated
International consensus: no competing classification
Accepted by the renal transplant community
Uniformly used in routine clinical care, clinico-pathologic studies, clinical trials, and drug testing
Weaknesses
Kidney transplant biopsy sampling limitation (biopsy 10x2x2mm/kidney 12x5x 2cm = 0.03%)
Morphologic criteria/scoring/threshold arbitrary, need independent validation, some criteria difficult to apply
The controversial "borderline' lesion
Limited use of cell phenotyping for classification
No clear guidance for application of the Banff in surveillance biopsies, follow-up biopsies, acute changes superimposing on chronic changes
Rejection injury may precede morphologic changes
Limited utilization of molecular parameters

CONCLUSION

The Banff classification of kidney transplant pathology is a comprehensive classification of diseases causing human renal allograft dysfunction, with an emphasis on transplant rejection. First introduced in the year 1991, the classification had multiple updates based on the evolution of pathogenetic understanding of disease. While building on its strengths, the weaknesses have inspired a constant refinement of this classification. It has a profound implication in the diagnosis, treatment, and prognosis of renal transplant rejection. It also serves as a foundation for further research advancement in this area. As the transplant science matures, the Banff classification has and will well serve the transplant community of patients and physicians.

REFERENCES

[1] Solez K. History of the Banff classification of allograft pathology as it approaches its 20th year. *Curr Opin Organ Transplant.* 2010;15(1):49-51.

[2] Solez K, Axelsen RA, Benediktsson H, Burdick JF, Cohen AH, Colvin RB, et al. International standardization of criteria for the histologic diagnosis of renal allograft rejection: the Banff working class ification of kidney transplant pathology. *Kidney Int.* 1993;44(2):411-22.

[3] Solez K, Benediktsson H, Cavallo T, Croker B, Demetris AJ, Drachenberg C, et al. Report of the Third Banff Conference on Allograft Pathology (July 20-24, 1995) on classification and lesion scoring in renal allograft pathology. *Transplant Proc.* 1996;28(1):441-4.

[4] Racusen LC, Solez K, Colvin RB, Bonsib SM, Castro MC, Cavallo T, et al. The Banff 97 working class ification of renal allograft pathology. *Kidney Int.* 1999;55(2):713-23.

[5] Racusen LC, Solez K, Colvin R. Fibrosis and atrophy in the renal allograft: interim report and new directions. *Am J Transplant.* 2002;2(3):203-6.

[6] Racusen LC, Halloran PF, Solez K. Banff 2003 meeting report: new diagnostic insights and standards. *Am J Transplant.* 2004;4(10):1562-6.

[7] Solez K, Colvin RB, Racusen LC, Sis B, Halloran PF, Birk PE, et al. Banff '05 Meeting Report: differential diagnosis of chronic allograft injury and elimination of chronic allograft nephropathy ('CAN'). *Am J Transplant.* 2007;7(3):518-26.

[8] Solez K, Colvin RB, Racusen LC, Haas M, Sis B, Mengel M, et al. Banff 07 classification of renal allograft pathology: updates and future directions. *Am J Transplant.* 2008;8(4):753-60.

[9] Sis B, Mengel M, Haas M, Colvin RB, Halloran PF, Racusen LC, et al. Banff '09 meeting report: antibody mediated graft deterioration and implementation of Banff working groups. *Am J Transplant.* 2010;10(3):464-71.

[10] Mengel M, Sis B, Haas M, Colvin RB, Halloran PF, Racusen LC, et al. Banff 2011 Meeting report: new concepts in antibody -mediated rejection. *Am J Transplant.* 2012;12(3):563-70.

[11] Haas M. The Revised (2013) Banff Classification for Antibody-Mediated Rejection of Renal Allografts: Update, Difficulties, and Future Considerations. *Am J Transplant.* 2016;16(5):1352-7.

[12] Loupy A, Haas M, Solez K, Racusen L, Glotz D, Seron D, et al. The Banff 2015 Kidney Meeting Report: Current Challenges in Rejection Classification and Prospects for Adopting Molecular Pathology. *Am J Transplant.* 2017;17(1):28-41.

[13] Haas M, Loupy A, Lefaucheur C, Roufosse C, Glotz D, Seron D, et al. The Banff 2017 Kidney Meeting Report: Revised diagnostic criteria for chronic active T cell -mediated rejection, antibody -mediated rejection, and prospects for integrative endpoints for next-generation clinical trials. *Am J Transplant.* 2018;18(2):293-307.

[14] Mengel M, Loupy A, Haas M, Roufosse C, Naesens M, Akalin E, et al. Banff 2019 Meeting Report: Molecular diagnostics in solid organ transplantation -Consensus for the Banff Human Organ Transplant (B-HOT) gene panel and open source multicenter validation. *Am J Transplant.* 2020;20(9):2305-17.

[15] Haas M, Sis B, Racusen LC, Solez K, Glotz D, Colvin RB, et al. Banff 2013 meeting report: inclusion of c4d-negative antibody -mediated rejection and antibody-associated arterial lesions. *Am J Transplant.* 2014;14(2):272-83.

[16] Sumitran-Holgersson S. Relevance of MICA and other non-HLA antibodies in clinical transplantation. *Current opinion in immunology*. 2008;20(5):607-13.

[17] Wang S, Zhang C, Wang J, Yang C, Xu M, Rong R, et al. Endothelial Cells in Antibody-Mediated Rejection of Kidney Transplantation: Pathogenesis Mechanisms and Therapeutic Implications. *Journal of Immunology Research*. 2017;2017: 8746303.

[18] Haas M, Mirocha J. Early ultrastructural changes in renal allografts: correlation with antibody -mediated rejection and transplant glomerulopathy. *Am J Transplant.* 2011;11(10):2123-31.

[19] Torres IB, Salcedo M, Moreso F, Sellarés J, Castellá E, Azancot MA, et al. Comparing transplant glomerulopathy in the absence of C4d deposition and donor-specific antibodies to chronic antibody -mediated rejection. *Clin Transplant.* 2014;28(10):1148-54.

[20] Filippone EJ, McCue PA, Farber JL. Transplant glomerulopathy. *Mod Pathol.* 2018;31(2):235-52.

[21] Wavamunno MD, O'Connell PJ, Vitalone M, Fung CL, Allen RD, Chapman JR, et al. Transplant glomerulopathy: ultrastructural abnormalities occur early in longitudinal analysis of protocol biopsies. *Am J Transplant.* 2007;7(12):2757-68.

[22] Roufosse C, Simmonds N, Clahsen-van Groningen M, Haas M, Henriksen KJ, Horsfield C, et al. A 2018 Reference Guide to the Banff Classification of Renal Allograft Pathology. *Transplantation.* 2018;102(11):1795-814.

[23] Mengel M, Reeve J, Bunnag S, Einecke G, Jhangri GS, Sis B, et al. Scoring total inflammation is superior to the current Banff inflammation score in predicting outcome and the degree of molecular disturbance in renal allografts. *Am J Transplant.* 2009;9(8):1859-67.

[24] Mannon RB, Matas AJ, Grande J, Leduc R, Connett J, Kasiske B, et al. Inflammation in areas of tubular atrophy in kidney allograft biopsies: a potent predictor of allograft failure. *Am J Transplant.* 2010;10(9):2066-73.

[25] Sis B, Halloran PF. Endothelial transcripts uncover a previously unknown phenotype: C4d-negative antibody -mediated rejection. *Curr Opin Organ Transplant.* 2010;15(1):42-8.

[26] Haas M. Evolving criteria for the diagnosis of antibody -mediated rejection in renal allografts. *Curr Opin Nephrol Hypertens.* 2018;27(3):137-43.

In: Issues in Kidney Disease – Transplantation
Editors: B. V. R. Murthy and S. Z. Fadem
ISBN: 978-1-53619-960-4

Chapter 8

MANAGEMENT OF KIDNEY TRANSPLANT REJECTION

Nidhi Aggarwal**, *MD
Selzman Institute for Kidney Health, Section of Nephrology,
and Michael E. DeBakey Veterans Affairs Medical Center,
Baylor College of Medicine, Houston, TX, USA

ABSTRACT

Advances in the field of transplantation over the last few decades have led to significant decline in acute rejection rates in kidney transplant recipients. Despite significant improvement in short-term graft survival, ongoing alloimmune injury remains a major cause of chronic allograft dysfunction and graft loss. Understanding the risk factors and mechanisms of graft rejection can help determine the probability of immunologic injury and guide management decisions. Kidney allograft biopsy remains the gold standard for diagnosis of graft rejection, and treatment decisions are guided by the type, severity, and chronicity of rejection as determined by the biopsy. While treatment of T-cell mediated rejection is well-established and usually effective, newer strategies continue to evolve for the treatment of antibody -mediated rejection. Chronic rejection is insidious, often irreversible, and even more challenging to manage.

Keywords: acute T-cell mediated rejection, acute antibody -mediated rejection, chronic rejection, donor-specific antibodies

INTRODUCTION

The prevalence of end-stage kidney disease (ESKD) is increasing, and kidney transplant remains the treatment of choice for most patients with advanced chronic kidney

* Corresponding Author's Email: Nidhi.Aggarwal@bcm.edu.

disease due to improvement in quality of life and survival advantage when compared to dialysis. Since 1988, close to half a million people have undergone kidney transplantation in the United States. Early attempts at kidney transplantation were only successful between HLA -identical twins. Shortened graft survival, mainly due to acute rejection, was a major concern in HLA non-identical individuals. Better understanding of the immune system, development of tissue typing techniques, enhanced matching protocols, and introduction of newer, more potent induction and maintenance immunosuppressive agents have led to significant reduction in acute rejection rates, with consequent improvement in allograft survival. Regardless, acute rejection remains one of the top differential diagnoses when dealing with allograft dysfunction. In this chapter, different types of kidney transplant rejection and their pathophysiological mechanisms are discussed, as well as their diagnostic criteria and management strategies.

Epidemiology

Episodes of clinical acute rejection in the first-year post-transplant ation are associated with shortened long-term graft survival, both among living-donor and deceased-donor renal transplants [1]. Currently, the overall incidence of acute rejection among kidney transplant recipients within first-year post-transplantation is about 8% [2]. Living-donor kidney transplants, when compared to deceased-donor transplants, have lower rates of acute rejection and better long-term graft survival. Despite significant improvement in short-term graft survival, ongoing alloimmune insult remains a major cause of chronic allograft injury and graft loss.

Pathophysiology

The major antigenic differences between a donor and recipient which cause transplant rejection are differences in HLA alleles. HLA genes are highly polymorphic, such that there are always some differences between individuals (except, identical twins). Transplantation of organs between non-HLA identical individuals triggers an immunological response due to recognition of allograft by the recipient's immune system as foreign (non-self). This causes an inflammatory reaction with certain specific pathological changes in the transplanted organ. This process, which may or may not be associated with allograft dysfunction, is termed as *allograft rejection.*

Rejection of allograft results from a complex series of interactions and coordination between both the innate and adaptive immune system s, with recipient T-cells performing the primary role in this process. Even though the adaptive immune response plays the major role in causing allograft rejection, early inflammation in the graft is caused by innate immune response. Ischemic reperfusion injury that occurs during transplantation can activate the innate immune system and trigger acute rejection, as well as contribute to chronic allograft nephropathy. Reactive oxygen species formed during ischemic reperfusion injury lead to activation and migration of dendritic cells to secondary lymphoid tissues and initiation of adaptive alloimmune response.

T-cells recognize the donor antigens from the graft, a process called *allorecognition.* T-cell receptor present on the surface of T-cells interacts with donor peptides bound in the groove of major histocompatibility complex (MHC) on the surface of antigen -presenting cells (APCs) (i.e., dendritic cell s, macrophages, and B-cells). There are two distinct pathways of allorecognition: *the direct pathway,* when T cells directly recognize intact non-self MHC molecules present on the surface of donor antigen presenting cells; and *the indirect pathway*, when donor proteins are processed and presented to T-cells by self-MHC molecules on the surface of recipient antigen presenting cells. These pathways lead to activation of T cells, which then undergo clonal expansion, differentiation into effector cells, and migration into the allograft where they lead to tissue destruction *(cellular rejection).* In addition, CD4+ T cells help B-cells produce alloantibodies, leading to *humoral rejection.*

Sensitization to foreign MHC antigens can occur as a result of exposure to these antigens, either from prior organ transplant, blood transfusion, or pregnancies. Presence of preexisting antibodies against donor MHC antigens or blood group (ABO) antigens can cause rapid rejection of the allograft in a complement -dependent reaction that can occur within minutes of transplantation. Various donor and recipient characteristics in the pre- as well as post-transplant period are associated with an increased risk of rejection, as listed in Table 1.

Table 1. Donor and recipient factors associated with increased risk of rejection

• HLA mismatch
• ABO incompatibility
• Prior sensitization with high panel reactive antibodies
• Presence of donor-specific antibodies (preformed or *de novo*)
• Positive crossmatch
• Deceased donor (higher risk than living donor transplant)
• Prolonged cold ischemia time
• Delayed graft function
• Older donor
• Younger recipient age
• African American recipient (higher risk than White race)
• Non-adherence to immunosuppression
• Inadequate immunosuppression
• Prior episodes of rejection

Classification of Transplant Rejection

Renal transplant rejection can be broadly classified into three major types, depending on the immunological characteristics and histopathology:

1. **Hyperacute rejection** – can occur within minutes to hours of transplantation
2. **Acute rejection** – can happen at any time after transplant, most commonly within the first-year post-transplant. Two major types of acute rejection are:
   (a) Acute T-cell mediated rejection or acute cellular rejection
   (b) Active antibody -mediated rejection
      (i) HLA antibody -mediated
      (ii) Non-HLA antibody -mediated
3. **Chronic rejection** – usually develops later, often 6 months post-transplant
   (a) Chronic antibody -mediated rejection – active and inactive
   (b) Chronic T-cell mediated rejection – active and inactive

Hyperacute Rejection

Hyperacute rejection occurs due to presence of high titers of preformed circulating alloantibodies (anti-HLA, anti-ABO blood group antibodies) to donor antigens in the recipient at the time of transplantation. When an organ is transplanted into such a recipient, these alloantibodies attack the graft immediately, bind to the vascular endothelial cells, and activate the complement and blood clot ting cascades. This results in an irreversible vascular rejection, intravascular thrombosis, and graft necrosis. The allograft becomes engorged and purple-colored due to deoxygenated, hemorrhaged blood. This leads to immediate loss of graft, usually within minutes to hours of transplantation, and often necessitates immediate graft nephrectomy. Histological examination reveals widespread endothelial damage, glomerular capillary thrombosis, fibrinoid necrosis, interstitial hemorrhage and polymorphonuclear leukocyte infiltration.

Hyperacute rejection was more prevalent when advanced ABO compatibility and crossmatching techniques were not available. It has become a rare occurrence due to the availability of sensitive crossmatching assays and ABO compatibility tests that are performed prior to transplantation. With crossmatching, one can determine if the recipient has antibodies against the donor antigens. A positive crossmatch indicates the presence of such antibodies. Hyperacute rejection can be prevented by avoiding transplant if there is a positive crossmatch between the donor and the intended recipient.

ACUTE REJECTION

Acute rejection occurs due to the immune response of the host to the allograft. It can happen any time after transplant, usually within days to weeks and generally in the first year after transplant. It is clinically suspected when there is a decline in kidney allograft function, when other causes such as volume depletion, obstructive uropathy, drug toxicities, infections have been excluded. Kidney biopsy is required for definitive diagnosis, and the type and severity of acute rejection is determined based on the Banff Working Group classification [3]. Untreated acute rejection inevitably leads to loss of allograft function. Depending on the immunological mechanism of injury, acute rejection can be classified into two major types: acute T-cell mediated rejection and acute antibody -mediated rejection .

Acute T-Cell Mediated Rejection

Acute T-cell mediated rejection, also called acute cellular rejection, occurs when the recipient lymphocytes become activated by the presentation of donor antigens by self-MHC or by recognition of foreign MHC on donor antigens, which leads to proliferation and infiltration of the T cells in the allograft, causing damage. It can manifest as allograft dysfunction (rise in serum creatinine, oliguria, hypertension, graft tenderness, or fever), or may be subclinical (as noted on protocol biopsies). It usually occurs in the early weeks to months after transplant, but can present later, especially if there is reduction in immunosuppression, either intentional as in the setting of an infection, or while switching immunosuppressive agent s, or due to non-adherence to the regimen.

Diagnosis

On a kidney biopsy, acute T-cell mediated rejection is characterized by diffuse infiltration by lymphocytes, monocytes, and plasma cells in the interstitium (interstitial inflammation) and in the tubules (tubulitis, *t*). In severe cases, lymphocytes, monocytes and macrophages invading the subendothelium and intima of the vessels (intimal arteritis, *v*) can be seen, and extreme cases reveal transmural arterial fibrinoid necrosis. The grading of acute T-cell mediated rejection, based on the Banff classification of renal allograft biopsy [3], is shown in Table 2. The Banff classification for kidney transplant rejection is discussed in detail elsewhere in this book.

Table 2. Banff classification of acute T-cell mediated rejection

Grade 1a	>25% Interstitial inflammation with moderate tubulitis (*t2*, 5-10 mononuclear cells/tubule)
Grade 1b	>25% Interstitial inflammation with severe tubulitis (*t3*, >10 mononuclear cells/tubule)
Grade IIa	Mild-to-moderate intimal arteritis (*v1*, <25% lumen), with or without interstitial inflammation and/or tubulitis
Grade IIb	Severe intimal arteritis (*v2*, >25% lumen), with or without interstitial inflammation and/or tubulitis
Grade III	Transmural arteritis and/or arterial fibrinoid necrosis (*v3*), with or without interstitial inflammation and/or tubulitis

Treatment

Treatment of acute T-cell mediated rejection is based on the severity of the acute lesion and degree of background chronicity as seen on the allograft biopsy. Grade I rejections usually respond to treatment with pulse glucocorticoids alone, either as intravenous methylprednisolone (250 to 500 mg/day for 3-5 days) or high dose oral prednisone, tapered over several days to maintenance dose. Severe T-cell mediated rejection (Grade II and III) generally respond poorly to steroids alone; therefore, T-cell depletion therapy is used in conjunction with glucocorticoids for the treatment of such rejections [4, 5]. Most centers now use rabbit anti-thymocyte globulin (rATG) dosed at 1.5 mg/kg/day for 5-7 doses, due to superior effectiveness over horse anti-thymocyte globulin (hATG) in reversing acute rejection [6]. In addition to these measures, optimization of the doses and levels of baseline maintenance immunosuppression is common to the treatment of all types of rejection (Figure 2). Occasionally, rATG may have to be given for Banff 1b rejection when response to intravenous methylprednisolone is sub-optimal.

Antibody-Mediated Rejection

Antibody-mediated rejection (ABMR) occurs due to graft injury caused by alloantibodies directed against donor antigens. These donor specific antibodies (DSA) can be pre-existing at a low level at the time of transplant, or develop *de novo* in the post-transplant period due to B-cell and plasma cell activation. The DSAs are usually directed against donor HLA antigens. However, in some cases non-HLA antigens, such as ABO blood antigens in cases of ABO-incompatible transplants, H-Y minor histocompatibility antigens encoded by the Y chromosome of male donors, MHC class I polypeptide -related chain A and B, angiotensin II type 1 receptor, can be the cause of alloantibody production and antibody mediated rejection [7, 8]. As mentioned previously, high levels of preexisting DSAs can cause hyperacute rejection, which is an extreme case of antibody-mediated rejection.

Donor specific antibodies cause rejection through complement -dependent or complement-independent mechanisms. Binding of DSAs to class I HLA expressed on allograft endothelial cells activates the classic complement cascade and causes *complement-dependent cytotoxicity,* a major pathologic process leading to acute antibody -mediated rejection. C4d, a degradation product of the complement pathway, binds covalently to the endothelium, and can be detected on biopsy specimens by immunofluorescence or immunohistochemistry in some cases of antibody mediated rejection.

Complement non-binding DSAs cause *antibody -dependent cytotoxicity* by recruiting innate immune cells (NK cells, macrophages and neutrophils), which trigger degranulation and release lytic enzymes, causing tissue injury and cell death. In addition, these DSAs can cause direct stimulation and have pleotrophic effects that lead to tissue injury, cellular recruitment, and endothelial proliferation. Complement-independent pathways are the major pathogenic mechanisms that lead to subclinical and chronic antibody mediated rejection [9].

Diagnosis

Diagnosis of antibody -mediated rejection is made using the Banff classification [3], which requires three criteria to be met for diagnosis: morphologic changes, including microvascular inflammation characterized by neutrophils and mononuclear cells in glomeruli (glomerulitis, *g*) and peritubular capillaries (peritubular capillaritis, *ptc*), thrombotic microangiopathy, acute tubular injury, or intimal or transmural arteritis (*v*); evidence of complement activation by C4d deposition in the peritubular capillaries or within arterial fibrinoid necrosis; and presence of DSAs (Table 3).

Table 3. Diagnostic criteria for active antibody -mediated rejection (Banff classification)

All three criteria below are required.
Morphologic evidence of acute tissue injury, including one or more of the following: • *Microvascular inflammation (g > 0 and/or ptc > 0)* • *Arteritis (v > 0)* • *Thrombotic microangiopathy* • *Acute tubular injury*
Evidence of current/recent antibody interaction with endothelium including one or more of the following: • *Positive linear C4d staining in peritubular capillaries* • *Moderate microvascular inflammation (g + ptc ≥ 2)* • *Increased expression of gene transcripts in biopsy tissue strongly associated with AMR*
Serologic evidence of donor-specific antibodies (DSA) • *Positive C4d staining or presence of ABMR-associated gene transcripts may substitute for DSA*

Treatment

The optimal treatment of antibody -mediated rejection is not clearly defined. It usually involves a combination of therapies targeted at either removing preformed circulating DSA, inhibiting the residual antibody, limiting its reformation by depleting antibody-producing B-cells or plasma cells, and/or inhibiting the complement binding or activation that can damage the graft (Figure 1). Following are some of the currently available therapies used in prevention and treatment of antibody mediated rejection:

Plasmapheresis

Removes the circulating preformed DSA but does not suppress antibody production.

Intravenous Immunoglobulin (IVIG)

IVIG contains pooled serum immunoglobulin G fractions and are considered natural modulators of inflammation and immunity. Their possible mechanisms of action include direct binding and neutralization of DSAs, inhibition of complement binding or activation by acting as a complement sink, suppression of DSA production, and increased catabolism of circulating antibodies.

Rituximab

Rituximab is a chimeric monoclonal IgG antibody directed at CD20 antigen present on the surface of B-cells. It causes rapid and sustained depletion of both pre-B and mature B-cells, thus reducing their transformation to plasma cells. It does not have activity against plasma cells or memory B cells, which do not express CD20. Common adverse reactions to rituximab are infusion reactions and increased susceptibility to infections

Glucocorticoids

Glucocorticoids are potent inhibitors of macrophage activation and NK-cell effector function.

Antithymocyte Globulin

ATG plays a role in prevention of AMR as it controls B-cell response directly by inducing B-cell apoptosis as well as indirectly by depleting helper T cell s. In addition, it depletes preexisting donor-reactive memory T-cells, NK cells and macrophages.

Bortezomib

Bortezomib is a proteosome inhibitor that induces apoptosis of plasma cells and can directly decrease DSA production.

Eculizumab

Eculizumab is a humanized monoclonal IgG antibody that binds to complement protein C5, and thus blocks terminal complement activation. It is used for treatment of resistant

AMR and in some cases, as part of the desensitization protocol for prevention of antibody-mediated rejection.

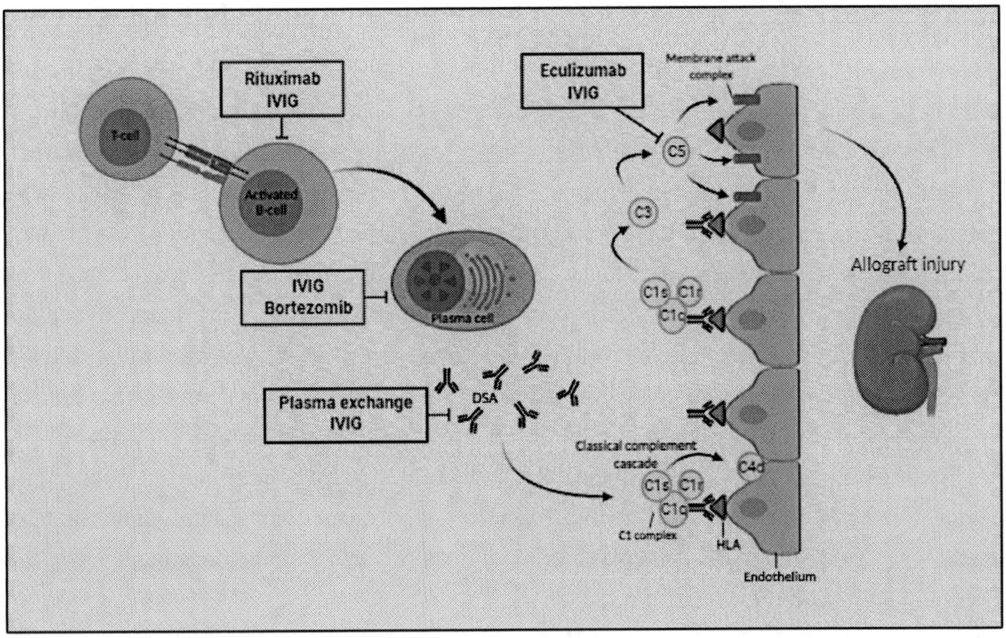

Figure 1. Therapeutic targets for antibody mediated allograft rejection. (DSA, Donor specific antibody; HLA, Human leukocyte antigen; IVIG, Intravenous immunoglobulin). Image created with BioRender.com.

Tocilizumab

Tocilizumab is a humanized monoclonal antibody against interleukin-6 receptor, which is involved in the differentiation of B-cells into plasmablasts and plasma cells.

The current mainstay of therapy for active antibody -mediated rejection is the use of plasma exchange and/or IVIG, in conjunction with glucocorticoids, with or without the addition of rituximab [4, 8, 10]. Combination of plasma exchange and IVIG has shown improvement in short-term outcomes of antibody-mediated rejection. A typical treatment includes 3-5 daily or alternate day plasma exchanges with 1.5 plasma-volume removal, followed by IVIG (sucrose free) at 100-200 mg/kg dose given after each plasma exchange session. A single dose of rituximab at 375 mg/m^2 is given after the last session of plasma exchange. The DSAs are serially monitored along with allograft function, and additional sessions of plasma exchange/IVIG are given if required. Eculizumab is given in cases that are resistant to standard treatment [11]. Bortezomib can be given in cases of plasma-cell rich acute rejection [12]. T-cell mediated rejection can often co-exist with antibody mediated rejection and will require treatment with T-cell directed therapies (Figure 2). After treatment of acute rejection episode, intensification of baseline immunosuppression should be done. In addition, anti-infective prophylaxis may also need to be added or extended depending on the type of treatment received. *Prognosis of Acute Rejection*

Alloimmune processes can cause progressive graft injury, and are a major cause of graft failure [13]. Presence of any episode of acute rejection, whether cell-mediated or antibody -mediated, clinical, or even subclinical, can lead to development of fibrosis, inflammation and transplant glomerulopathy over time, thus reducing graft survival [14-16]. Acute rejection in the first year after kidney transplantation is associated with worse long-term allograft outcomes [1]. Early stages of acute T cell -mediated rejection usually respond well to treatment and have good prognosis. However, poor response to treatment in acute T cell-mediated rejection is associated with reduced allograft function and poor long-term allograft survival. In addition, there is increased incidence of de novo donor specific anti-HLA antibody development, thus increasing the risk of active and chronic active ABMR [17-19]. Antibody mediated rejection is more challenging to treat and has worse long-term prognosis when compared to T-cell mediated rejection. Presence of pre-existing anti-HLA DSA alone, especially at high titers, is associated with a poorer graft survival even in the absence of active ABMR [20]. DSAs with complement -binding capacity are associated with an increased risk of antibody-mediated rejection, severe tissue injury, and subsequent graft failure [21].

CHRONIC REJECTION

Chronic rejection usually occurs later in the post-transplant period and is the major cause of long-term graft failure. While it can be T-cell mediated, the major cause of chronic rejection is antibody -mediated injury. Chronic active antibody-mediated rejection results from ongoing allograft injury despite treatment of early antibody-mediated rejection. It can also be detected on surveillance biopsies when circulating DSAs cause subclinical allograft injury. DSAs can be preexisting at the time of transplantation or can develop de novo due to inadequate immunosuppression, which is either due to physician-directed reduction in drugs, or patient non-adherence, or due to variability in drug metabolism. Clinically, chronic active ABMR can present as slow and progressive allograft dysfunction, worsening proteinuria and ultimately allograft loss.

Diagnosis

Histopathologic examination is the key to determining the chronicity and extent of allograft injury. On biopsy, chronic active ABMR is characterized by changes, such as expansion and duplication of the glomerular basement membrane, designated as transplant glomerulopathy (cg), peritubular basement membrane multilayering, and interstitial fibrosis and tubular atrophy. Other features that may be present are C4d positivity and vascular lesions, and occasionally concomitant T-cell mediated rejection. Criteria used for diagnosis of chronic active T cell -mediated rejection and chronic active antibody -mediated rejection are based on Banff classification, and are shown in Tables 4 and 5, respectively [3].

Table 4. Banff classification of chronic active T-cell mediated rejection

Grade 1a	>25% Interstitial inflammation (ti 2 or 3) and >25% of sclerotic cortical parenchyma (i-IFTA score 2 or 3) with moderate tubulitis (t2); exclude other causes of i-IFTA*
Grade 1b	>25% Interstitial inflammation and >25% of sclerotic cortical parenchyma (i-IFTA score 2 or 3) with severe tubulitis (t3); exclude other causes of i-IFTA*
Grade II	Chronic allograft arteriopathy (arterial intimal fibrosis with mononuclear cell inflammation in fibrosis and formation of neointima)

i-IFTA; Interstitial fibrosis and tubular atrophy

*BK virus infection, active AMR, recurrent glomerulonephritis, or obstruction

Table 5. Diagnostic criteria for chronic active antibody -mediated rejection (Banff classification)

All three criteria below are required:
Morphologic evidence of chronic tissue injury, including one or more of the following: • *Transplant glomerulopathy (cg>0), without evidence of thrombotic microangiopathy or glomerulonephritis (de novo or recurrent)* • *Severe peritubular basement membrane multilayering* • *New-onset arterial intimal fibrosis*
Evidence of current/recent antibody interaction with endothelium including one or more of the following: • *Positive linear C4d staining in peritubular capillaries* • *Moderate microvascular inflammation (g+ptc ≥2)* • *Increased expression of gene transcripts in biopsy tissue strongly associated with AMR*
Serologic evidence of donor-specific antibodies (DSA) • *Positive C4d staining or presence of ABMR-associated gene transcripts may substitute for DSA*

Treatment

The main goal of treatment of chronic rejection is to stabilize or reduce the rate of decline of renal allograft function, avoid worsening of proteinuria and DSA titers. Like treatment of early antibody -mediated rejection, IVIG and plasma exchange, with or without Rituximab, Eculizumab and bortezomib have been used for treatment of a chronic antibody-mediated rejection but these therapies have not been shown to improve outcomes [22-24]. Use of Tocilizumab, an interleukin-6 receptor antibody, has shown reductions in DSA, stabilization of graft function, as well as improved long-term graft and patient survival [25, 26]. Overall, treatment mainstay is optimization of maintenance immunosuppression, with higher target levels of calcineurin inhibitors, reintroduction of anti-metabolite (if previously held), and/or addition of steroids (if on steroid-free regimen). Risk of adverse drug events, such as infections, must be weighed against the potential benefit to be gained from use of additional immunosuppression. Treatment should also focus on medication management and optimization of blood pressure, diabetes, and lipids.

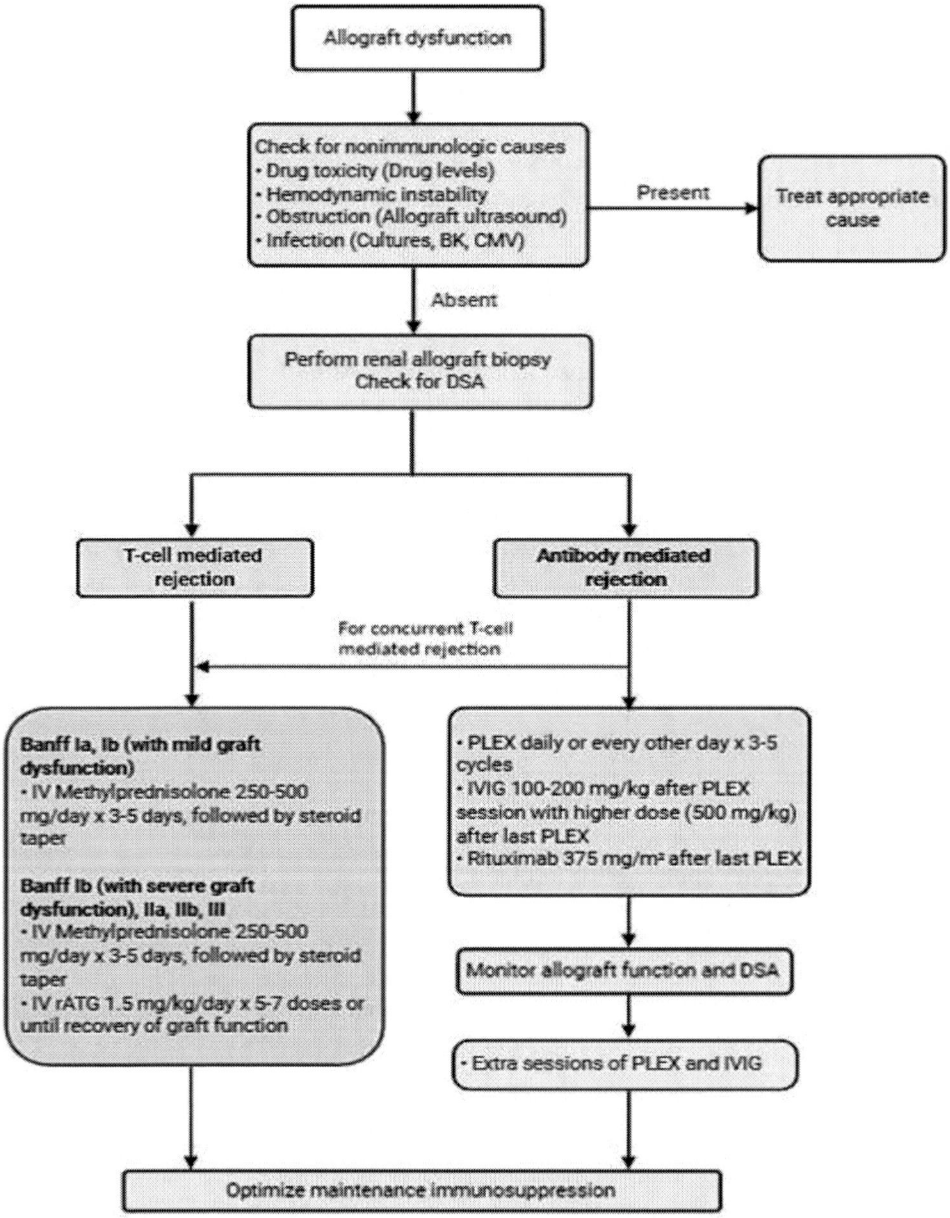

Figure 2. Algorithm for management of biopsy -proven acute kidney allograft rejection. (BK, BK virus; CMV, Cytomegalovirus; DSA, donor-specific antibody; IV, intravenous; IVIG, intravenous immunoglobulin; PLEX, plasma exchange; rATG, rabbit antithymocyte globulin). Image created with BioRender.com.

NEWER DIAGNOSTIC TECHNIQUES

Current monitoring techniques for allograft rejection rely on serial measurement of serum creatinine and urinary protein, which are non-specific markers of allograft dysfunction. Measurement of circulating anti-HLA DSA levels, determination of its strength, as well as its capacity to activate complement, may improve the ability to predict antibody -mediated rejection. As mentioned previously, renal allograft biopsy is the gold standard for diagnosis of rejection. However, frequent biopsies for surveillance of acute rejection are not performed at most centers due to cost involved, logistics, potential patient discomfort and complications due to its invasive nature. In addition, biopsy may be associated with sampling error and variable pathological interpretation. Even for diagnostic purposes, allograft biopsy may occasionally be difficult to perform. As such, several non-invasive biomarkers in blood and urine are being tested to assess the immune risk, monitor allograft function, diagnose acute rejection, and predict long-term outcomes.

Cytotoxic T lymphocyte-induced apoptosis is mediated by the perforin/granzyme B pathway and the Fas-Fas ligand lytic pathway (Fas-L). Urinary measurement of perforin and granzyme B mRNA as well as Fas-L was studied and shown to have high accuracy in predicting acute rejection [27]. However, in subsequent studies, these markers were shown to be non-specific, and were noted to be upregulated in other causes of allograft injury as well [28]. When granzyme B and perforin were used together, the likelihood of detecting acute rejection improved [29].

Regulatory T cell (Tregs) play an important role in maintaining T cell homeostasis and may help antagonize the inflammation associated with kidney transplantation. Tregs express FOXP3 (the X-linked forkhead/winged helix transcription factor). Higher levels of urinary FOXP3 mRNA levels are associated with successful reversal of rejection and lower risk of graft failure [30]. Some other urinary biomarkers are chemokines CXCL9 and CXCL10, but these are non-specific for acute rejection, and may be elevated in other conditions such as BK virus nephropathy [31].

MicroRNA (miRNA) act as key regulators of B- and T-cell differentiation, maturation and proliferation, and play a role in Treg function and antigen signaling. Urinary miRNA has been investigated as a biomarker of acute rejection. Certain miRNA can be downregulated during acute rejection, and increase to stable levels after treatment of rejection [32, 33]. Some other non-invasive tests utilize changes in leukocyte or whole-blood gene expression to predict rejection.

Donor-derived cell-free DNA (dd-cfDNA), measured as a fraction of total cell-free DNA in the blood of transplant recipients, is a non-invasive marker of graft rejection that can allow for more frequent and safer assessment of rejection. The basis of this biomarker test is that rejection causes injury to the allograft and therefore, increased cell death, causing increased dd-cfDNA to be released into the bloodstream of the recipient. In the DART (Circulating Donor-Derived Cell-Free DNA in Blood for Diagnosing Active

Rejection in Kidney Transplant Recipients) study, a cut-off value of 1% dd-cfDNA had a high negative predictive value in discriminating antibody -mediated rejection from absent ABMR [34]. In addition, levels >1% were also associated with type 1B T cell -mediated rejection and transplant glomerulopathy. Given high negative predictive value, dd-cfDNA, despite its inability to distinguish immune from non-immune mechanisms of graft injury, can be used to 'rule out' rejection in the setting of levels below threshold.

Conclusion

Despite improvements in acute rejection rates due to better tissue typing techniques and potent immunosuppression, alloimmune injury continues to affect long-term graft survival. Prompt recognition of allograft dysfunction and performance of tissue biopsy allows for diagnosis and classification of allograft rejection. Management decisions should be based on the type, severity, and chronicity of rejection. Treatment strategies for acute rejection continue to evolve. Chronic rejection continues to have limited treatment choices and a poor prognosis, often leading to graft failure.

References

[1] Hariharan S, Johnson CP, Bresnahan BA, Taranto SE, McIntosh MJ, Stablein, D. Improved Graft Survival after Renal Transplantation in the United States, 1988 to 1996. *New England Journal of Medicine*., 2000, 342(9), 605-12.

[2] Hart A, Smith JM, Skeans MA, Gustafson SK, Wilk AR, Castro S, et al. OPTN/SRTR 2018 Annual Data Report: Kidney. *American Journal of Transplantation*., 2020, 20(s1), 20-130.

[3] Haas M, Loupy A, Lefaucheur C, Roufosse C, Glotz D, Seron D, et al. The Banff 2017 Kidney Meeting Report: Revised diagnostic criteria for chronic active T cell -mediated rejection, antibody -mediated rejection, and prospects for integrative endpoints for next-generation clinical trials. *Am J Transplant*., 2018, 18(2), 293-307.

[4] KDIGO clinical practice guideline for the care of kidney transplant recipients. *Am J Transplant*., 2009, 9 Suppl 3, S1-155.

[5] Webster AC, Wu S, Tallapragada K, Park MY, Chapman JR, Carr SJ. Polyclonal and monoclonal antibodies for treating acute rejection episodes in kidney transplant recipients. *Cochrane Database of Systematic Reviews*., 2017(7).

[6] Gaber AO, First MR, Tesi RJ, Gaston RS, Mendez R, Mulloy LL, et al. Results of the double-blind, randomized, multicenter, phase III clinical trial of Thymoglobulin versus Atgam in the treatment of acute graft rejection episodes after renal transplantation. *Transplantation*., 1998, 66(1), 29-37.

[7] Dragun D, Müller DN, Bräsen JH, Fritsche L, Nieminen-Kelhä M, Dechend R, et al. Angiotensin II Type 1–Receptor Activating Antibodies in Renal-Allograft Rejection. *New England Journal of Medicine.*, 2005, 352(6), 558-69.

[8] Loupy A, Lefaucheur C. Antibody-Mediated Rejection of Solid-Organ Allografts. *N Engl J Med.*, 2018, 379(12), 1150-60.

[9] Zhang R. Donor-Specific Antibodies in Kidney Transplant Recipients. *Clin J Am Soc Nephrol.*, 2018, 13(1), 182-92.

[10] Burton SA, Amir N, Asbury A, Lange A, Hardinger KL. Treatment of antibody - mediated rejection in renal transplant patients: a clinical practice survey. *Clin Transplant.*, 2015, 29(2), 118-23.

[11] Stegall MD, Diwan T, Raghavaiah S, Cornell LD, Burns J, Dean PG, et al. Terminal complement inhibition decreases antibody -mediated rejection in sensitized renal transplant recipients. *Am J Transplant.*, 2011, 11(11), 2405-13.

[12] Eskandary F, Regele H, Baumann L, Bond G, Kozakowski N, Wahrmann M, et al. A Randomized Trial of Bortezomib in Late Antibody-Mediated Kidney Transplant Rejection. *J Am Soc Nephrol.*, 2018, 29(2), 591-605.

[13] El-Zoghby ZM, Stegall MD, Lager DJ, Kremers WK, Amer H, Gloor JM, et al. Identifying specific causes of kidney allograft loss. *Am J Transplant.*, 2009, 9(3), 527-35.

[14] Loupy A, Vernerey D, Tinel C, Aubert O, Duong van Huyen JP, Rabant M, et al. Subclinical Rejection Phenotypes at 1 Year Post-Transplant and Outcome of Kidney Allografts. *J Am Soc Nephrol.*, 2015, 26(7), 1721-31.

[15] Lefaucheur C, Gosset C, Rabant M, Viglietti D, Verine J, Aubert O, et al. T cell - mediated rejection is a major determinant of inflammation in scarred areas in kidney allografts. *Am J Transplant.*, 2018, 18(2), 377-90.

[16] Hoffman W, Mehta R, Jorgensen DR, Sood P, Randhawa P, Wu CM, et al. The Impact of Early Clinical and Subclinical T Cell–mediated Rejection After Kidney Transplantation. *Transplantation,* 2019, 103(7), 1457-67.

[17] Wiebe C, Gibson IW, Blydt-Hansen TD, Karpinski M, Ho J, Storsley LJ, et al. Evolution and clinical pathologic correlations of de novo donor-specific HLA antibody post kidney transplant. *Am J Transplant.*, 2012, 12(5), 1157-67.

[18] El Ters M, Grande JP, Keddis MT, Rodrigo E, Chopra B, Dean PG, et al. Kidney allograft survival after acute rejection, the value of follow-up biopsies. *Am J Transplant.*, 2013, 13(9), 2334-41.

[19] Bouatou Y, Viglietti D, Pievani D, Louis K, Duong Van Huyen JP, Rabant M, et al. Response to treatment and long-term outcomes in kidney transplant recipients with acute T cell -mediated rejection. *Am J Transplant.*, 2019, 19(7), 1972-88.

[20] Lefaucheur C, Loupy A, Hill GS, Andrade J, Nochy D, Antoine C, et al. Preexisting donor-specific HLA antibodies predict outcome in kidney transplantation. *J Am Soc Nephrol.,* 2010, 21(8), 1398-406.

[21] Loupy A, Lefaucheur C, Vernerey D, Prugger C, van Huyen J-PD, Mooney N, et al. Complement-Binding Anti-HLA Antibodies and Kidney-Allograft Survival. *New England Journal of Medicine*., 2013, 369(13), 1215-26.

[22] Kulkarni S, Kirkiles-Smith NC, Deng YH, Formica RN, Moeckel G, Broecker V, et al. Eculizumab Therapy for Chronic Antibody-Mediated Injury in Kidney Transplant Recipients: A Pilot Randomized Controlled Trial. *Am J Transplant*., 2017, 17(3), 682-91.

[23] Cooper JE, Gralla J, Klem P, Chan L, Wiseman AC. High dose intravenous immunoglobulin therapy for donor-specific antibodies in kidney transplant recipients with acute and chronic graft dysfunction. *Transplantation*., 2014, 97(12), 1253-9.

[24] Macklin PS, Morris PJ, Knight SR. A systematic review of the use of rituximab for the treatment of antibody -mediated renal transplant rejection. *Transplant Rev (Orlando)*., 2017, 31(2), 87-95.

[25] Choi J, Aubert O, Vo A, Loupy A, Haas M, Puliyanda D, et al. Assessment of Tocilizumab (Anti-Interleukin-6 Receptor Monoclonal) as a Potential Treatment for Chronic Antibody-Mediated Rejection and Transplant Glomerulopathy in HLA - Sensitized Renal Allograft Recipients. *Am J Transplant*., 2017, 17(9), 2381-9.

[26] Shin BH, Everly MJ, Zhang H, Choi J, Vo A, Zhang X, et al. Impact of Tocilizumab (Anti–IL-6R) Treatment on Immunoglobulins and Anti-HLA Antibodies in Kidney Transplant Patients With Chronic Antibody-mediated Rejection. *Transplantation*., 2020, 104(4), 856-63.

[27] Li B, Hartono C, Ding R, Sharma VK, Ramaswamy R, Qian B, et al. Noninvasive diagnosis of renal-allograft rejection by measurement of messenger RNA for perforin and granzyme B in urine. *N Engl J Med.,* 2001, 344(13), 947-54.

[28] Yannaraki M, Rebibou JM, Ducloux D, Saas P, Duperrier A, Felix S, et al. Urinary cytotoxic molecular markers for a noninvasive diagnosis in acute renal transplant rejection. *Transpl Int.,* 2006, 19(9), 759-68.

[29] Heng B, Li Y, Shi L, Du X, Lai C, Cheng L, et al. A Meta-analysis of the Significance of Granzyme B and Perforin in Noninvasive Diagnosis of Acute Rejection After Kidney Transplantation. *Transplantation.,* 2015, 99(7), 1477-86.

[30] Muthukumar T, Dadhania D, Ding R, Snopkowski C, Naqvi R, Lee JB, et al. Messenger RNA for FOXP3 in the urine of renal-allograft recipients. *N Engl J Med.,* 2005, 353(22), 2342-51.

[31] Jackson JA, Kim EJ, Begley B, Cheeseman J, Harden T, Perez SD, et al. Urinary chemokines CXCL9 and CXCL10 are noninvasive markers of renal allograft rejection and BK viral infection. *Am J Transplant*., 2011, 11(10), 2228-34.

[32] Lorenzen JM, Volkmann I, Fiedler J, Schmidt M, Scheffner I, Haller H, et al. Urinary miR-210 as a mediator of acute T-cell mediated rejection in renal allograft recipients. *Am J Transplant*., 2011, 11(10), 2221-7.

[33] Anglicheau D, Sharma VK, Ding R, Hummel A, Snopkowski C, Dadhania D, et al. MicroRNA expression profiles predictive of human renal allograft status. *Proc Natl Acad Sci U S A.*, 2009, 106(13), 5330-5.

[34] Bloom RD, Bromberg JS, Poggio ED, Bunnapradist S, Langone AJ, Sood P, et al. Cell-Free DNA and Active Rejection in Kidney Allografts. *J Am Soc Nephrol.* 2017, 28(7), 2221-32.

In: Issues in Kidney Disease – Transplantation
Editors: B. V. R. Murthy and S. Z. Fadem

ISBN: 978-1-53619-960-4

Chapter 9

INFECTIOUS COMPLICATIONS AFTER TRANSPLANTATION

Marion Hemmersbach-Miller**, MD, PhD and Tyler M. Lambing, MD
Section of Infectious Diseases, Department of Medicine,
Baylor College of Medicine, Houston, TX, USA

ABSTRACT

Infectious complications after kidney transplantation impact morbidity and graft function in the initial years after surgery. They are a well-known cause of long-term mortality. This chapter presents an overview of donor, candidate, and recipient evaluation from the infectious disease perspective. The evaluation of the candidate focuses on required and recommended testing as well as immunization practices. In the donor section, universal screening is highlighted as well as special scenarios as they relate to geographic and risk factors for transmissible diseases. Donor-derived infections are highlighted. The kidney transplant recipient section features frequent post-transplant infectious complications, such as urinary tract infections and cytomegalovirus but also less frequent ones, such as fungal and other viral infection s. Finally, post-transplant antimicrobial prophylaxis and vaccinations are discussed.

INTRODUCTION

Infectious complications after kidney transplantation impact morbidity and graft function in the initial years after surgery. They are a well-known cause of long-term

* Corresponding Author's Email: dr_mhm@hotmail.com.

mortality. Presented here is a brief overview of donor and recipient evaluation as well as common post-transplant infectious complications.

Pre-Transplant Evaluation of the Kidney Transplant Recipient

The pre-transplant evaluation of the kidney transplant recipient is essential to achieve optimal outcomes after transplantation. This involves a thorough history of infectious diseases, exposures, and immunizations. While some of the workup is determined by center-specific protocols, this evaluation might need to be expanded based on the result of the candidates ' history. Generally, active infections should be appropriately treated and ideally resolved prior to transplant surgery. As per the American Society of Transplantation Guidelines [1], the candidate should be screened for the following: human immunodeficiency virus (HIV), cytomegalovirus (CMV), Hepatitis B virus (HBV) with HBV surface Ag (HBsAg), HBV core antibody (HBcAb-IgM and IgG, or total core antibody), Hepatitis C (HCV), Epstein-Barr virus (EBV) antibodies, Toxoplasma IgG, syphilis, varicella-zoster virus (VZV), measles (rubeola), mumps and rubella immunity. If the patient is from an endemic area, the following screenings are recommended as well: Strongyloides IgG, Coccidioides, and *Trypanosoma cruzi* serology. Human T-cell lymphotropic virus (HTLV) deserves special consideration. HTLV-1 is the most oncogenic of its family; it is endemic in the Caribbean, parts of South America, West Africa, Asia, Australia, and the Pacific. Long-term effects of immunosuppression on HTLV-1 are not known, and if screening is performed, a positive result should be confirmed [2].

For the screening of tuberculosis (TB), interferon -gamma-release assays (IGRA) may have advantages over tuberculin skin testing (TST) in patients with end-stage renal disease (ESRD). Neither of these tests can distinguish active from latent infection. A positive test should be reviewed, and the patient considered for latent TB infection (LTBI) treatment once active TB is ruled out. There are several regimens available for the treatment of LTBI: 9 months of isoniazid (INH), 4 months of rifampin (RIF), or the 3 HP regimen (weekly INH and rifapentine for 12 doses). Additionally, there is a series of alternative regimens. Each of these has its limitations due to toxicities and drug-drug interactions and requires close laboratory monitoring after initiation of therapy. Rifamycin-based regimen continuation post-transplant is preferably avoided, if possible, due to the interactions with immunosuppressive medications; and alternatives are preferred. Recent TB exposures or TST conversion should be considered for treatment once active TB is ruled out. Kidney transplant candidates should begin treatment prior to transplantation due to the risk of TB reactivation with ESRD [3].

Pre-transplant serology and immunization history review needs close attention. If possible, immunizations should be completed prior to transplantation. Candidates should be up to date on their tetanus and pneumococcal vaccines (PSV13 and PPSV23). If no immunity is present to hepatitis A and B, vaccination should be initiated. If there is no immunity to measles, mumps, rubella (MMR) and/or varicella, vaccines should be given. However, the MMR and varicella vaccines are live vaccines, requiring that the transplant needs to be put on hold for 4-weeks after the last live vaccine is given. Candidates 50 years or older that are VZV IgG positive, should get the recombinant zoster vaccine. Human papillomavirus (HPV) vaccination is indicated in adult candidates up to 45 years of age. This is especially important as transplant recipients are at increased risk of malignancies related to HPV [4].

The pre-transplant period is an ideal time to counsel the candidate and her/his family about food handling, lifestyle, travel, pet ownership, safe sexual practices, donor-derived infections, and infection prevention strategies [5, 6].

Evaluation of the Kidney Transplant Donor. Donor-Derived Infections

While improvements in surgical technique, immunosuppression, and antimicrobial prophylaxis have improved morbidity and mortality of kidney transplant recipients, donor-derived infections (DDIs) are common. DDIs are defined as any infection present in the donor that is transmitted to one or more recipients. Some are expected; e.g., cytomegalovirus (CMV), and dedicated post-transplant strategies are in place to avoid these. The Organ Procurement and Transplantation Network (OPTN) policy requires organ procurement organizations (OPOs) and transplant centers to report potential donor disease transmission events. These are then reviewed by the Disease Transmission Advisory Committee (DTAC). Donor disease transmission events are not limited only to infections but also include malignancies. This chapter focuses on the infections which can be divided into two categories: expected and unexpected. Expected transmission occurs when it is known that the donor is infected or colonized with a certain pathogen. Appropriate measures to prevent transmission should be in place for these scenarios: microbiological monitoring, pre-emptive therapy, and/or universal prophylaxis. This minimizes the impact of the DDI. Unexpected transmissions require a high index of suspicion; any early infection should be followed by an inquiry of the donor and status of other recipients. Unexpected transmissions occur when one or more recipients develop an infection from a donor when the donor was not known to be infected prior to donation; this happens in <0.2% [7] but can be very serious. Table 1 shows known pathogens that can be transmitted from the donor.

Table 1. Donor-derived infections by type of pathogen. MDROs: multi-drug resistant organisms; NTM: non-tuberculous mycobacteria; CMV: cytomegalovirus, HBV: hepatitis B virus, HCV: hepatitis C virus; HEV: hepatitis E virus: LCM: lymphocytic choriomeningitis; HSV: herpes simplex virus; HTLV: human T-lymphotropic virus; HHV-8: human herpesvirus-8; EEEV: eastern equine encephalitis virus

Category	Pathogen(s)	Comments
Bacterial	Gram-positives Gram-negatives *Mycoplasma* spp. Syphilis Other	Of growing importance in this category ar e MDROs
Fungal	Candidemia Endemic mycoses: blastomycosis, histoplasmosis, coccidioidomycosis Cryptococcal infection Aspergillus / mold infections Other	
Mycobacterial	Tuberculosis / NTM	Often require prolonged therapies and invasive therapeutic procedures
Viral	CMV HBV HCV HEV LCM Community respiratory viruses Parvovirus West Nile virus HSV HTLV Rabies HHV-8 EEEV	Very diverse group from preventable (e.g., intentional HCV mismatch transplantation), preventable (e.g., CMV), potentially requiring life-long therapy (e.g., HBV), associated with malignancies (e.g., HHV-8) to potentially lethal (e.g., LCM, rabies).
Parasitic	Strongyloidiasis Toxoplasmosis Trypanosomiasis Balamuthia Leishmania Plasmodium spp.	Donor exposure history is of utmost importance for many of these
Prion	Creutzfeldt-Jakob disease	

Adapted from the following main sources: Wolfe et al. *Clin Transplant* 2019; 33;e13547; Kaul et al. *Am J Transplant* 2020. doi: 10.1111/ajt.16178; *Transplant Infections*, 4th ed by Ljungman P et al. Chapter 8 Donor-derived Infections.

Universal Donor Screening

In order to avoid transmission of certain infections, universal donor screening helps identify some of these pathogens. OPTN policy requires screening for certain pathogens. Table 2 shows the required infectious diseases testing. Additionally, certain active infections are exclusion criteria for donation; these can be found in the OPTN document. The donor's medical and behavioral history must include any testing and lab results to identify the presence of transmissible disease or malignancies or any condition that might be transmitted to the recipient, whether the donor has risk factors that predispose him/her to an increased risk for disease transmission, and whether the donor has a history of prior exposure or treatment with non-recombinant human pituitary derived growth factor.

Table 2. Deceased donor testing as per OPTN. Additionally, certain active infection are exclusion criteria for donation; these can be found in the OPTN document. HIV: human immunodeficiency virus; Ab: antibody; Ag: antigen; RNA: ribonucleic acid; NAT: nucleic acid test; CMV: cytomegalovirus; EBV: Epstein-Barr Virus

Test
Cultures: – Urine – Blood
HIV Ab or HIV Ag/Ab combination test
Hepatitis B – Hepatitis B surface Ag – Hepatitis B core Ab
Hepatitis C – Hepatitis C Ab – Hepatitis C RNA or NAT
CMV Ab
EBV Ab
Syphilis
Toxoplasma IgG
HIV RNA or NAT or HIV Ag/Ab combination**

**This additional testing is only required for increased risk donors for HIV, HBV and HCV transmission according to the U.S. Public Health Services (PHS) Guideline, unless:

- the donor already has been tested for HIV using the Ag/Ab combination test, OR.
- the donor's only risk factor is having received hemodialysis within the past 12 months.

Adapted, Source: *Organ Procurement and Transplantation Network.* https://optn.transplant .hrsa.gov/ media /1200/ optn_policies.pdf. Effective date 09/10/2020; accessed 10/27/2020.

Special Scenarios

Special scenarios represent situations where an organ from a donor with a known infection is used. Some of these situations have become increasingly more prevalent and require special attention; e.g., the use of hepatitis B or C positive donors, or even HIV positive donors. The latter is only allowed under a research umbrella provided by the HIV Organ Policy Equity (HOPE) Act.

Another special scenario is hemodilution. At times, upon evaluation of deceased donors, the only available blood sample for serological screening is a hemodiluted sample. In this case, the OPO must treat the donor as presenting an increased risk for disease transmission .

Donor Screening for Endemic Infections

New pathogens have become more prevalent over the last decades and screening for these should be considered based on local prevalence of the disease and origin of the donor. Ideally, the donor risk assessment interview (DRAI) form should help guide some of these tests in deceased donors. Some pathogens that have been described as are: West Nile Virus, *Trypanosoma cruzi* (Chagas disease), *Strongyloides stercolaris* and coccidioidomycosis .

West Nile Virus

West Nile Virus (WNV) is a mosquito-borne flavivirus. Most patients develop no or only mild symptoms, but about 1 out of 150 (CDC data) develop a serious, sometimes fatal, illness including meningoencephalitis. It is a seasonal disease found throughout the United States. It has no specific treatment. Serologic testing does not predict risk for infection and Health Resources and Services Administration (HRSA) recommends testing of all prospective live donors with nucleic acid testing (NAT), although there have been transmissions with negative NAT [8]. This is challenging in deceased donors and universal screening is not recommended due to concern of underusage of organs attributable to false positive s, although the same authors also state that screening would be preferable for kidney donors in areas of high disease prevalence and high tests specificity [9]. It is prudent in general to avoid organs from donors with unexplained encephalitis.

Trypanosoma cruzi

Chagas diseases is caused by the parasite *Trypanosoma cruzi.* It is transmitted to humans by insect vectors, triatomine bugs; it is found mainly in Latin America, but is now also seen in the Southern part of the U.S. It is estimated that 300,000 persons with this infection live in the U.S. (CDC) and its transmission via organ transplantation has been clearly documented. Hearts from infected donors should not be used for transplantation, but kidneys and livers can be considered with informed consent from the recipient and preemptive monitoring by polymerase chain reaction (PCR) and microscopy of buffy coat for detection of early infection and initiation of therapy [1].

Strongyloides stercolaris

Strongyloides is a parasite that exists worldwide but is most common in the tropics, subtropics, and temperate regions. Its importance resides in the significant morbidity and mortality in transplant recipients; hyperinfection syndrome can occur in the setting of immunosuppression. Living donors should be screened by serology as well as deceased donors if feasible, especially those with epidemiologic risk factors. Transplant candidates can be screened as well [1]. Pre-transplant treatment with a short course of ivermectin is warranted if the living donor or transplant candidate tests positive. Treatment is also indicated if a patient received an organ from a deceased donor that screened positive.

Coccidioidomycosis

Coccidioidomycosis, also known as Valley fever, is a fungal infection. The fungus lives in the soil in the Southwestern part of the U.S., Central and South America. Most people do not know that they have been exposed to this disease as it can be self-limited. Transmission of coccidioidomycosis by transplantation has been reported as well as reactivation of the infection in a previously infected recipient; this latter scenario seems to be more frequent. Screening should be therefore recommended in endemic areas, ideally with enzyme immunoassays (EIAs) [10]. Results of this test have an impact on post-transplant prophylaxis which might include fluconazole for varying durations.

SURGICAL SITE INFECTIONS

Surgical site infections (SSI) are infections that occur after surgery at the part of the body where the surgery took place. In transplant patients these infections are frequent and have increased clinical significance. The most common infection in the peri-transplant period is a SSI. Rates of SSI for kidney transplant patients range from 3-11%. Reduced graft survival is associated with SSIs. Risk factors that have been associated with SSI in kidney transplant recipients are diabetes, obesity, chronic glomerular nephritis, re-operation, ureteral leak, hematoma at the surgical site, blood transfusion, use of antithymocyte globulin, azathioprine, mycophenolate, and sirolimus [11].

The criteria for the CDC definition of SSI:

- Occurs within 30 days of operation
- One of the following: purulent drainage, positive cultures from the site from an aseptically obtained specimen

- One of the following: localized pain or tenderness, localized swelling, erythema, heat, diagnosis of a superficial incisional SSI by a surgeon, physician, or physician designee [12].

The CDC differentiates SSI into three entities: superficial, deep, and organ /space. Superficial involves only the skin and the subcutaneous tissue of the incision. Deep involves the deep soft tissues such as the fascial and muscle layers. Organ or space SSI involves any layer of the body that is deeper than the muscle layer that is opened or manipulated during the procedure. Cultures should be taken at the appropriate level that the infection is suspected at [11, 12].

Prevention

To prevent SSIs, it is recommended to have hemoglobin at appropriate levels to provide oxygenation to tissue, a chlorhexidine gluconate bath prior to surgery, tight glycemic control, and peri-operative antibiotics. There is no universal regimen for peri-op antibiotic for kidney transplants. The most commonly used agent is a first-generation cephalosporin s. Studies have found no difference in the rate of SSIs when comparing first generation cephalosporins to anti-staphylococcal penicillins or third generation cephalosporins. A fluoroquinolone or aztreonam can be given as an alternative if there is a severe cephalosporin allergy. If the recipient is known to be colonized with a resistant organism, the peri-operative prophylaxis should be expanded to cover that [11].

Treatment

Treatment of SSI in kidney transplant patients should include a multifaceted approach with source control and antimicrobial agents. Clearly infected wounds should be opened to be irrigated, debrided, and to ensure there is no fascial dehiscence, drainage that extends to the organ, or enteric fistula. Empiric antibiotic coverage should cover the most common causative organisms. For kidney transplant patients the most common organisms for SSIs after transplant are gram positive cocci and flora from the area. A first-generation cephalosporin or an anti-staphylococcal penicillin are appropriate first line agents. If patient is known to be colonized with methicillin-resistant *Staphylococcus aureus* coverage should be expanded to cover for that. Coverage for multidrug resistant organisms can be considered if the patient is considered high risk. Risk factors for multidrug resistant organism in this setting include pre-transplant colonization, long term hospitalization, urologic manipulation, post-transplant urinary obstruction, recurrent urinary tract infections (UTIs), and renal replacement therapy needed after transplant [11].

Urinary Tract Infections

Urinary tract infections (UTIs) are the most common infection in kidney transplant patients. Up to 80% of recipients will be diagnosed with a UTI after transplant [13]. The risk for UTI is greatest during the first three to six months after transplant. Increased age, female gender, need for immediate post-transplant dialysis, rejection, deceased donor kidney, post-transplant catheterization, neurogenic bladder, renal calculi, ureteral stent, vesicoureteral reflux (VUR), and urological abnormalities all increase the risk of UTI. Use of antithymocyte globulin for induction is associated with higher incidence of UTI compared to basiliximab. A difference in UTI rates between different maintenance immunosuppression agents has not been described [14].

Previously there was no consensus on how to define UTIs. Numerous criteria were used to define UTI and how to treat it. To make treatment uniform, societal guidelines have now defined distinct clinical entities. The terms currently used are asymptomatic bacteriuria, acute simple cystitis, acute pyelonephritis /complicated UTI, and recurrent UTI. These definitions are based on urinary culture and clinical symptoms [14].

Testing

Getting an appropriate specimen for culture is critical for the correct diagnosis. If inappropriate technique is used the results may be altered by contamination. Antiseptic wipes should be used to clean the perineum or glans and a midstream urine sample should then be obtained in a sterile container. If a midstream collection cannot be obtained, then a straight catheterization can be attempted. Indwelling catheters should be removed and urine should be collected from a midstream void or by a new urinary catheter [14].

Asymptomatic Bacteriuria

Asymptomatic bacteriuria (ASB) is the presence of 10^5 colony forming units (CFU) without urinary or systemic symptoms. This can be with or without pyuria. Treatment of ASB post-transplant has not clearly been shown to be beneficial. The majority of studies have shown lack of benefit and potential harm in ASB treatment. Studies evaluating the benefit of antimicrobial treatment in kidney transplant patients found no difference in progression to symptomatic UTI or pyelonephritis compared to no treatment. Some studies have indicated that there may be harm in treating ASB as treatment was associated with increased incidence in symptomatic UTI, decreased clearance of pathogens, and increased pathogen resistance. As of yet no study has evaluated ASB treatment before two months post-transplant. Current societal guidelines recommend against treating ASB two months beyond transplant [14, 15].

Simple Cystitis

Simple cystitis is defined as the growth of an uropathogen in urine culture with accompanying lower urinary symptoms (dysuria, frequency, urgency) but without fever, allograft pain, hemodynamic instability, or indwelling device (ureteral stent, nephrostomy tube, chronic urinary catheter). If a urinary catheter is in place, it should be removed or replaced. Empiric treatment in the outpatient setting typically consists of a third-generation cephalosporin, amoxicillin-clavulanate, or a fluoroquinolone. Nitrofurantoin is not recommended if creatinine clearance is <30 ml/min. When susceptibility data is obtained, the narrowest spectrum antibiotic should be used to complete a course. Duration is generally a 5 to 7 day course but can be extended to a 7 to 10 day course if it occurs within the first 6 months after transplant [14].

Complicated UTI

Complicated UTI (pyelonephritis, upper tract UTI) is growth of an uropathogen and at least one of the following; fever, chills, malaise, hemodynamic instability, leukocytosis, bacteremia with same organism, pain over the allograft, or costovertebral angle tenderness. UTIs are also considered complicated if there is a chronic indwelling foley, prostatitis, indwelling ureteric stent, or a percutaneous nephrostomy in place. Blood cultures should be obtained if symptoms of pyelonephritis are present given high rates of bacteremia. Renal ultrasound or non-contrast computerized tomography should be considered to evaluate for possible structural abnormalities such as abscess, strictures or obstruction. Patients with mild cases of pyelonephritis that are clinically stable can be empirically started on ceftriaxone, ampicillin-sulbactam, or ciprofloxacin. In more severe cases or hemodynamic instability piperacillin-tazobactam, cefepime, or a carbapenem should be used. Speciation and susceptibilities from cultures should guide antimicrobial selection. Complicated UTIs should be treated with 14 to 21 days of antimicrobial therapy [14].

Recurrent UTI

Recurrent UTI is defined as greater than or equal to three UTIs in a 12-month span or greater than 2 in a 6-month span. Preventing recurrent UTIs involves a multifaceted approach that includes evaluating underlaying structural abnormalities, lifestyle modifications, and medications. Structural urological malformations, bladder atony, complex renal cysts, vesicoureteral reflux, ureteric stenosis, urinary fistulas, urinary catheters, or ureteric stents can all contribute to recurrent UTIs. Post void residual volume quantification and imaging should be considered to help evaluate for these. Voiding cystourethrograms, urodynamic studies, and cystoscopy may also be helpful. Lifestyle modifications include keeping adequately hydrated, frequent and timed voiding, double voiding, females wiping front to back, and voiding after sexual intercourse. Good glycemic control in diabetic patients is essential. If UTIs can be connected to sexual activity stand by post coital antibiotics can be attempted. Antibiotics for UTI prophylaxis can be considered but must be weighed against potential side effects. Trimethoprim / Sulfamethoxazole (TMP/SMX) given for Pneumocystis pneumonia prophylaxis may also help prevent development of UTIs and bacteremia. If unable to tolerate TMP/SMX, alternative UTI prophylaxis may be considered in high-risk patients for the first month after transplant. Typical agents used are cephalosporins or nitrofurantoin. Fluoroquinolones are generally not recommended because of their side effect profile and studies showing increased resistance. Nitrofurantoin use may be limited as it is not recommended for use in patients with creatinine clearance <30 ml/min [14].

Microbiology

The most common cause of UTI in kidney transplant patients is gram negative bacteria with *Escherichia coli* accounting for roughly 70%. *Pseudomonas aeruginosa,* coagulase-negative Staphylococci, and *Enterobacter cloacae* are frequently found in urine cultures in the first several months after kidney transplantation. Enterococcus species and *Escherichia coli* become more common a few months after transplant. *Staphylococcus epidermidis*, Gardnerella, Candida are unlikely to be invasive pathogens. Candida is frequently an asymptomatic colonizer and generally should not be treated unless symptoms are clearly present. It rarely can lead to ascending infection or obstruction at ureterovesical junction. High rates of clearance of candiduria occur without antimicrobial intervention. There is a higher chance for antibiotic resistance in kidney transplant recipients because of host factors. They are more likely to have numerous previous hospitalizations and antibiotic exposures. There are high rates of extended spectrum beta lactamase (ESBL) producers in this population and the chance of this increases with each subsequent UTI [13, 14, 16].

Cytomegalovirus

Cytomegalovirus (CMV) is a herpesvirus that infects the majority of humans. Primary infection is generally asymptomatic in immunocompetent hosts and occurs during childhood. After primary infection, CMV becomes a lifelong latent infection with little clinical significance in immunocompetent hosts. In transplant recipients, CMV has far greater implications and is associated with high morbidity and mortality. CMV infection is strongly associated with allograft dysfunction and rejection. After immunosuppression, CMV can reactivate from its latent phase if the recipient had been infected at some time prior to transplant. Primary infection can occur if the recipient was not infected with CMV prior to transplant. Primary infection in kidney transplant recipients is associated with high symptom burden and organ dysfunction when compared to immunocompetent patients. One of the most common ways for a primary infection to occur after transplant is via donor transmission. This can occur when the donor has been infected with CMV and the recipient never was [17, 18].

Clinical Entities

CMV infections are described in three separate ways; infection, disease, and asymptomatic. Asymptomatic is when there is CMV replication without signs or symptoms. CMV infection describes presence of CMV replication in blood, tissue or body fluid regardless of symptoms. CMV disease is defined as CMV infection but with clinical signs and symptoms. A subset of CMV disease is CMV syndrome which includes fever, malaise, atypical lymphocytosis, leukopenia /neutropenia, thrombocytopenia, and elevated liver function tests [17, 18].

Risk

The risk for CMV infection /reactivation after transplant is determined by donor and recipient CMV IgG serostatus. The highest risk is when the donor is CMV IgG positive and the recipient is CMV IgG negative. If the recipient is CMV IgG positive, it is considered moderate risk regardless of donor status. The lowest risk is when both the recipient and the donor are both CMV IgG negative. If the CMV IgG testing is borderline or indeterminate, risk determination should error on the side of whatever gives the highest risk [17, 18].

Testing

Laboratory testing for CMV includes viral culture, histopathology, pp65 antigen testing, and molecular assays. The preferred method for detecting CMV is nucleic acid testing (NAT) for DNA. Quantitative testing is preferred over qualitative. While higher viral loads are associated with end organ damage, the kinetics of viral replication is more important than a single viral load number. There can be variation in viral load values between different labs as they can have different gene targets, extraction techniques, and amplicon sizes. This can lead to significantly different values. The testing of whole blood instead of plasma may also result in different values with whole blood values generally higher. End organ disease can occur even with a negative blood polymerase chain reaction (PCR) so histopathology remains gold standard for diagnosing end organ disease. Histopathology can help differentiate between rejection which clinically can appear near identical to CMV disease; immunohistochemical stains for CMV are helpful for this. More recently cellular immunity assays have been used to monitor treatment and risk stratify after transplant. These tests measure CMV specific T-cell quantity and function. Clinically, they have been used to determine if further treatment is needed, whether secondary prophylaxis is needed, or if primary prophylaxis can be stopped. If there is adequate CMV specific T-cells with good function it is theorized the host will be able to control the infection on their own [17, 18].

CMV Prevention

Strategies for preventing CMV vary between centers, but the two major approaches are pre-emptive monitoring and antiviral prophylaxis. Pre-emptive therapy involves monitoring CMV viral loads and starting anti-viral medications when CMV viral load exceeds a certain threshold. In this approach, CMV levels are measured weekly for at least the first three months. There is no agreed upon cut off value at which to start therapy. When therapy is started it should be continued until there are two undetectable CMV viral loads at least a week apart. If pre-emptive therapy is selected, acyclovir should be started to prevent HSV. Prophylactic therapy involves giving an antiviral medication to prevent disease for a period of time. CMV prophylaxis should be started within 10 days of the transplant. Medications generally used are valganciclovir and ganciclovir. Valganciclovir is preferred as it is oral and has good bioavailability. Oral formulation of ganciclovir is not commercially available in the United States and intravenous ganciclovir is used. Letermovir is not currently approved for solid organ transplant recipients but trials are ongoing. Duration for CMV prophylaxis varies but is generally between 3-6 months for kidney transplant recipients. Post prophylaxis delayed-onset CMV disease can occur after completing prophylaxis. This is more common in higher risk patients (CMV IgG donor +/ recipient -) and occurs about 3-6 months after finishing prophylaxis. To monitor for this, CMV PCR surveillance can be done for a period of time (generally 3 months) after finishing prophylaxis. CMV prophylaxis should be restarted if the patient is treated for rejection with lymphodepleting agents. There is no consensus for how long but is generally given for 1-3 months. When comparing pre-emptive against prophylactic therapy some small studies have shown similar efficacy. More recent studies favor pre-emptive monitoring with recipients having lower rates of CMV disease [17, 18].

Treatment

First line therapy for CMV treatment is intravenous ganciclovir or oral valganciclovir. In mild to moderate cases, valganciclovir is preferred. Second line agents include foscarnet and cidofovir but their use is limited by side effects. Letermovir is not approved for treatment. Duration of therapy is individualized and is based on symptom resolution and virologic clearance. Therapy is generally given until viral load is undetectable on two different tests a week apart. Immunoglobulin therapy (CMV specific Ig or IVIG) can be considered in severe disease, CMV pneumonitis, resistant disease, or hypogammaglobulinemia but evidence for its use is limited. Immunosuppression reduction should also be considered. While on treatment, complete blood counts and serum creatinine should be monitored for side effects and need for dose adjustment. Leukopenia is a common side effect of treatment with both ganciclovir and valganciclovir and can be exacerbated when given with other immunosuppression. Foscarnet and cidofovir are associated with significant metabolic and renal toxicity. Recurrence after treatment is common (35%) and many centers give secondary prophylaxis for 1-3 months after finishing treatment. The efficacy of this approach is not proven [17, 18].

Resistant/Refractory Disease

Within two weeks of treatment, there should be at least a one log decrease in viral load. If this decrease does not occur, the concern for refractory or resistant disease should be raised and resistance testing should be sent. Two major resistance mutations that occur are UL97 and UL54. UL97 mutations can confer resistance to ganciclovir. Treatment options include foscarnet, cidofovir, and high dose ganciclovir. UL54 mutations can include resistance to ganciclovir, foscarnet, and cidofovir. Treatment options may be limited in this setting and consideration may have to be given to clinical trial drugs such as maribavir and letermovir. Immunoglobulin therapy and CMV specific T cells can also be considered. Antiviral drug choice should be guided by the results of the genotypic assays showing exact drug resistances [17, 18].

Other Viral Infections and Considerations

BK Polyomavirus

BK Polyomavirus will be addressed elsewhere in this book.

Adenovirus

Adenoviruses are non-enveloped, double stranded DNA viruses. They are classified in seven subgroups (A-G) which can be further divided into over 60 distinct serotypes. They are present throughout the year and cause mostly self-limited disease: conjunctival, respiratory, and gastrointestinal. Infection can be asymptomatic, defined as detection of adenovirus by culture, antigen test or polymerase chain reaction (PCR) in the absence of signs or symptoms. On the contrary, adenovirus disease is defined as virus detection in biopsy specimens (with immunohistochemical stain) or from bronchoalveolar lavage (BAL) or cerebrospinal fluid (CSF) by culture, antigen detection, or PCR in the absence of another diagnosis that explains the symptoms. Disseminated disease is present if two or more organs are involved, not including viremia. Reported adenovirus incidence in adult kidney transplant recipients varies between 4.1-6.5% [19].

One entity that deserves special attention in this population is hemorrhagic cystitis due to adenovirus which can accompany adenovirus nephritis and be confused with renal rejection. Adenovirus nephritis usually presents as persistent fever, hematuria (microscopic or macroscopic) and elevated creatinine. Biopsies can show granulomatous features. Immunohistochemical stains are essential as other viruses, such as CMV or HSV among others, can present similarly. Any organ can be affected, with the most severe presentation being interstitial pneumonia which is associated with a high mortality rate and is usually seen in cases of disseminated disease. Antiviral treatment options are limited with no antiviral agents approved by the Food and Drug Administration (FDA) for the treatment of adenovirus infection. The first step in management consists of reduction of immunosuppression, if possible. There are some proposed treatments with cidofovir but no randomized trials exist; side effects are important and often limit its prolonged use. Ribavirin might have antiviral activity against certain subtypes of group C adenoviridae but available information is limited to case reports.

Kidney Transplantation in the HIV -Positive Recipient

Due to improvements in the survival of individuals infected with the human immunodeficiency virus (HIV), life expectancy of this population approaches that of the general population. However, the number of patients with well controlled HIV yet end-stage-kidney disease is increasing. Potential candidates should undergo routine pre-transplant evaluation as well as an infectious diseases consultation. In addition to center-specific listing criteria, the usual pre-transplant labs, the CD4 count should be >200 cells/mcl and the HIV viral load undetectable for three months prior to transplantation [20]. Evaluation should include a good history, physical, and focus on history of certain opportunistic infections (OIs) that might preclude a transplant as well as to ensure absence of active OIs. There are several treatment considerations in this patient population. Certain antiretrovirals interact with immunosuppressive medications and can make the post-transplant follow up challenging. Ritonavir or cobicistat-boosted regimens are not ideal, and attempts should be made to avoid their use because of interactions. Single tablet regimens are usually not an option as they do not allow for dose adjustment in the setting of underlying altered renal function. There are no standardized immunosuppressive regimens for HIV-positive kidney transplant recipients. It is known that rejection rates are higher than in the HIV-negative recipient. There is a tight balance between over-immunosuppression risking OIs or other infectious complications against under-immunosuppression with the risk of organ rejection. In 2013, the HIV Organ Policy Equity (HOPE) Act was signed into law in the U.S., allowing organs from HIV-positive donors to be transplanted into HIV-positive recipients under the National Institute of Health-stipulated research umbrella [21]. Consequently, there is the opportunity for people with HIV to become organ donors, living or deceased. These organs can only be used for HIV-positive recipients. Additionally, it requires the centers to fulfill certain criteria and submit for research approval. Transplant Infectious Diseases should be involved in donor and recipient evaluation in these scenarios.

Viral Hepatitis

We will focus on hepatitis B and C in the pre-and post-transplant setting. Both of these diseases are included in the donor and candidate screening.

Hepatitis B

The prevalence of chronic hepatitis B in dialysis patients has decreased over the last decades thanks to stricter infection control measures in dialysis centers as well as universal vaccination. Transplant candidates that are not immune should be vaccinated. HBsAg-positive patients have lower survival rates after kidney transplant. This can be mitigated by HBV DNA suppression with antivirals. Recommended regimens for kidney patients are either tenofovir disoproxil fumarate or entecavir. Data on tenofovir alafenamide is lacking. Therapy should be continued indefinitely after transplant as long as the patient remains immunosuppressed. Pre-transplant evaluation by a specialist in the management of HBV is recommended. Surveillance should follow Hepatology guidelines.

Special mention should be made to HBsAg- or anti-HB core-positive donors, especially if the recipient is not immune to hepatitis B. The optimal management of non-liver transplant recipients from a HBsAg-positive donor remains unknown. Combinations that have been used include hepatitis B immunoglobulin (HBIg), antiviral prophylaxis with consideration of HBIg for at least the first 6-12 months if anti-HBs titers are <100 IU/ml, and indefinite antiviral (entecavir or tenofovir disoproxil fumarate). Although there's still a risk of transmission of hepatitis B with a kidney transplant from an anti-HB core-positive donor, it is lower than for liver transplants. Center-specific protocols should be in place for this scenario. Historically, lamivudine has been used in the post-transplant setting but more centers now use entecavir or tenofovir due to the high rates of resistance development to lamivudine [22].

Hepatitis C

Prevalence of hepatitis C (HCV) among patient with end-stage renal disease is higher than the general population with variability between countries, regions, and even dialysis centers. It is important to differentiate between positivity for HCV antibodies and actual viremic patients. A positive HCV Ab in a candidate should be followed by an HCV viral load. A positive HCV RNA confirms active infection. Additional workup includes a genotype and a Hepatology referral to assess the degree of liver damage. The presence of cirrhosis can be a consideration for combined liver-kidney transplantation. Outcomes from HCV positive donors have been historically worse in terms of survival and graft function. That said, UNOS has not collected the viral load status on these patients, and it is not known if these were viremic donors or simply hepatitis C antibody positive donors. The availability of well-tolerated direct-acting antivirals (DAAs) will likely change this scenario. In kidney transplant candidates and recipients, the main hurdle for the use of DAA remains kidney function, although we now have several safe and effective regimens even in the setting of ESRD. Timing of treatment should be carefully selected with the input of an expert in the field considering options, anticipated wait-time on the list, severity of liver disease, drug access and coverage and the potential of utilizing a HCV viremic donor [23]. The utilization of HCV viremic donors has increased over the last years, not only for HCV viremic candidates but also for HCV-negative recipients (HCV mismatch kidney transplantation). This can be offered to selected patients in the setting of a detailed informed consent and under a potential research umbrella. Timing of optimal post-transplant treatment initiation remains unknown but most centers opt for an early initiation.

Epstein-Barr Virus. Post-Transplant Lymphoproliferative Disorder

Epstein-Barr Virus (EBV) is a herpesvirus of the gamma genus that infects the majority of people and persists during the lifetime of its host. Acquisition usually happens in childhood and often goes unnoticed. As such, most kidney transplant recipients have been infected with EBV pre-transplant. Some will experience primary EBV infection after transplant, either as primary infection or DDI, most commonly seen in the case of EBV mismatch. Its spectrum of clinical conditions is broad and is characterized by lymphoproliferation. EBV viremia is usually self-limited. It can be an indicator of over-immunosuppression. Other manifestations include infectious mononucleosis, organ - specific diseases, hemophagocytic lymphohistiocytosis, and macrophage activation syndrome. Fortunately, post-transplant lymphoproliferative disorder (PTLD) remains a rare complications of kidney transplantation. Oncological evaluation is indicated in those cases. Management of PTLD is covered in more detail elsewhere in this book.

Fungal Infections

In addition to endemic fungal infections mentioned also under donor evaluation: histoplasmosis, coccidioidomycosis and blastomycosis, invasive fungal infections with *Candida species* or molds and cryptococcal infection can be seen in kidney transplant recipients.

Candida

Infectious complications after kidney transplantation include candidemia, oropharyngeal or esophageal candidiasis, UTIs and surgical site infections. The latter are described elsewhere in this chapter. Infectious disease consultation is recommended in cases of candidemia as further workup is required. Guidelines for treatment of these infections are available from the American Society of Transplantation [23] and the Infectious Diseases Society of America [16].

Cryptococcosis

Cryptococcosis deserves special mention as it is the third most common cause of invasive fungal infections in solid organ transplant recipients. In kidney transplant recipients it is usually of late onset. It can be caused by *C. neoformans* or *C. gattii*. The single most important part of the patient with suspected or confirmed cryptococcosis is the thorough evaluation of pulmonary and extrapulmonary sites of infection, which includes a lumbar puncture with measurement of an opening pressure and cultures of other sites as indicated [24]. Choice of antifungal treatment will depend on affected sites and severity of infections but should continue for at least a minimum of 6-12 months. Pulmonary disease might be managed with fluconazole while CNS, disseminated disease or moderate-severe disease might need induction therapy with liposomal amphotericin or amphotericin B lipid complex followed by consolidation and maintenance with fluconazole. Serial lumbar punctures might be indicated in patients with meningitis and elevated intracranial pressure. If possible, reduction of the net state of immunosuppression is part of the treatment approach. This should happen in a gradual fashion in order to not compromise the graft function and to avoid an immune reconstitution syndrome (IRIS) which can emerge after treatment initiation. IRIS is due to an overwhelming immune response as the immune system recovers and results in a paradoxical worsening of the previous infectious process, in this case cryptococcosis.

Invasive Aspergillosis (IA)

Aspergillus is most commonly acquired through inhalation and the majority of infections are limited to the lungs. Risk factors for early IA include older age, renal failure, CMV disease, bacterial co-infection and neoplasms. Specific risk factors in kidney transplant recipients include COPD, acute rejection in the last 3 months, graft failure and high and prolonged duration of corticosteroids. Late IA is often related to over-immunosuppression [25]. Pulmonary colonization can be difficult to distinguish from infection. Serum galactomannan (GM) has good specificity but lacks sensitivity in this patient population. A galactomannan in BAL has better sensitivity and is the preferred sampling method for the diagnosis of pulmonary aspergillosis in transplant recipients. Aspergillus PCR can also be used in combination with other diagnostic modalities such as GM and CT chest. Aspergillus PCR will not be able to differentiate colonization from disease. Additionally, it has the possibility of yielding false positive results due to cross-reactivity with other mold species. Prompt treatment is indicated with voriconazole being the drug of choice. Duration of therapy should be guided by clinical response, with 12 weeks of therapy being the minimum recommended duration. The use of azole requires close monitoring of the QTc interval, hepatic function, and calcineurin or mTOR inhibitors. Reduction of immunosuppression is recommended if possible, and adjuvant surgical therapy might be necessary.

Antimicrobial Prophylaxis

In the months after transplant there is increased risk for infection given the high levels of immunosuppression. Antimicrobial prophylaxis is used to prevent common and serious infections in this time period. Recipients get antimicrobials for a predetermined set of time when immunosuppression is thought to be the greatest. For kidney transplant recipients, prophylaxis is most frequently given for CMV, *Pneumocystis jirovecii* pneumonia (PJP), and candida. CMV prophylaxis is further described in the CMV section.

Pneumocystis Pneumonia

Pneumocystis jirovecii is a fungal pathogen that is an important cause of pneumonia in immunocompromised patients. Universal prophylaxis for PJP in kidney transplant recipients is recommend as high rates of infection are seen in the first 6 months after transplant when prophylaxis is not given. It is very rare for PJP to occur when on prophylaxis. Prophylaxis is recommended for the first 6 to 12 months after transplant. First line therapy is TMP/SMX. This is preferred as it has the strongest clinical evidence supporting its use. The side effects of TMP/SMX include hyperkalemia, renal dysfunction, and leukopenia. If the side effects are severe enough, another agent may have to be used. In the setting of hyperkalemia, it is recommended that TMP/SMX use be attempted again once hyperkalemia has resolved. Dapsone is second line therapy for PJP prophylaxis. Before starting dapsone, a Glucose-6-phosphate dehydrogenase (G6PD) must be checked as a G6PD deficiency greatly increases the risk of dapsone-induced hemolytic anemia. Dapsone is not recommend as alternative agent for recipients who have had severe side effects to TMP/SMX such as neutropenia, desquamating rash, nephritis, or hepatitis. Atovaquone is available as another agent for prophylaxis when TMP/SMX and dapsone cannot be used. Inhaled pentamidine can also be used but is associated with increased rates of breakthrough and bronchospasm. Consideration for restarting prophylaxis should occur if the patient is being treated for rejection [26, 27].

Coccidioidomycosis

Coccidioidomycosis is a fungal infection that is endemic in the southwestern US and areas of US bordering Mexico. Incidence has been increasing in the US over the recent years and is thought to be related to climate change. Infections in transplant recipients can be severe with high rates of mortality. Prophylaxis is recommended for recipients who live in endemic regions with fluconazole for a minimum of 6-12 months. For seronegative recipients, fluconazole 200mg daily is adequate; for seropositive recipients, fluconazole

400mg daily is recommended; doses might need adjustment to renal function. For the latter (seropositive recipient) some authors consider lifelong prophylaxis [10, 27]. Any evidence of prior or active infection should be evaluated pre-transplant by an infectious diseases specialist.

Candida

There is no consensus for universal candida prophylaxis after kidney transplant. The American Society of Transplant recommends against prophylaxis unless patients are high risk for infection. In that circumstance, prophylactic fluconazole can be considered. The Kidney Disease Improving Global Outcomes guidelines recommend oral and esophageal Candida prophylaxis for 1 to 3 months after transplant with oral clotrimazole lozenges, nystatin, or fluconazole [10, 27].

Antimicrobial Interactions with Anti-Rejection Medication

Antimicrobials can interact with immunosuppression via a pharmacokinetic or pharmacodynamic effect. Pharmacokinetic involves alerted drug concentrations and interacts with absorption, distribution, metabolism, and elimination. Pharmacodynamic is when drugs increase or decrease the toxicity of each other. Commonly used antimicrobials that may interact with immunosuppression are macrolides, antifungals, antiretroviral agents, and rifamycins. Macrolides are moderate inhibitors of CYP3A4 and decrease the metabolism of calcineurin inhibitors (CNI) and mTOR inhibitors. Concentrations can increase 3 to 10 fold when starting macrolides. The exception to this is azithromycin which has a far less of an interaction effect. If macrolides must be used, daily CNI monitoring and every third day monitoring of mTORs should occur. Azoles decrease the metabolism of CNI and mTORs as well. Ketoconazole has the most potent effect followed by itraconazole and posaconazole. Fluconazole and voriconazole have the least effect and the fluconazole interaction is dose dependent. Voriconazole and Posaconazole are contraindicated with sirolimus as they can rapidly increase sirolimus levels. A variety of HIV antiretrovirals can interact with immunosuppression and HIV expert should be consulted with their use. Rifamycins are strong inducers of CYP3A4 and decrease levels of CNIs and mTORs. They also have some effect on mycophenolate. If they must be used with these drugs, a multidisciplinary approach including pharmacy to manage dosing should occur. This dose may have to be increased until appropriate levels are achieved [28].

Post-Transplant Vaccination

Prevention is an important pillar of the care of kidney transplant recipients. This is not limited to antimicrobial prophylaxis but also includes continuing appropriate vaccinations in the post-transplant setting.

As a general recommendation, live vaccines should not be given after transplant due to the risk of inducing the disease. Inactivated vaccines can be given starting 3-6 months post-transplant with the exception of the inactivated influenza vaccine that can be given as early as one-month post-transplant during flu season [4].

Vaccination should be guided by missed vaccines pre-transplant, available serologies (e.g., hepatitis A or B), routine vaccinations (e.g., Td/TdaP every 10 years, pneumococcal polysaccharide vaccine), age (e.g., recombinant adjuvanted Zoster vaccine, pneumococcal polysaccharide vaccine, human papillomavirus vaccine), comorbidities or special circumstances (e.g., meningococcal vaccination in patients receiving eculizumab, HiB & pneumococcal vaccines in splenectomized patients etc.) and season (influenza).

Dosing of vaccines can be different in the transplant recipient. As such, post-transplant hepatitis B vaccine series should be high-dose (40µg). In certain situations, titers can be monitored to assess vaccine response and the need for revaccination. For post-transplant vaccines where there is no clear data, recommendations are made by national advisory committees. In the U.S., this is the Advisory Committee on Immunization Practices (ACIP), also available on the website of the Centers for Disease Control and Prevention (CDC).

Conclusion

Donor and candidate evaluation includes the assessment of past and active infections, as well as serological testing. Infectious complications in the kidney transplant recipient affect morbidity, mortality and graft function. A good armament exists to prevent some opportunistic infections.

References

[1] Malinis M, Boucher HW. Screening of donor and candidate prior to solid organ transplantation -Guidelines from the American Society of Transplantation Infectious Diseases Community of Practice. *Clin Transplant*. 2019;33(9):e13548.

[2] Kaul DR, Sharma TS. Human T-cell lymphotrophic virus in solid-organ transplant recipients: Guidelines from the American society of transplantation infectious diseases community of practice. *Clin Transplant*. 2019;33(9):e13575.

[3] Subramanian AK, Theodoropoulos NM. Mycobacterium tuberculosis infections in solid organ transplantation: Guidelines from the infectious diseases community of practice of the American Society of Transplantation. *Clin Transplant*. 2019;33(9): e13513.

[4] Danziger-Isakov L, Kumar D. Vaccination of solid organ transplant candidates and recipients: Guidelines from the American society of transplantation infectious diseases community of practice. *Clin Transplant*. 2019;33(9):e13563.

[5] Avery RK, Michaels MG. Strategies for safe living following solid organ transplantation -Guidelines from the American Society of Transplantation Infectious Diseases Community of Practice. *Clin Transplant*. 2019;33(9):e13519.

[6] Wolfe CR, Ison MG. Donor-derived infections: Guidelines from the American Society of Transplantation Infectious Diseases Community of Practice. *Clin Transplant*. 2019;33(9):e13547.

[7] Echenique IA, Ison MG. Update on donor-derived infections in liver transplant ation. *Liver Transplant* 2013;19(6):575-85.

[8] West Nile virus infections in organ transplant recipients --New York and Pennsylvania, August-September, 2005. *Morb Mortal Wkly Rep*. 2005;54(40):1021-3.

[9] Kiberd BA, Forward K. Screening for West Nile virus in organ transplantation: a medical decision analysis. *Am J Transplant*. 2004;4(8):1296-301.

[10] Miller R, Assi M. Endemic fungal infections in solid organ transplant recipients - Guidelines from the American Society of Transplantation Infectious Diseases Community of Practice. *Clin Transplant*. 2019;33(9):e13553.

[11] Abbo LM, Grossi PA. Surgical site infections: Guidelines from the American Society of Transplantation Infectious Diseases Community of Practice. *Clin Transplant*. 2019;33(9):e13589.

[12] Berríos-Torres SI, Umscheid CA, Bratzler DW, Leas B, Stone EC, Kelz RR, et al. Centers for Disease Control and Prevention Guideline for the Prevention of Surgical Site Infection, 2017. *JAMA surgery*. 2017;152(8):784-91.

[13] Vidal E, Torre-Cisneros J, Blanes M, Montejo M, Cervera C, Aguado JM, et al. Bacterial urinary tract infection after solid organ transplantation in the RESITRA cohort. *Transpl Infect Dis*. 2012;14(6):595-603.

[14] Goldman JD, Julian K. Urinary tract infections in solid organ transplant recipients: Guidelines from the American Society of Transplantation Infectious Diseases Community of Practice. *Clin Transplant*. 2019;33(9):e13507.

[15] Arencibia N, Agüera ML, Rodelo C, López I, Sánchez-Agesta M, Hurtarte A, et al. Short-Term Outcome of Untreated Versus Treated Asymptomatic Bacteriuria in Renal Transplant Patients. *Transplant Proc*. 2016;48(9):2941-3.

[16] Pappas PG, Kauffman CA, Andes DR, Clancy CJ, Marr KA, Ostrosky-Zeichner L, et al. Clinical Practice Guideline for the Management of Candidiasis: 2016 Update by the Infectious Diseases Society of America. *Clin Infect Dis*. 2016;62(4):e1-50.

[17] Razonable RR, Humar A. Cytomegalovirus in solid organ transplant recipients - Guidelines of the American Society of Transplantation Infectious Diseases Community of Practice. *Clin Transplant*. 2019;33(9):e13512.

[18] Kotton CN, Kumar D, Caliendo AM, Huprikar S, Chou S, Danziger-Isakov L, et al. The Third International Consensus Guidelines on the Management of Cytomegalovirus in Solid-organ Transplantation. *Transplantation*. 2018;102(6): 900-31.

[19] Florescu DF, Schaenman JM. Adenovirus in solid organ transplant recipients: Guidelines from the American Society of Transplantation Infectious Diseases Community of Practice. *Clin Transplant*. 2019;33(9):e13527.

[20] Blumberg EA, Rogers CC. Solid organ transplantation in the HIV -infected patient: Guidelines from the American Society of Transplantation Infectious Diseases Community of Practice. *Clin Transplant*. 2019;33(9):e13499.

[21] HRS Administration. *Final Human Immunodeficiency Virus Organ Policy Equity (HOPE) Act safeguards and research criteria for transplantation of organs infected with HIV Fed Regis* 2015; 34912–349212015 [Available from: https://www.federalregister.gov/documents/2015/06/18/2015-15034/human -immunodeficiency -virus-hiv-organ -policy -equity -hope-act-safeguardsand-research-criteria-for.

[22] Te H, Doucette K. Viral hepatitis: Guidelines by the American Society of Transplantation Infectious Disease Community of Practice. *Clin Transplant*. 2019;33(9):e13514.

[23] Aslam S, Rotstein C. Candida infections in solid organ transplantation: Guidelines from the American Society of Transplantation Infectious Diseases Community of Practice. *Clin Transplant*. 2019;33(9):e13623.

[24] Baddley JW, Forrest GN. Cryptococcosis in solid organ transplantation -Guidelines from the American Society of Transplantation Infectious Diseases Community of Practice. *Clin Transplant*. 2019;33(9):e13543.

[25] Husain S, Camargo JF. Invasive Aspergillosis in solid-organ transplant recipients: Guidelines from the American Society of Transplantation Infectious Diseases Community of Practice. *Clin Transplant*. 2019;33(9):e13544.

[26] Fishman JA, Gans H. *Pneumocystis jiroveci* in solid organ transplantation: Guidelines from the American Society of Transplantation Infectious Diseases Community of Practice. *Clin Transplant*. 2019;33(9):e13587.

[27] KDIGO clinical practice guideline for the care of kidney transplant recipients. *Am J Transplant*. 2009;9 Suppl 3:S1-155.

[28] Sparkes T, Lemonovich TL. Interactions between anti-infective agents and immunosuppressants-Guidelines from the American Society of Transplantation Infectious Diseases Community of Practice. *Clin Transplant*. 2019;33(9):e13510.

In: Issues in Kidney Disease – Transplantation
Editors: B. V. R. Murthy and S. Z. Fadem
ISBN: 978-1-53619-960-4

Chapter 10

Malignancies after Transplantation

Stephen Blake Tanner, MD and Mohanram Narayanan*, MD
Division of Nephrology and Hypertension, Department of Medicine,
Texas A&M Health Science Center College of Medicine,
Baylor Scott & White Medical Center, Temple, TX, US

Abstract

Transplant recipients in general are at higher risk of developing malignancy which comprises an increasingly common cause of morbidity and mortality in this population. Familiarity with the common types of cancer and their management is essential for the nephrology practitioner. In this chapter, various cancers frequently seen in transplant recipients are discussed with particular attention dedicated to the rate of occurrence, risk factors, screening recommendations, and management decisions.

Keywords: malignancy, transplantation, immunosuppression

Introduction

Kidney transplant recipients (KTRs) are at a significantly higher risk of multiple different forms of cancer compared with the general population. KTRs have a 2-4-fold increased risk of cancer and cancer-related death compared to gender and age -matched counterparts in the general population [1]. Along with heart disease and infection, cancer is one of the leading causes of death in KTRs [2]. Posttransplant malignancies account for up to 47% of deaths in organ transplant recipients with progressive increase in mortality as

* Corresponding Author's Email: Mohanram.Narayanan@BSWHealth.org.

graft survival increases [3]. Aside from Non-Hodgkin's Lymphoma (NHL) no cancers have shown decline in the relative risk of death over the last 30 years despite significant advances in oncologic therapies [2].

Risk Factors

Multiple factors are at play when determining cancer risk in organ transplant recipients. Differences in cancer risk depend on the type of cancer. Compared with the general population, non-melanoma skin cancer, particularly cutaneous squamous cell carcinoma, and cancers associated with oncogenic viruses demonstrate the highest relative risk. Most registries show no particular increase in breast or prostate cancer [1]. The underlying cause of end stage renal disease (ESRD) affects the risk of malignancy. In the general population, diabetes mellitus is associated with an increased risk of liver, pancreas, breast, and colorectal cancer (4) though risk of malignancies is lower in transplant patients with ESRD due to diabetes mellitus compared with other causes [5]. While a decrease in malignancy is observed in patients with polycystic kidney disease after kidney transplant, likely owing to more frequent native nephrectomies [6], acquired cystic kidney disease is associated with a significant increase in renal cell carcinoma [7]. Other factors that increase risk of malignancy after transplant include age greater than 50 years, male sex, smoking, longer dialysis vintage (>54 months vs <18 months) and increasing number of HLA -DR mismatches [1]. The increase in cancer risk after transplantation is often attributed, at least in part, to immunosuppression with associated reduction in immunosurveillance or increased susceptibility to DNA damage. This risk is not uniform and different immunosuppressive agents present different risks [1]. Induction therapies have been linked to increased risk of malignancy. Muromonab-CD3, while no longer used, has been associated with increased risk of multiple malignancies including NHL, particularly when used to treat acute rejection [8, 9]. Alemtuzumab (anti CD52) and anti-thymocyte globulin (ATG) have variable associations with cancer. In an evaluation of registry data with 111, 857 kidney transplant recipients (1987-2009), ATG was associated with an increased risk of melanoma in non-Hispanic whites but was not associated with development of other malignancies. In the same study, alemtuzumab was associated with increased risk of NHL, colorectal, and thyroid cancer [8, 10]. Basiliximab and daclizumab (IL-2 receptor antagonists) are not associated with increased risk of cancer [8, 10]. Chronic immunosuppressive regimens are also implicated in increased cancer risk. In general, calcineurin inhibitors (CNIs), inhibit production of IL-2 and downstream T-cell activation. This results in impaired immunosurveillance. In addition, CNIs also upregulate vascular endothelial growth factor (VEGF) and tumor growth factor beta (TGF -β) which promote tumor growth. Azathioprine inhibits DNA replication, T-cell proliferation and limits DNA repair mechanisms leading to increased risk of cutaneous squamous cell cancer specifically

[11]. Mycophenolate mofetil (MMF), an inhibitor of inosine monophosphate dehydrogenase leading to reduced lymphocyte proliferation, has not been consistently shown to increase risk of malignancy generally [11, 12]. Belatacept, an inhibitor of the CD28-B7 costimulatory pathway, increases risk of posttransplant lymphoproliferative disorder (PTLD), particularly in the central nervous system [11, 13]. There is no clear data on the oncogenic potential of corticosteroids [11]. Common cancers occurring after transplantation will be addressed individually throughout the rest of this chapter.

Table 1. Risk factors for posttransplant malignancy

Cause of ESRD
Older age
Male gender
Tobacco use
Longer dialysis vintage
Increased HLA- DR mismatches
Immunosuppression

Skin Cancer

Skin cancers account for the majority of post-transplant ation malignancies and tend to be more aggressive in the transplant recipient population [14]. Based on registry data of more than 100,000 patients, both melanoma with standardized incidence ratio (SIR) of 2.38 (95% CI, 2.14-2.63) and non-melanoma skin cancer (SIR of 13.85, 95% CI 11.92-16.00) are more common in transplant recipients [15]. In a review of ten clinical practice guidelines for skin cancer screening, nine recommended annual skin examination. Four of the guidelines recommended primary care provider screening while the other 5 recommended specialist screening. Patients with increased risk due to skin type, sun exposure history, or other risk factors may require more frequent screening [16].

Squamous Cell Carcinoma

Squamous cell carcinoma (SCC) is the most common malignancy among solid organ transplant (SOT) recipients. Typical presentation includes nodules with ulceration or bleeding in sun-exposed areas [17]. The histology is more commonly poorly differentiated with behavior more aggressive than in the general population [15].

Risk Factors

Risk factors for development of SCC include sun exposure, male sex, older age, smoking, history of sunburns, increased age at transplantation, intensity and duration of immunosuppression. In 20% of SCC occurring in SOT recipients, there is a spindle cell component which indicates epithelial–to–mesenchymal transformation which is believed to be due to immunosuppression. Furthermore, patients with heart or lung transplants, who require higher levels of immunosuppression, have a higher incidence of SCC compared to those with renal or hepatic allografts [17]. In addition, the choice of immunosuppressive agents can affect risk of SCC. Cyclosporine-A (CsA) has been shown to induce resistance to human keratinocyte apoptosis and inhibit DNA repair following exposure to UV associated damage. CsA has also been shown to stimulate epithelial-to-mesenchymal transformation and tumor progression via induction of TGF -β [18]. The observed incidence of SCC with use of belatacept is similar to that of CsA [14, 19]. Azathioprine induces sensitization to UV-A radiation and increases frequency of mutations in the gene encoding p53 leading to promotion of carcinogenesis [14, 20]. Tacrolimus is not known to induce resistance to apoptosis and demonstrates a reduced risk of skin cancer compared to CsA [14]. Mycophenolate mofetil is associated with a reduced incidence of SCC compared to those taking Azathioprine [14]. Mammalian target of rapamycin (mTOR) inhibitors are associated with decreased risk of non-melanoma skin cancers compared to calcineurin inhibitors. In a meta-analysis of 21 randomized trials including 5876 kidney transplant patients, use of sirolimus was associated with a 56% reduction in the risk of non-melanoma skin cancer compared with controls. Despite the reduction in malignancy, mortality was increased with sirolimus use compared to controls (HR 1.43, 95% CI 1.21-1.71). Cardiovascular and infectious complications were the primary causes of mortality [21]. Other medications used for management of coexisting chronic disease may also increase risk of SCC. For instance, a recent single center cohort study of 2496 kidney (n = 2155), pancreas (n = 59) or combined kidney-pancreas (n = 282) transplant recipients, exposure to hydrochlorothiazide was associated with a statistically significant increased risk of SCC (HR 2.04; 95% CI 1.27-3.28) [20]. The exact mechanism for increased SCC risk is not clear but may be related to a photosensitizing effect of hydrochlorothiazide [22].

Management

Management of cutaneous SCC is determined by risk of metastasis. High risk features are size (>2 cm), multiple lesions, high risk locations (ear, scalp, temple), recurrent lesions, poorly differentiated with perineural or deep invasion [23]. Low risk and localized cancers can be treated with local cryotherapy, topical chemotherapy, photodynamic therapy or excision under the guidance of a dermatologist [14]. With high risk features, aggressive surgical therapy is the mainstay of treatment for amenable cases; however, radiation therapy, particularly if there is perineural disease, and chemotherapy can be considered [14, 23]. Alteration in immunosuppression to reduce risk of recurrent or new cancers must be balanced with the risk of graft loss. In general, as morbidity and mortality from skin malignancy increases, the risk of graft loss from reduced immunosuppression becomes more acceptable. Mild reduction in immunosuppression can be considered if multiple skin cancers develop or if individual skin cancers are high risk. Moderate reductions in immunosuppression are appropriate if more than 25 skin cancers develop per year or if 3-year mortality risk is >10%. If skin cancer is life-threatening, severe reductions in immunosuppression may be required. Options for reduction of immunosuppression include dose reduction, elimination of one drug from a multidrug regimen or change from one class of drug to another [24].

Basal Cell Carcinoma

SOT recipients are at 10-fold greater risk of basal cell carcinoma (BCC) compared with the general population, but BCC is approximately 10-fold less common than SCC in SOT recipients [14]. BCC in SOT recipients tend to be the superficial histologic subtype and occur in younger patients. Lesions are typically found in sun-exposed areas with variable description including pink, scaly, or scar-like plaques, or pearly, translucent nodules [25].

Risk Factors

Innate risk factors include fair skin and light color eyes and hair. The strongest environmental risk factor is UV radiation exposure. Other risk factors include childhood sun burns, intense intermittent sun exposure, tanning bed use, arsenic exposure, family history of skin cancer, and immunosuppression. Constitutive activation of the Hedgehog signaling pathway leads to development of BCC [25].

Management

BCC management in SOT recipients is similar to that in the general population. Most cases can be managed with local surgical or topical therapies. In rare cases, locally advanced or metastatic disease may require systemic therapy. In 2012, FDA approval was granted for vismodegib, a hedgehog pathway inhibitor, for treatment of locally advanced and metastatic BCC [14, 25]. Data from Hedgehog pathway inhibitor use in SOT recipients is sparse, but they have been used in a heart transplant recipient without allograft failure [26].

Kaposi Sarcoma

Kaposi Sarcoma (KS) is a tumor of endothelial cell origin associated with human herpes virus 8 (HHV 8), that usually involves skin or mucosa and is typically composed of papules and nodules with color variation that includes purple, red, blue, brown and black [27].

Risk Factors

Based on registry data of more than 100,000 patients, Kaposi Sarcoma (KS) is more common in transplant recipients with SIR of 61.46 (95% CI, 50.95-73.49) [15]. In patients seropositive for HHV 8 prior to transplant, the risk of developing KS is 23% following transplantation compared to 0.7% for those who are seronegative prior to transplantation [14, 28]. Visceral involvement is reported as high as 25% in renal transplant patients who develop KS after transplantation [14].

Management

The initial step in management of KS in SOT recipients is reducing immunosuppression and/or substituting Sirolimus for CNIs. If there is inadequate response to revision of the immunosuppression regimen, patients can be managed similar to classic KS with local surgical or topical therapies applied to focal disease. For extensive or progressive mucocutaneous disease or visceral disease, commonly prescribed chemotherapeutic regimens include doxorubicin, vinblastine, paclitaxel, and etoposide [14].

Merkel Cell Carcinoma

Merkel cell carcinoma (MCC) is a tumor of neuroendocrine origin and is associated with Merkel cell polyoma virus which is detected in over 80% of MCC [10]. MCC typically presents with firm, red, rapidly expanding nodules in sun exposed areas; however, a minority of cases may present as a tumor positive lymph node without a discernible cutaneous manifestation. Biopsy is necessary to confirm the diagnosis [29].

Risk Factors

In a registry study that included 189,498 SOT recipients, the risk of MCC in transplant population was 24-fold greater than that of the general population [30]. General risk factors include advancing age (greater than 65 years) and sun exposure [29]. Risk factors among transplant recipients included older age at transplant (older than 50 years), increasing transplant vintage, and use of cyclosporine, azathioprine, or mTOR inhibitors. The combination of Cyclosporine and azathioprine was associated with highest risk among combination therapies while tacrolimus and MMF use was associated with decreased risk [30].

Management

Current management is informed by staging and treatment guidelines in the general population. PET -CT can be used for staging and detecting distant metastases. Although efficacy is not firmly established, sentinel lymph node biopsy is a consideration for patients with clinically negative lymph nodes [14]. The primary therapy for MCC is wide local excision. Radiation therapy can be considered as either adjuvant or as palliative treatment if cases are inoperable. With advanced MCC, cytotoxic therapies are commonly used, and the most common regimens involve either platinum -based regimens or combination of cyclophosphamide, doxorubicin, and vincristine. MCC is typically responsive to initial cytotoxic therapy, but the response is not durable with tumor recurrence typically occurring in less than 15 months. Immunotherapy is emerging as a treatment modality but use in transplant patients is likely to increase risk of graft loss [29].

Malignant Melanoma

Malignant melanoma (MM) is a neoplasm that develops from melanocytes found in the basal layer of the epidermis. MM is usually identified by clinician assessment of skin lesions that follow the ABCDE rule for asymmetry, irregular border, color variation, diameter > 6mm, and elevated surface and diagnosis is determined by biopsy [31]. Based on registry data of more than 100,000 patients, MM is more common in transplant recipients with standardized incidence ratio (SIR) of 2.38 (95% CI, 2.14-2.63) [15].

Risk Factors

Risk factors for MM in the SOT recipient population include history of pretransplant MM, white race, age greater than 50 years, UV radiation exposure [32, 33]. There are several pathogenic mutations identified. Activating mutations in the proto-oncogene BRAF (Rapidly Activating Fibrosarcoma oncogene coding for serine -threonine protein kinase B) is present in the majority of MM cases. BRAF mutations result in uncontrolled cell growth and proliferation. NRAS (Neuroblastoma RAS viral oncogene homolog) is an oncogene which exhibits mutations in approximately 20% of metastatic melanomas and may allow for initiation or propagation of MM. The oncogene cyclin-dependent kinase 4 (CDK4), which promotes G1 to S phase progression, has been implicated in MM with familial predisposition. Cyclin-dependent kinase inhibitor 2A (CDKN2A), a tumor suppressor gene which encodes p16INK4a, responsible for halting G1 to S progression, is shown to have an inactivating mutation in some cases of familial melanoma. The melanocortin 1 receptor (MC1R) acts as a G-protein coupled receptor that plays a role in determining pigmentation and protection against UV radiation. In those with MC1R variants, there is decreased melanin and increased susceptibility to UV damage [14, 31].

Management

Management of MM in SOT recipients is similar to management in immunocompetent patients. Primary treatment is surgical and should follow established guidelines for margins. Systemic therapies that target some of the molecular pathways noted above are in use in the general population and, in limited cases, within the SOT recipient population [14]. For example, a heart transplant patient with MM and BRAF mutation was treated with BRAF inhibitor dabrafenib. She was maintained on cyclosporine during this time with no apparent graft complications. She remained without disease recurrence for 15 months [34]. Decisions regarding adjustment of immunosuppression should be individualized based on the severity of melanoma [14]. In a large study evaluating United States registry data, mortality from malignant melanoma was demonstrated to be higher in SOT recipients compared to nonrecipients (HR 2.98, 95% CI 2.26-3.93) [32].

Renal Cell Carcinoma

Renal Cell Carcinoma (RCC) accounts for approximately 85% of all kidney cancers and approximately 5% of all malignancies occurring after renal transplant. More than 90% of RCCs are found in native kidneys [35, 36]. RCC is diagnosed at earlier stages in the transplant population compared with the general population. Earlier diagnosis is likely due to more frequent exposure to abdominal imaging [37].

Risk Factors

Risk factors for RCC in the ESRD population include male sex and African American ancestry; however, tobacco use is not associated with increased RCC risk in the ESRD population. Additional risk factors for RCC among ESRD patients include acquired cystic kidney disease (ACKD), ESRD due to tuberous sclerosis, focal segmental glomerulosclerosis, or urinary obstruction [38]. Risk factors for developing RCC post-transplant ation include male sex, age greater than 60 years, and greater than 3 years on dialysis [39]. African descent is associated with increased risk of developing RCC, but whether the APOL1 risk alleles contribute to this association is unknown [40]. Transplant patients with glomerulonephritis, hypertensive nephrosclerosis, or vascular disease as a cause of ESRD have an increased risk of RCC compared to other etiologies. On the other hand, patients with ESRD due to ADPKD or diabetes mellitus have a lower risk of RCC. A biphasic pattern of RCC risk occurs post-transplantation. Risk of RCC is high in the immediate post-transplantation period and declines for the next 2 to 3 years. This decline is followed by a steady increase in risk for the next 15 years [39]. Impaired DNA repair mechanisms and accumulation of toxic, carcinogenic substances have been implicated as the cause of increased cancer risk in ESRD patients [35]. Finally, BK virus has been implicated in the development of RCC in renal allografts, though the exact role the virus plays in its genesis is yet to be elucidated [41].

Screening

The European Association of Urologists (EAU) recommends annual screening of native and allograft kidneys for RCC in specific high-risk scenarios. The American Society of Transplantation (AST) and Kidney Disease Improving Global Outcomes (KDIGO) do not recommend routine surveillance imaging after renal transplantation [42]. More study is needed to reach a consensus.

Management

Management of post-transplant ation RCC depends on the stage and location of the mass. Radical nephrectomy is the standard of care for RCC in the native kidney [35]. Management of RCC in the transplant kidney is akin to management of RCC in a patient with a single native kidney with prioritization of nephron sparing strategies [43]. T-cell depleting agents have been associated with an increased risk of malignancy including malignancy of the genitourinary tract [44]; however, a recent study with greater than 100,000 patients found no association between any induction agent and development of RCC [8]. Mammalian Target of Rapamycin (mTOR) inhibitors have been hypothesized to reduce the risk of malignancy after transplantation by attenuating expression of carcinogenic cytokines and chemokines [35]. A recent meta-analysis reviewed 11 RCTs and included over 1600 patients. This study found no difference in cancer diagnoses in patients treated with everolimus compared with patients treated with CNIs [45]. Management of immunosuppression in the setting of RCC remains unclear.

Urothelial Carcinoma and Bladder Cancer

Bladder cancer arises from the epithelium covering the inner surface of the bladder, and urothelial carcinomas represent the most common type of bladder cancer [46]. Gross or microscopic hematuria are typical findings that lead to imaging and cystoscopy for diagnosis [47].

Risk Factors

A recent meta-analysis found a significantly increased risk of bladder cancer among KTRs compared with the general population with a standardized incidence ratio (SIR) of 3.18 (95% CI: 1.34–7.53, $P = 0.008$). Asian transplant recipients, primarily those of Chinese descent, had an even greater risk with SIR of 14.74 (95% CI: 3.66–59.35, $P < 0.001$) while those of European descent had a more modest elevation in risk with SIR 2.00 (95% CI: 1.51–2.65, $P = 0.001$). The increased risk among those of Chinese descent may be attributable to genetic or environmental factors such as exposure to aristolochic acid in Chinese herbs [48]. The exact cause of increased bladder cancer is not known. Implicated risk factors include direct cellular damage and impaired DNA repair mechanisms in the setting of long-term immunosuppression. Viral and environmental factors have also been suggested [48]. Multivariate analysis in a group of KTRs determined that the presence of polyoma virus infection and history of smoking were significant risk factors for development of bladder cancer with risk ratios (RR) of 11.6 and 6.1, respectively. Proposed oncogenic mechanisms include inhibition of tumor suppressors p53 and pRB likely in concert with environmental carcinogenic events such as smoking and ongoing immunosuppression [49].

Screening

There are no standard screening recommendations [16].

Management

In general, treatment of urothelial carcinoma is guided by tumor stage with superficial bladder cancer treated with transurethral resection and consideration of local instillation of mitomycin or Bacillus Calmette-Guerin (BCG). Muscle invasive disease is treated with radical cystectomy and neoadjuvant chemotherapy [35]. In a case series of 17 KTRs with bladder cancer diagnosed after renal transplant, standard therapy was followed, and immunosuppression regimens were not altered. BCG was given to 4 patients. None of these patients had direct adverse events related to BCG; however, 3 of the 4 developed recurrence including development of upper tract urothelial carcinoma in one case which may indicate reduced efficacy in immunosuppressed population [50]. There are no guidelines to direct management of immunosuppression in the setting of urothelial cancer and continuation of the regimen may be appropriate in localized disease [35].

Gynecologic Cancers

Gynecologic cancers can be divided into those that are primarily hormone related, uterine and ovarian cancer s, and those associated with human papilloma virus (HPV), namely cervical, vulvar and vaginal cancers. The virally mediated cancers are more common among SOT recipients [51]. A recent US study of greater than 185,000 SOT recipients, of which 64% were kidney recipients, demonstrated no increased risk of invasive cervical cancer s, but did show increased incidence of in situ cancer of the cervix (SIR 3.3, 95% CI 2.6-4.2). This study also showed increased risk of in situ vaginal cancer (SIR 10.6, 95% CI 7.4-14.8) and invasive vulvar cancer (SIR 7.3, 95% CI 5.6-9.2) [52]. Multiple analyses of uterine cancer in SOT recipients demonstrate an SIR of 0.9 to 2.1;

however, no recent large studies have demonstrated statistical significance. Most studies show no statistically significant increase in risk for ovarian cancer in SOT recipients [51].

Risk Factors

Persistent infection with oncogenic Human Papilloma Virus (HPV) is associated with development of cervical cancer. There are 12 oncogenic HPV types, but types 16 and 18 account for 70% of all cervical cancers [53]. Worldwide, HPV is associated with 78% of vaginal cancers and 25% of vulvar cancers with HPV types 16 and 18 accounting for most virus mediated cases [54]. Oncogenicity of the higher risk HPV types is related to expression of viral oncogenes and high-risk types are associated with increased expression of early E genes (E6 and E7) [51, 53]. E6 and E7 genes increase virion production and genome amplification in the epithelial cell layers. These effects are more pronounced in the high-risk HPV types and limited in the low-risk HPV types [53]. In addition to infection with high-risk HPV types, risk factors for malignancy of the cervix, vagina, and vulva include multiple sexual partners, tobacco use, presence of other sexually transmitted infections, and immune deficiency. There is minimal data regarding the impact of specific immunosuppressive medications on gynecologic cancers. Decisions regarding alteration of immunosuppression in the setting of gynecologic malignancy should be individualized [51].

Screening

A review of cervical cancer screening guidelines revealed variable recommendations. KDIGO and Renal Association Clinical Practice guidelines are consistent with guidelines for the general population with recommendation for cytology with pelvic examination every 3 years. More frequent screening, with annual cytology and pelvic examination, is recommended by the American Society of Transplantation, Canadian, Australian, and European guidelines [16].

A panel of healthcare professionals involved in cancer research assembled and published the following screening guidelines for SOT recipients in 2019 [55].

Cytology is recommended for patients <30 years

Cytology + HPV testing is preferred for patients ≥ 30 years

Cytology Alone – annual testing

If 3 consecutive cytology tests are normal, continue with cytology every 3 years

Cytology + HPV testing

Perform baseline co-testing. If initial test is normal, repeat co-testing every 3 years

If transplanted prior to age 21 years, start screening within 1-year of sexual debut.

Continue screening throughout lifetime. Discontinue screening based on shared decision making considering expected life span and quality of life .

Pelvic examination is performed with cytology and HPV testing to screen for vulvar and vaginal cancer. No effective screening modalities have been established for ovarian or uterine malignancy. Those with known or suspected genetic syndromes such as BRCA 1 or BRCA 2, Lynch Syndrome or other syndromes should be referred to a medical geneticist for evaluation [51].

Management

Cancer of the cervix, uterus, vagina or vulva are diagnosed by biopsy and staged per International Federation of Gynecology and Obstetrics guidelines. Ovarian cancer is identified by imaging studies and is associated with elevated CA-125 levels. Surgery, chemotherapy and radiation therapy are considerations for gynecologic cancer in consultation with specialists in those fields [51].

Breast Cancer

Among women in the general population in developed countries, breast cancer is the most common solid organ malignancy [56]. Overall risk of developing breast cancer is not significantly altered by organ transplantation or immunosuppression [10, 15]; however, a large population cohort study did show an increased risk of breast cancer at younger ages and in males [5]. While the risk of developing breast cancer may not be increased, SOT recipients are more likely to present with more advanced disease and have reduced survival [10, 37].

Risk Factors

Traditional risk factors for breast cancer include early menopause or late menarche, nulliparity, obesity, prolonged or increased estrogen exposure, smoking and alcohol use [56].

Screening

The majority of guidelines advocate that breast cancer screening for transplant recipients follow general population screening guidelines. Most recommend mammography for women aged 50 to 69 years of age who are at average cancer risk at annual or biennial screening intervals [16, 57]. Guidelines suggest that women aged 40 to 49 years of age could undergo screening but there is insufficient evidence to recommend for or against this practice in the renal transplant population [57].

Management

There is minimal data on management of breast cancer in SOT recipients. Management is similar to that of the general population. Surgical and radiation therapy approaches are similar. Hormonal therapy, while data are limited, is likely to be safe in appropriate cases. For more advanced cases, immunotherapy is under investigation. Most trials of immune checkpoint inhibitors in breast cancer have excluded transplant patients, but increased T-cell activation with these drugs would be expected to cause cellular rejection in the allograft [56, 58]. If immune checkpoint inhibitors are deemed necessary, risk of graft loss should be conveyed and weighed against the burden of malignancy.

Colorectal Cancer

Colorectal Cancer (CRC) is the third most common cancer in the United States and accounts for just under 10% of worldwide cancer cases in the general population. There is significant variability in the incidence of CRC in SOT recipients [59]. While the incidence is variable, the prognosis is worse for SOT recipients. Transplant registry 5-year survival for SOT recipients is approximately half that of the general population, 30.7% and 63.5%, respectively [60]. This decreased survival has been demonstrated across all stages of CRC [61]. Decreased survival may also be due to the increased risk of infection, cardiovascular disease, and kidney disease among SOT recipients [59].

CRC develops and progresses in a stepwise fashion. There are four pathways with identified mutations leading to development of CRC in the general population: chromosomal instability pathway involving the adenomatous polyposis coli gene (APC), mutations in DNA mismatch repair genes MLH1 and MLH2, protooncogene pathway with mutations of RAS, and upregulation of PI3K. The development of colorectal adenocarcinoma in SOT recipients is thought to occur through similar pathways as no others have been discovered [59].

Risk Factors

Traditional risk factors for colon cancer include family history of CRC, polyps >1 cm or with villous and tubulovillous histology or high-grade dysplasia, CRC syndromes such as familial adenomatous polyposis (FAP), hereditary nonpolyposis colorectal cancer (HNPCC) and other hereditary syndromes, inflammatory bowel disease, primary sclerosing cholangitis, African-American race obesity, diabetes mellitus, smoking, alcohol use, and consumption of processed meats [59]. In addition to traditional risk factors, the immunosuppression regimen may affect risk of CRC development and progression. CNIs, particularly cyclosporine, increase tumor cell proliferation in animal models through a direct cellular effect linked to stimulation of TGF -β production [62, 63]. MMF has been shown to reduce gastrointestinal cancer cell adhesion [64] and may lead to a lower risk of colorectal cancer in transplant recipients [65]. It is postulated that stimulation of mTOR complex 1 (mTORC1) pathway stimulates polyp formation [66] and there is evidence that mTOR inhibition can prevent polyp formation and expansion in mouse models [67]. More recent data focused on colorectal cancer showed a trend toward reduced incidence with sirolimus use, but the results were not statistically significant [68].

Screening

Standard screening guidelines are recommended for SOT recipients without increased risk and screening intervals are determined by presence of traditional risk factors [16].

Management

The chemotherapeutic and surgical management of transplant recipients is similar to that of the general population. There are no major drug interactions between the standard chemotherapy agents, 5-fluorouracil, oxaliplatin, leucovorin, and standard immune-suppression regimens [59].

Post-Transplant Lymphoproliferative Disorder

Post-transplant lymphoproliferative disorders (PTLDs) manifest as abnormal lymphoid lineage proliferation in the context of immunosuppression after SOT, of which the most common is NHL [69]. Clinical presentation is variable and may include constitutional symptoms and symptoms related to the affected organs. Anemia, thrombocytopenia, and leukopenia are typical abnormalities along with elevated lactate dehydrogenase (LDH), hypercalcemia, and hyperuricemia in some cases [10]. The incidence of PTLD is bimodal with a peak incidence within the first 1-2 years (early PTLD) and another peak at 10 years after transplantation [10, 69].

Risk Factors

A strong risk factor for PTLD is activation of oncogenic Epstein-Barr virus (EBV). The highest risk situation involves an EBV seropositive donor with an EBV seronegative recipient [69]. EBV invades oropharyngeal or nasopharyngeal mucosal tissue where it causes a lytic infection of naïve B cells in lymphoid tissue. It then switches to a latent replication cycle and persists through avoidance of immune surveillance by hindering expression of all its latency proteins. In the setting of immunosuppression, lytic reactivation and infection of nearby B cells results in activation of signaling cascades leading to lymphoproliferation and progression from early lesions to polymorphic to monomorphic PTLD [70]. Additional risk factors for PTLD include increased potency and duration of immunosuppression, extremes of age, Caucasian race, and increased number of HLA mismatches [69]. Early PTLD is commonly EBV positive whereas later onset PTLD has a higher proportion of EBV negative cases [10].

The immunosuppressive regimen can contribute to PTLD risk. Unlike skin malignancies, use of mTOR inhibitors is associated with increased risk of PTLD [71]. Belatacept, an inhibitor of the CD28-B7 costimulatory pathway, increases risk of PTLD, particularly in the central nervous system and is contraindicated for use in EBV seronegative SOT recipients [10, 69].

Screening

A complete history and physical exam every 3 months, particularly in the first year after transplant and annually thereafter is the recommended screening for lymphoma. Patients at increased risk may benefit from more frequent screening [16]. There are several different recommendations that suggest monitoring of EBV-PCR in the posttransplant period. Most recommend more frequent monitoring over the first year and in those at increased risk (EBV seronegative recipients) though many centers have individual protocols [72]. No strong data support EBV surveillance after SOT [70].

Management

Tissue diagnosis is preferred and allows for classification by the WHO classification of hematological malignancies [69]. Computed tomography (CT) and positron emission tomography (PET) scans are the preferred imaging modalities for initial staging [69]. The various treatment options are shown in table 2. Initial management involves reduction in immunosuppression with additional management depending on the clinical circumstances [73]. Current treatment strategies are based on a randomized controlled trial of SOT recipients with CD20+ PTLD who failed to respond to 30 to 50% reduction in calcineurin inhibitor dose and cessation of azathioprine and mycophenolate mofetil, were treated with four doses of rituximab 375 mg/m2 once weekly followed by four cycles of CHOP (Cyclophosphamide, Hydroxydaunorubicin, or doxorubicin, Oncovin or Vincristine, Prednisone) every 3 weeks. 90% of patients had a complete or partial response to therapy with medial overall survival of 6.6 years [74]. In a follow-up clinical trial, those who achieved a complete response to rituximab induction utilized rituximab consolidation while those who did not achieve a complete response received CHOP. In this study, 25% were able to avoid CHOP therapy due to complete response to Rituximab alone. The combined complete and partial response rate was 88% while 70% achieved a complete response [75].

Table 2. Treatment options for PTLD

Reduction of immunosuppression
Antiviral therapy
Anti B-cell antibodies
Combination chemotherapy
Surgical excision
Radiation therapy
Adoptive immunotherapy

Donor-Transmitted Cancer

Unintended transmission of cancer cells from a donor is a rare event but may result in metastatic cancer in the immunosuppressed SOT. Estimates of incidence range from 0.01 to 0.05% [1]. In a systematic review of 128 articles, 234 cases of KTRs with donor-transmitted malignancy were identified. The most common malignancies in descending order were lymphomas (n = 48), renal cancer (n = 42), malignant melanoma (n = 40), non-small cell lung cancer (n = 13), choriocarcinoma (n = 10), leukemia (n = 9), small cell lung cancer (n = 7), glioblastoma (n = 6), breast cancer (n = 5), others with less than 5 cases each (n = 50). The median time to cancer diagnosis was 7 months with 84% of cases diagnosed within 2 years. Transmitted melanoma and non-small cell lung cancer had the worst prognosis with 2-year survival of 43 and 19%, respectively. Donor-transmitted renal carcinoma had the best overall survival (5-year survival of 93%). The majority of renal carcinomas were managed by transplant nephrectomy. Since KTRs can still return to dialysis, more aggressive reduction in immunosuppression, chemotherapy, and transplant nephrectomy are warranted [76].

Living kidney donor candidates are screened using general population guidelines for common malignancies such as breast, colon, prostate, and cervical cancer [10]. The use of organs from any donor with a known malignancy depends on risk of transmission and requires use of clinical judgment to determine appropriate use. Low transmission risk lesions include skin limited non-melanoma skin cancer s, cervical cancer in situ, resected solitary RCC that is 1.0 cm in size or less [1, 10].

Conclusion

There is an increased risk of a wide range of cancers associated with SOT. The ability to prevent and diagnose early-stage malignancies relies upon periodic exams and strict adherence to prophylactic measures. Specifically, excessive immunosuppression or repeated exposure to lymphocyte-depleting drugs should be avoided. Reduction or withdrawal of immunosuppression is used mainly in KTRs since loss of the graft to rejection is not a fatal event. Identification of risk factors, initiation of appropriate screening practices, and implementation of appropriate management will be critical for driving improvement in the management of post-transplant malignancy in transplant recipients.

References

[1] Au E, Wong G, Chapman JR. Cancer in kidney transplant recipients. *Nat Rev Nephrol.* 2018 Aug; 14(8): 508-520.

[2] Blosser CD, Haber G, Engels EA, Changes in cancer incidence and outcomes among kidney transplant recipients in the United States over a thirty-year period. *Kidney Int* 2021, 99(6):1430-38.

[3] Katabathina VS, Menias CO, Tammisetti VS, Lubner MG, Kielar A, Shaaban A et al. Malignancy after solid organ transplantation: comprehensive imaging review. *Radiographics.* 2016 Oct; 36(5): 1390-1407.

[4] Vigneri P, Frasca F, Sciacca L, Pandini G. Diabetes and cancer. *Endocr Relat Cancer;* 2009 Dec; 16(4): 1103-1123.

[5] Webster AC, Craig JC, Simpson JM, Jones MP, Chapman JR. Identifying high risk groups and quantifying absolute risk of cancer after kidney transplantation: a cohort study of 15183 recipients. *Am J Transplant.* 2007 Sep; 7(9): 2140-2151.

[6] Wetmore JB, Calvert JP, Yu ASL, Lynch CF, Wang CJ, Kasiske BL et al. Polycystic kidney disease and cancer after renal transplantation. *J Am Soc Nephrol.* 2014 Oct; 25(10): 2335-2341.

[7] Schwarz A, Vatandaslar S, Merkel S, Haller H. Renal cell carcinoma in transplant recipients with acquired cystic kidney disease. *Clin J Am Soc Nephrol.* 2007 Jul; 2(4): 750-756.

[8] Hall EC, Engels EA, Pfeiffer RM, Segev DL. Association of antibody induction immunosuppression with cancer after kidney transplantation. *Transplantation.* 2015 May; 99(5): 1051-1057.

[9] Caillard S, Dharnidharka V, Agodoa L, Bohen E, Abbott K. Posttransplant lymphoproliferative disorders after renal transplantation in the United States in era of modern immunosuppression. *Transplantation.* 2005 Nov. 80(9): 1233-1243.

[10] Rossi AP, Klein CL. Posttransplant malignancy. *Surg Clin North Am.* 2019 Feb; 99(1): 49-64.

[11] Krisl JC, Doan VP. Chemotherapy and transplantation: the role of immunosuppression in malignancy and a review of antineoplastic agents in solid organ transplant recipients. *Am J Transplant.* 2017 Aug; 17: 1974-1991.

[12] Robson R. Cecka JM, Opelz G, Budde M, Sacks S. Prospective registry-based observational cohort study of the long-term risk of malignancies in renal transplant patients treated with mycophenolate mofetil. *Am J Transplant.* 2005 Dec; 5 (12): 2954-2960.

[13] Grinyo J, Charpentier B, Pestana JM, Vanrenterghem Y, Vincenti F, Reyes-Acevedo R et al. An integrated safety profile analysis of belatacept in kidney transplant recipients. *Transplantation.* 2010 Dec; 90(12): 1521-1527.

[14] Mittal A, Colegio OR. Skin cancers in organ transplant recipients. *Am J Transplant.* 2017 Oct; 17: 2509 – 2530.

[15] Engels EA, Pfeiffer RM, Fraumeni JF, Kasiske BL, Israni AK, Snyder JJ et al. Spectrum of cancer risk among U.S. solid organ transplant recipients: the transplant center match study. *JAMA*. 2011 Nov; 306(17): 1891-1901.

[16] Acuna SA, Huang JW, Scott AL, Micic S, Daly C, Brezden-Masley, C et al. Cancer screening recommendations for solid organ transplant recipients: a systematic review of clinical practice guidelines. *Am J Transplant*. 2017 Jan; 17(1): 103-114.

[17] Chockalingam R, Downing C, Tyring SK. Cutaneous squamous cell carcinomas in organ transplant recipients. *J Clin Med*. 2015 Jun; 4(6): 1229-1239.

[18] Walsh SB, Xu J, Xu H, Kurundkar AR, Maheshwari A, Grizzle WA et al. Cyclosporine A mediates pathogenesis of aggressive cutaneous squamous cell carcinoma by augmenting epithelial-mesenchymal transition: role of TGF -β signaling pathway. *Mol Carcinog*. 2011 Jul; 50(7): 516-527.

[19] Rostaing L, Vincenti F, Grinyo J, Rice KM, Bresnahan B, Steinberg S. Long-term belatacept exposure maintains efficacy and safety at 5 years: results from long-term extension of the BENEFIT study. *Am J Transplant*. 2013 Nov; 13(11): 2875-2883.

[20] Letellier T, Leborgne F, Kerleau C, Gaultier A, Dantal, Ville S. Association between use of hydrochlorothiazide and risk of keratinocyte cancers in kidney transplant recipients. *Clin J Am Soc Nephrol*. 2020 Dec: 15 (12):1804-1813.50(7): 516-527.

[21] Knoll GA, Kokolo MB, Mallick R, Beck A, Buenaventura CD, Ducharme, R. Effect of sirolimus on malignancy and survival after kidney transplantation: systematic review and meta-analysis of individual patient data. *BMJ*. 2014 Nov; 349: g6679.

[22] Shin D, Lee ES, Kim J, Guerra L, Naik D, Prida X. Association between the use of thiazide diuretics and the risk of skin cancer s: a meta-analysis of observational studies. *J Clin Med Res*. 2019 Apr; 11(4): 247-255.

[23] Zwald FO, Brown M. Skin cancer in solid organ transplant recipients: advances in therapy and management – Part II. *J Am Acad Dermatol*. 2011 Aug; 65(2): 263-279.

[24] Otley CC, Griffin MD, Charlton MR, Edwards BS, Neuburg M, Stasko T et al. Reduction in immunosuppression for transplant associated skin cancer: expert consensus survey. *Br J Dermatol*. 2006 Mar; 154(3): 395 – 400.

[25] Kim DP, Kus KJB, Ruiz E. Basal cell carcinoma review. *Hematol Oncol Clin North Am*. 2019 Feb; 33(1): 13-24.

[26] Cusack CA, Nijhawan R, Miller B, Henien M, Malat G, Doyle A et al. Vismodegib for local advanced basal cell carcinoma in a heart transplant recipient. *JAMA Dermatol*. 2015 Jan; 15(1): 70-72.

[27] Vangipuram R, Tyring SK. Epidemiology of Kaposi sarcoma: review and description of the nonepidemic variant. *Int J Dermatol*. 2019 May; 58(5): 538-542.

[28] Cattani P, Capuano M, Graffeo R, Ricci R, Cerimele F, Cerimele D et al. Kaposi's sarcoma association with previous human herpesvirus 8 infection in kidney transplant recipients. *J Clin Microbiol*. 2001 Feb; 39(2): 506-508.

[29] Villani A, Fabbrocini G, Costa C, Annunziata MC, Scalvenzi M. Merkel cell carcinoma: therapeutic update and emerging therapies. *Dermatol Ther* (Heidelb). 2019 Jun; 9(2): 209-222.

[30] Clarke CA, Robbins HA, Tatalovich Z, Lynch CF, Pawlish KS, Finch JL et al. Risk of merkel cell carcinoma after solid organ transplantation. *J Natl Cancer Inst*. 2015 Jan; 107(2): dju382.

[31] Liu Y, Sheikh MS. Melanoma: molecular pathogenesis and therapeutic management. *Mol Cell Pharmacol*. 2014 Mar; 6(3): 228.

[32] Robbins HA, Clarke CA, Arron ST, Tatalovich Z, Kahn AR, Hernandez BY et al. Melanoma risk and survival among organ transplant recipients. *J invest dermatol*. 2015 Aug; 135(11): 2657-2665.

[33] Garrett GL, Blanc PD, Boscardin J. Incidence of and risk factors for skin cancer in organ transplant recipients in the United States. *JAMA Dermatol*. 2017 Mar; 153(3): 296-303.

[34] Garrett GL, He SY, Sabouni N, Daud A, Arron ST. Combined dabrafenib and trametinib therapy in metastatic melanoma and organ transplantation: case report and review of the literature. *JAAD Case Rep*. 2015 Nov; 1(6): S23-S25.

[35] Hickman LA, Sawinski D, Guzzo T, Locke JE. Urologic malignancies in kidney transplantation. *Am J Transplant*. 2018 Jan;18: 13-22.

[36] Cohen H, McGovern F. Renal-Cell Carcinoma. *N Engl J Med*. 2005;353 (23):2477-2490.

[37] Miao Y, Everly JJ, Gross TG, Tevar AD, First MR, Alloway RR et al. De novo cancers arising in organ transplant recipients are associated with adverse outcomes compared with the general population. *Transplantation*. 2009 May; 87(9): 1347-1359.

[38] Hurst FP, Jindal RM, Fletcher JJ, Dharnidharka V, Gorman G, Lechner B et al. Incidence, predictors, and associated outcomes of renal cell carcinoma in long-term dialysis patients. *Urology*. 2011 Jun; 77(6): 1271-1276.

[39] Karami S, Yanik EL, Moore LE, Pfeiffer RM, Copeland G, Gonsalves L et al. Risk of renal cell carcinoma among kidney transplant recipients in the United States. Am *J Transplant*. 2016 Dec; 16(12): 3479-3489.

[40] Hofmann JN, Schwartz K, Chow WH, Ruterbusch JJ, Shuch BM, Karami S et al. The association between chronic renal failure and renal cell carcinoma may differ between black and white Americans. *Cancer Causes Control*. 2013 Jan; 24; 167-174.

[41] Neirynck V, Claes K, Naesens M, De Wever L, Pirenne J, Kuypers D et al. Renal cell carcinoma of native kidneys in the allograft: what is the role of the polyomavirus. *Case Rep Nephrol Urol*. 2012 Jul; 2(2): 125 – 134.

[42] Moris D, Kakavia K, Argyrou C, Garbis N, Bokos J, Vernadakis S et al. De novo renal cell carcinoma in renal transplant recipients: a single-center experience. *Anticancer Res*. 2017 Feb; 37(2): 773-779.

[43] Warren H, Olsburgh J. Management of renal cell carcinoma and other renal masses in the kidney graft. *Curr Urol Rep*. 2020 Feb; 21(1): 8.

[44] Lim WH, Turner RM, Chapman JR, Ma MKM, Webster AC, Craig JC. Acute rejection, T-cell depleting antibodies, and cancer after transplantation. *Transplantation*. 2014 Apr; 97(8): 817-825.

[45] Liu J, Liu D, Li, J, Lan Z, Chengliang Z, Lei K, et al. Efficacy and safety of everolimus for maintenance immunosuppression of kidney transplantation: a meta-analysis of randomized controlled trials. *PLoS One*. 2017 Jan; 12(1): e0170246.

[46] Sanli O, Dobruch J, Knowles MA, Burger M, Alemozaffar M, Nielsen ME et al. Bladder cancer. *Nat Rev Dis Primer*. 2017 Apr; 3: 17022.

[47] Ardelt PU, Rieken M, Ebbing J, Bonkat G, Vlajnic T, Bubendorf L et al. Urothelial cancer in renal transplant recipients: incidence, risk factors, and oncological outcome. *Urology*. 2016 Feb; 88: 104-110.

[48] Yan L, Chen P, Chen EZ, Gu A, Jiang ZY. Risk of bladder cancer in renal transplant patients: a meta-analysis. *Br J Cancer*. 2014 Feb; 110(7): 1871-1877.

[49] Liu S, Chaudhry M, Berrebi A, Papadimitriou JC, Drachenberg CB, Haririan A, et al. Polyomavirus replication and smoking are independent risk factors for bladder cancer after renal transplantation. *Transplantation.* 2017 June; 101(6): 1488-1494.

[50] Prabharasuth D, Moses KA, Bernstein M, Dalbagni G, Herr HW. Management of bladder cancer after renal transplantation. *Urology*. 2013 Apr; 81(4): 813-819.

[51] Liao JB, Fisher CE, Madeleine MM. Gynecologic cancers and solid organ transplantation. *Am J Transplant*. 2019 May; 19 (5): 1266-1277.

[52] Madeleine MM, Finch JL, Lynch CF, Goodman MT, Engels EA. HPV -related cancers after solid organ transplantation in the US. *Am J Transplant*. 2013 Dec; 13(12): 3202-3209.

[53] Schiffman M, Doorbar J, Wentzensen N, de SanJose S, Fakhry C, Monk BJ et al. Carcinogenic human papillomavirus infection. *Nat Rev Dis Primers*. 2016 Dec; 2:16086.

[54] De Martel, C, Plummer M, Vignat J, Franceschi S. Worldwide burden of cancer attributable to HPV by site, country and HPV type. *Int J Cancer*. 2017 Aug; 141(4): 664-670.

[55] Moscicki AB, Flowers L, Huchko MJ, Long ME, MacLaughlin KL, Murphy J, et al. Guidelines for cervical cancer screening in immunosuppressed women without HIV infection. *J Low Genit Tract Dis*. 2019 Apr; 23(2): 87-101.

[56] Wong G, Au E, Badve SV, Lim WH. Breast cancer and transplantation. *Am J Transplant.* 2017 May; 17: 2243-2253.

[57] Wong G, Chapman JR, Craig JC. Cancer screening in renal transplant recipients: what is the evidence ? *Clin J Am Soc Nephrol*. 2008 Mar; 3 (supplement 2): S87-S100.

[58] Alhamad T, Venkatachalam K, Linette GP, Brennan DC. Checkpoint inhibitors in kidney transplant recipients and the potential risk of rejection. *Am J Transplant*. 2016 Apr; 16(4): 1332-1333.

[59] Prenner S, Levitsky J. Comprehensive review on colorectal cancer and transplant. *Am J Transplant*. 2017; 17(11): 2761-2774.

[60] Johnson EE, Leverson GE, Pirsch JD, Heise CP. A 30-year analysis of colorectal adenocarcinoma in transplant recipients and proposal for altered screening. *J Gastrointest Surg.* 2007; 11: 272-279.

[61] Papaconstantinou HT, Sklow B, Hanaway MJ, Gross TG, Beebe TM, Trofe J, et al. Characteristics and survival patterns of solid organ transplant patients developing de novo colon and rectal cancer. *Dis Colon Rectum*. 2004 Nov; 47(11): 1898-1903.

[62] Hojo M, Morimoto T, Maluccio M, Asano T, Morimoto K, Lagman M, et al. Cyclosporine induces cancer progression by a cell-autonomous mechanism. *Nature.* 1999 Feb; 397(6719): 530-534.

[63] Suthanthiran M, Hojo M, Maluccio M, Boffa DJ, Luan FL. Post-transplantation malignancy: a cell autonomous mechanism with implications for therapy. *Trans Am Clin Climatol Assoc*. 2009; 120: 369-388.

[64] Leckel K, Beecken WD, Jonas D, Oppermann E, Coman MC, Beck KF. The immunosuppressive drug mycophenolate mofetil impairs adhesion capacity of gastrointestinal tumor cells. *Clin Exp Immunol*. 2003 Nov; 134(2): 238-245.

[65] Safaeian M, Robbins HA, Berndt SI, Lynch CF, Fraumeni JF, Engels EA. Risk of colorectal cancer after solid organ transplant in the United States. *Am J Transplant.* 2016; 16 (3): 960-967.

[66] Aoki K, Tamai Y, Horiike S, Oshima M, Taketo MM. Colonic polyposis caused by mTOR-mediated chromosomal instability in APC +/delta716 cdx2+/- compound mutant mice. *Nat Genet*. 2003 Dec; 35(4): 323-330.

[67] Fujishita T, Aoki K, Lane HA, Aoki M, Taketo MM. Inhibition of the mTORC1 pathway suppresses intestinal polyp formation and reduces the mortality in APC Delta716 mice. *Proc Natl Acad Sci U S A*. 2008 Sep; 105(36): 13544-13549.

[68] Yanik EL, Gustafson SK, Kasiske BL, Israni AK, Snyder JJ, Hess GP. Sirolimus use and cancer incidence among US kidney transplant recipients. *Am J Transplant*. 2015 Jan; 15(1): 129-136.

[69] Dharnidharka VR. Comprehensive review of post-organ transplant hematologic cancers. *Am J Transplant*. 2018 Nov; 18: 537-549.

[70] DeStefano CB, Desai SH, Shenoy AG, Catlett JP. Management of post-transplant lymphoproliferative disorders. *Br J Haematol*. 2018 Aug; 182(3): 330-343.

[71] Kirk AD, Cherikh WS, Ring M, Burke G, Kaufman D, Knechtle S et al. Dissociation of T-cell depletion and post-transplant lymphoproliferative disease in kidney recipients treated with alemtuzumab. *Am J Transplant*. 2007 Nov; 7(11): 2619-2625.

[72] Dharnidharka VR. Peripheral blood Epstein-Barr viral nucleic acid surveillance as a marker for posttransplant cancer risk. *Am J Transplant*. 2017 Mar; 17(3): 611-616.

[73] Dierickx D, Vergote V. Management of post-transplant lymphoproliferative disorders. *HemaSphere*. 2019; 3: S2 – 74-77.

[74] Trappe R, Oertel S, Leblond V, Mollee P, Sender M, Reinke P et al. Sequential treatment with rituximab followed by CHOP chemotherapy in adult B-cell post-transplant lymphoproliferative disorder (PTLD): the prospective international multicenter phase 2 PTLD-1 trial. *Lancet Oncol*. 2012 Feb; 13(2): 196-206.

[75] Trappe RU, Dierickx D, Zimmerman H, Morschhauser F, Mollee P, Zaucha JM et al. Response to rituximab induction is a predictive marker in B-cell post-transplant lymphoproliferative disorder and allows stratification into rituximab or R-CHOP consolidation in an international, prospective, multicenter phase II trial. *J Clin Oncol*. 2017 Feb; 35(5): 536-543.

[76] Eccher A, Girolami I, Motter JM, Marletta S, Gambar G, Momo REN et al. Donor-transmitted cancer in kidney transplant recipients: a systematic review. *J Nephrol*. 2020: 33(6):1321-1332.

In: Issues in Kidney Disease – Transplantation
Editors: B. V. R. Murthy and S. Z. Fadem
ISBN: 978-1-53619-960-4

Chapter 11

RECURRENT DISEASE IN THE KIDNEY ALLOGRAFT

Pascale Khairallah*[*,1], MD, Taquiddin Khaja[2], MD and Bhamidipati V. R. Murthy[3], MD, DM

[1]Selzman Institute for Kidney Health, Section of Nephrology, and Michael E. DeBakey Veterans Affairs Medical Center, Baylor College of Medicine, Houston, TX, USA
[2]Selzman Institute for Kidney Health, Section of Nephrology, Baylor College of Medicine, Houston, TX, USA
[3]Selzman Institute for Kidney Health, Section of Nephrology, and Division of Abdominal Transplantation, Department of Surgery, Baylor College of Medicine, Houston, TX, USA

ABSTRACT

Despite significant improvements in allograft survival, allograft failure is currently the 4th most common cause of kidney failure in the US. Glomerular diseases represent one of the most common causes of allograft failure in kidney transplant recipients. Most glomerular diseases in the allograft represent recurrence of glomerular diseases of the native kidney. The rate of recurrence after transplantation, time to recurrence, donor and recipient risk factors, and specific management considerations differ among these diseases. This chapter reviews the most commonly occurring recurrent glomerular diseases post-transplantation.

Keywords: kidney transplantation, glomerular diseases, recurrent disease, allograft failure

[*] Corresponding Author's Email: Pascale.khairallah@bcm.edu.

Introduction

Kidney transplantation is currently the best treatment for end-stage kidney disease (ESKD) [1]. There have been improvements in both short-term [2] and long-term allograft survival [3], albeit the latter has lagged as compared to the former. Despite significant improvements in allograft survival, allograft failure is currently the 4th most common cause of kidney failure in the US [4]. Glomerular diseases are one of the main causes of native kidney failure in kidney transplant recipients [5]. Glomerular diseases are also one of the most common causes of allograft failure in kidney transplant recipients [6, 7]. The incidence of glomerular diseases is reported to be as high as 42% at 10 years post-transplant ation [8]. Glomerular disease in the allograft can rarely be donor-derived, most commonly due to recurrent glomerulonephritis (GN), and less commonly *de novo* [9]. The incidence ranges from 2.6% to 50%, the disparity being caused by varying follow-up times, incomplete biopsy data, variable thresholds for transplantation, and inconsistent reporting [9]. Different primary GNs have different rates of recurrence [8, 10-12]. This chapter addresses incidence, pathogenesis, and management of recurrent glomerular diseases in the allograft.

IgA Nephropathy

Overview

IgA nephropathy is deemed to be the most common glomerular disease globally [13]. The disease presents with higher prevalence in Eastern and Pacific Asian populations and has a low prevalence among African populations [14, 15]. The key pathophysiology of IgA Nephropathy involves defects in glycosylation on the hinge region of IgA1 to which circulating immune complexes form [16]. These complexes deposit in the glomerular tissue and activate the complement system which leads to nephritic syndrome in such patients. There is currently no serum marker to diagnose IgA nephropathy. Kidney biopsy confirms the diagnosis. Key findings in the biopsy consist of mesangial proliferation under light microscopy, positive IgA deposits in the mesangium on Immunofluorescence, and mesangial electron -dense deposits on electron microscopy.

Clinical manifestations of IgA are very broad ranging from asymptomatic microscopic hematuria, hematuria with proteinuria, rapidly progressive renal failure, or a slowly progressive proteinuric renal disease. Progression to ESKD is generally slow over one or two decades but rapid progression is seen in patients with uncontrolled hypertension or patients with crescentic IgA [13].

Treatment of IgA nephropathy includes antiproteinuric and antihypertensive therapy in patients with proteinuria >1 g/day. Antiproteinuric therapy could be given with angiotensin converting enzyme inhibitor (ACEI) or angiotensin receptor blocker (ARB) drugs [17]. Steroid treatment is typically given for 6 months for patients with persistent proteinuria that have not responded to above therapy. Steroids are helpful especially in patients with proteinuria of greater than 3 g/day [13]. The use of cyclophosphamide or antiproliferative agents such as Mycophenolate mofetil or azathioprine are generally reserved for patients at high risk for kidney disease progression such as crescentic glomerulonephritis [18]. Mycophenolate mofetil has mixed efficacy. Unlike with other glomerular diseases, rituximab is not effective in IgA nephropathy [13]. While many trials with biologics are being conducted, a search for a safe and effective therapy targeting the pathogenetic mechanism continues. It is also imperative that patients control their weight since obesity can play a role in proteinuria as well.

IgA nephropathy can recur in the allograft. Recurrence is reported to occur in up to 60% of recipients with primary IgA nephropathy, but graft failure occurs over several years [9, 19, 20]. Risk factors for recurrence include living-related donor, the HLA alleles HLA-B35 and HLA-DR4 in recipient, well-matched and zero HLA mismatch between the donor and the recipient, high serum IgA concentrations, and crescentic disease in the native kidney [21-27]. It has been proposed that galactose-deficient-IgA1, IgG autoantibodies, and IgA–sCD89 complexes are valuable biomarkers to predict disease recurrence [23].

Diagnosis Post-Transplantation

Patients can present with unexplained graft dysfunction, proteinuria, hypertension, hematuria, or occasionally acute kidney injury. Some patients can also be asymptomatic, which can make reaching a diagnosis challenging. Diagnosis of IgAN recurrence is usually confirmed by kidney transplant biopsy. Histologic recurrence is identified in 50 to 60% of patients, but clinical recurrence is reported in only 7 to 30% of patients [28]. In general, recurrence of IgA nephropathy is a time-dependent phenomenon. Varying incidence is likely from differences in the indication for biopsy and post-transplant length of follow-up [29].

Management Post-Transplantation

There are no specific proven therapies for recurrent IgA nephropathy. The management options for IgA nephropathy in native kidneys also applies to recurrent disease – i.e., proteinuria control with ACEI/ARB and aggressive antihypertensive management [29]. In the absence of specific therapies, focus is being shifted to preventive strategies. In this context, steroid withdrawal has been observed with increased rates of recurrence [30], and induction with anti-thymocyte antibodies (ATG) has been observed to be associated with a lower recurrence of IgA nephropathy [31].

MEMBRANOUS NEPHROPATHY

Overview

Primary membranous nephropathy (MN), which constitutes 80% of all cases of MN, is associated with circulating autoantibodies against phospholipase A2 receptor (PLA2R) in 70% of patients, staining of PLA2R antibodies on biopsy despite a negative circulating antibody in 15%, and circulating antibody to thrombospondin type-1 domain-containing 7A (THSD7A) in another 3 to 5% of patients [32-34]. Primary MN is a major cause of nephrotic syndrome in adults of European ancestry [33]. Clinical presentation consists of nephrotic syndrome in 80%, and non-nephrotic proteinuria in the remaining 20%; microhematuria may be seen in up to 30% of patients [34]. Spontaneous remission is seen in about a third of patients. In patients treated with steroids /alkylating agents, 8 to 11% progress to ESKD, but untreated, 35-40% progress to ESKD [35].

Diagnosis is confirmed with positive PLA2R antibodies in the serum and/or on biopsy showing typical biopsy findings of MN with thickening of glomerular basement membrane and subepithelial spikes on light microscopy, IgG (usually IgG4) and C3 granular staining along glomerular capillaries, and subepithelial electron -dense deposits and effacement of podocyte foot processes on electron microscopy [33, 34, 36, 37]. Immune complexes of IgG-PLA2R that accumulate in the subepithelial space of the glomerular capillaries are responsible for the clinical and pathological findings associated with this disease.

Treatment of primary MN consists of supportive therapy with ACEI/ARB, and immunosuppressive therapy including steroids, cytotoxic agents (cyclophosphamide or chlorambucil), calcineurin inhibitors (cyclosporine or tacrolimus), Rituximab or adrenocorticotrophic hormone (ACTH) [34]. The most popular first line treatment is Modified Ponticelli regimen consisting of steroids alternating with cyclophosphamide monthly for a total of 6 months [34]. Anti-PLA2R antibody titers can guide treatment duration, inform treatment response, and prognosticate disease [38].

Recurrence Post-Transplant

MN recurrence in the allograft is relatively common, with a prevalence ranging from 7 to 44% [8, 39]. Therefore, patients being evaluated for transplantation and their donors should be notified about these risks. A previous confirmed diagnosis of MN helps to suspect the disease as recurrent MN. The clinical presentation is similar to that of primary

MN in native kidneys with proteinuria with or without nephrotic syndrome and a bland urinary sediment. The light microscopic picture in recurrent MN is similar to that of the original disease with diffuse membrane thickening, and sub-epithelial spikes on light microscopy, and polyclonal global granular staining of IgG along the glomerular capillary basement membrane on immunofluorescence. These represent immune complexes with PLA2R antigen and PLA2R antibodies (usually IgG4), as in the original disease. However, few differences are observed from primary MN in native kidneys. C4d staining is often detected with a diffuse granular pattern in recurrent MN. However, in contrast to native disease, C3 staining is not as prevalent in recurrent MN [40]. Thus, while alternate pathway complement activation is predominant in the primary MN, presence of C4d in recurrent MN argues in favor of classical complement pathway activation [41]. While the PLA2R antibody is directed against podocyte antigens in primary MN, in post-transplant MN, it is directed against brush border, or tubular epithelial or interstitial antigens [42]. In the early phases of the disease, membrane spikes may not be observed despite heavy proteinuria, but electron microscopy shows subepithelial electron-dense deposits, and is necessary to confirm the diagnosis in such cases [41]. It is important to note that in recurrent MN, electron dense deposits are sparse, and not as dense as seen in original disease.

Recurrence is detected more often in centers that perform protocol biopsies [43] with some cases diagnosed as early as 6 days after transplantation [44]. In the absence of a protocol biopsy, recurrence is generally reported 1 to 3 years after transplant, with a few reported years later. The factors associated with higher risk of recurrence include high levels of proteinuria pre-transplant, high anti-PLA2R titer prior to transplant, and possibly living-related donor transplant [45]. Additional risk factors for recurrence include use of steroid-free regimens [11, 46-49], recipient HLA -DR3, *HLA DQA1*0501* and HLA-A3 [47, 49, 50], and donor HLA-DRB1 and HLA-DQA1 [51]. Persistence of high anti-PLA2R titers after transplant heralds recurrent MN [40, 52]. Similarly, reappearance of anti-PLA2R antibodies or a rising titer is associated with recurrence. Re-emergence of anti-PLA2R antibodies could occur because of intercurrent infections or because of weaning of immunosuppression [45]. In case of living donors, the increased susceptibility stems from the higher probability of sharing target antigen (PLA2R) polymorphism or HLA polymorphism in related donors [53].

Management Post-Transplantation

As in the native kidney, supportive therapy with ACEI/ARB to minimize proteinuria is the cornerstone of therapy. High-dose steroids, alkylating agents, or mycophenolic acid do not provide any significant response in recurrent MN [45]. Rituximab has emerged as the first line therapy for these patients. It is recommended to institute Rituximab therapy early for patients with proteinuria > 1 g/d [11]. Dose of Rituximab has not been defined but a large series by Grupper et al., from Mayo Clinic used two doses of 1000 mg each 2 weeks apart, which seems to be reasonable [11]. Rituximab has been associated with reasonable success with 82% achieving partial or complete remission, and 40% of patients showing complete histological remission without a relapse over a follow-up period of 15 months [11]. The deposits may persist for weeks to months even after the circulating antibody is undetectable and new immune complex formation has ceased. In cases of complete remission, the deposits are gradually reabsorbed and eventually disappear. Most studies that have shown detrimental effects of recurrent MN on allograft survival were from previous era when the pathogenesis was not clearly understood, and Rituximab had not emerged as a therapy option [46, 54, 55]. Long term studies in the current era with Rituximab therapy are still pending.

De novo MN has some differences from the recurrent disease. MN occurring beyond 3 years after transplant could suggest *de novo* MN. A well-defined pathogenetic mechanism has not been defined. As in original disease, secondary causes such as hepatitis B infection, hepatitis C infection, and solid organ malignancies could be associated with *de novo* MN. However, secondary MN after transplant has also been observed with antibody -mediated rejection [56]. *De novo* MN after transplant is less often associated with PLA2R antibodies in serum or PLA2R staining on biopsies [43, 57]. While IgG4 subclass is detected in the immune deposits in primary MN, IgG1 is found to be dominant in *de novo* MN [58]. Thus, *de novo* MN may have a different pathogenetic mechanism compared to recurrent MN [45]. Treatment of *de novo* MN is similar to that of recurrent MN, and Rituximab is still the first line of therapy.

Focal Segmental Glomerulosclerosis

Overview

Focal Segmental Glomerulosclerosis (FSGS) is the most common primary glomerular disease associated with high-grade proteinuria and ESKD [59]. FSGS represents a non-specific histologic lesion with diverse causes leading to podocyte injury and depletion, and eventual sclerosis. Subclasses of FSGS include primary, genetic, and secondary forms. When a specific etiology cannot be defined, FSGS is considered primary and is thought to be a result of a circulating factor which compromises the integrity of the glomerular filtration barrier [60]. Secondary FSGS is linked to underlying etiologies such as infections, obesity, and drugs. Genetic FSGS results from a mutation in genes encoding podocyte proteins. These genetic mutations can be limited to the kidney causing FSGS or part of syndromes that involve multiple organs in addition to the kidney [61].

A kidney biopsy is used to determine the histological variants of FSGS, which include collapsing, perihilar, cellular, tip-variant, and not otherwise specified (NOS) lesions of

FSGS – termed as the Columbia classification of FSGS [60]. Each variant is associated with different prognosis and management considerations. NOS variant is the most common, and it is equally distributed among primary and secondary forms [62, 63]. Tip lesion, cellular, and collapsing variants usually share the presenting features of heavy proteinuria and the nephrotic syndrome, but they may also present with subnephrotic-range proteinuria [61]. Tip lesions tend to occur more frequently in white patients, are more likely to respond to therapy, and have overall the best prognosis [60]. The collapsing variant occurs in patients with primary FSGS, particularly malignant in its course, and is the characteristic lesion seen in HIV -associated nephropathy, FSGS associated with APOL1 alleles, parvo B19 virus infection, and pamidronate toxicity [61]. A general rule to distinguish primary from secondary FSGS is to observe foot process effacement by electron microscopy. Near complete foot process effacement ($\geq$ 80% of total glomerular capillary surface area s) is generally associated with primary FSGS [61, 63, 64].

Management of FSGS involves complete remission of proteinuria and preservation of renal function. Proteinuria is managed by use of ACEI/ARB; volume overload is managed by diuretics. KDIGO recommends treatment with high-dose corticosteroids for 16 weeks as first line therapy for Primary FSGS, and calcineurin inhibitors (CNI) and mycophenolate mofetil as second and third line therapies [65]. Rituximab is an emerging second-line therapy for primary FSGS that is steroid non-responsive, but results of a randomized trial are still pending. Management of secondary FSGS consists of cessation of offending drugs, treatment of viral infection s, and weight loss in obese patients.

According to the KDIGO Transplant Guidelines, patients with primary FSGS are not excluded as candidates for kidney transplantations [66]. Recurrence of primary FSGS in the kidney allograft manifests very early after transplantation, affects up to 40% of patients with FSGS, and is associated with high rates of allograft loss [12, 67]. The risk of graft loss increases incrementally with risk of recurrence reaching 45% for a second allograft and 100% for a third allograft if the first graft and second graft were lost to recurrent FSGS respectively [12]. Given these high risks, it is essential for the transplant nephrologist to discuss extensively the risks of recurrence and allograft loss with potential transplant recipients. Recipient risk factors for recurrence include European ancestry, younger age at diagnosis, FSGS recurrence with previous allograft, history of bilateral nephrectomy pre-transplantation, as well as some circulating antibodies [12, 67-73]. Donor risk factors for recurrence include African race, likely the result of the APOL1 risk variant, and older donor age [67, 68].

Evidence points to a circulating permeability factor in the pathogenesis of FSGS based on the speed at which proteinuria can occur after transplantation, and improvement of proteinuria after treatment with plasmapheresis in some patients. Although no single factor has been clearly identified that explains all manifestations of recurrent FSGS, studies have suggested the role of the soluble urokinase -type plasminogen activator receptor (suPAR), cardiotrophin-like cytokine factor-1 (CLCF-1), CD40 axis, and apolipoprotein A-Ib

(ApoA-Ib) in the pathogenesis of recurrent FSGS [74]. While animal studies support each one of these factors, human studies have been equivocal. Further research on these biomarkers is needed to clarify pathogenesis of FSGS, facilitate an earlier diagnosis of primary FSGS, predict recurrent FSGS, and facilitate the development of effective and novel therapies of primary as well as recurrent FSGS [74].

While not widely adopted yet, genetic testing for FSGS is becoming a cornerstone of diagnosis. This is important for treatment and prognostication since the majority of patients with monogenic forms of FSGS do not respond to corticosteroids and have a very low risk of recurrence in the allograft [61]. Further, identifying a monogenic cause in the recipient allows testing of potential donors ensuring that family members with a similar mutation are excluded from donation [61]. This is particularly useful in the case of APOL1 variant-associated FSGS. The likelihood of identifying a monogenic cause of FSGS correlates inversely with the age of disease onset. Pathogenic mutations are identified in 60%–100% during the first year of life, 40%–60% of young children, 25%–40% of older children, and 10%–25% of adolescents, with the yield higher in familial and in those with syndromic disease [61, 75-77]. In patients with adult-onset FSGS, a genetic cause can be established in only 8%–14% [61].

Diagnosis Post-Transplant

Recurrent Primary FSGS presents as proteinuria, often in the nephrotic-range, and can occur within first hours to weeks of a kidney transplantation. The patient can also have transplant dysfunction as well [59, 60]. The diagnosis is confirmed with an allograft kidney biopsy. There are no histologic findings that are specific for recurrent lesions compared to native disease. The likelihood of predicting recurrence based on the histological variant of FSGS in native kidneys is poor, and the correlation of the histological variant between the original lesions and recurrent lesions is also poor [78].

Management Post-Transplantation

Management of post-transplant ation FSGS depends on whether the recipient has primary, secondary or genetic FSGS. In secondary and monogenic causes of FSGS, risk of recurrence is very low and therefore targeted FSGS treatments are not needed. Plasmapheresis theoretically removes the podocyte-directed circulating factor from the blood. While pre-transplant plasmapheresis has not shown any benefits in prevention of FSGS recurrence post-transplantation [66], several case reports and case series have reported improvement in up to 70% of patients in prevention or treatment of recurrent FSGS post-transplantation [79, 80]. No controlled trials have been performed to date on any therapeutic interventions. Currently, plasmapheresis and rituximab are the most frequently used treatments by centers in the United States. Because of lack of homogeneity in the available studies, no firm treatment regimen for plasmapheresis can be provided at this time. Cyclophosphamide can be added if remission is not achieved. Ofatumumab, a monoclonal antibody to CD20, has been found to induce remission in cases resistant to plasmapheresis and Rituximab [81-83]. Two other therapies are being tried on an experimental basis in the treatment of recurrent FSGS – immunoadsorption and low density lipoprotein apheresis (LDL -A) [80]. These studies are isolated case reports or small case series and demonstrate reduction in proteinuria and improvement in lipid abnormalities in drug-resistant recurrent FSGS. Randomized controlled studies with long-term follow-up are needed to justify the beneficial health outcomes of either of these therapies. Overall, FSGS recurrence is challenging, and only 40-60% of patients achieve any response with any of these treatments. These responses are often incomplete and non-sustained [12].

MEMBRANOPROLIFERATIVE GN (MPGN)

Overview

Membranoproliferative GN (MPGN) is a progressive renal disease which can present as either nephritic syndrome, nephrotic syndrome or a combined (nephritic-nephrotic) picture. MPGN or mesangiocapillary glomerulonephritis, refers to a specific glomerular lesion that is characterized by mesangial expansion and hypercellularity, leading to an accentuated lobular appearance of the glomerular tuft, mesangial interposition into the capillary wall giving rise to duplicated or split glomerular basement membranes (tram-track appearance), and mesangial and subendothelial immune deposits on immunofluorescence. MPGN can be idiopathic or secondary to a variety of diseases. It is typically classified as immune complex-mediated, complement -mediated, and MPGN secondary to chronic thrombotic microangiopathy (TMA) [84]. Immune Complex-Mediated MPGN is caused by systemic diseases that produce immune complexes. As with other glomerular diseases, the presence of circulating and deposited immune complexes may result in tissue injury. Immune deposits in this category consist of immunoglobulins and C3 component of the complement. This type of MPGN is associated with hepatitis B, Hepatitis C and cryoglobulinemia, autoimmune disease (lupus and rheumatoid arthritis) and paraproteinemias. The so called idiopathic MPGN is classified in this category in the absence of a known cause.

Complement-mediated MPGN, otherwise called C3 Glomerulopathy, is caused by dysfunction in the complement pathway. The two types of diseases that fall under this category a re C3 Glomerulonephritis (C3GN) and Dense Deposit Disease (DDD). These two types of MPGN are distinguished on electron microscopy. DDD typically shows mesangial and intramembranous C3 deposits. On the other hand, C3GN has a more diffuse pattern of C3 deposits in the mesangium, subepithelial and subendothelial spaces [84]. Terminal complement components (C5-9) may also be present in these complement deposits. Of note, in these two conditions, no immunoglobulin deposits are seen. In C3 Glomerulopathy, the deposition predominantly of C3 suggests a dysregulated alternate complement pathway, resulting in the amplification and subsequent overproduction of C3 and related products of the terminal complement cascade. The exact cause of the complement dysregulation remains uncertain, although genetic mutations (e.g., mutations of Factor H or Factor I genes) or autoantibodies (e.g., C3 or C4 nephritic factor directed against C3 convertase or Factor H autoantibodies) resulting in dysfunctional complement regulatory proteins and, therefore, uncontrolled amplification of the C3 protein have been implicated in the pathogenesis [85].

MPGN pattern of injury in the absence of IC or complement deposits, in the setting of TMA such as with hemolytic uremic syndrome (HUS) or thrombotic thrombocytopenic purpura (TTP) is classified in the third category [84].

Thus, kidney biopsy is essential to differentiate the category of MPGN.

Treatment of MPGN usually consists of treating the underlying systemic disease or infection associated with MPGN. With complement -mediated MPGN, eculizumab, a humanized monoclonal antibody that binds to C5 proteins, inhibiting cleaving into C5a and C5b and blocking production of the C5b-9 membrane attack complex, has shown promise [84]. For idiopathic MPGN, treatment remains unclear, but steroids and cyclophosphamide have been used for rapidly progressive crescentic variant with variable results [86].

Every effort should be made to determine the primary cause of the patient's MPGN prior to transplantation. Patients with MPGN generally have no contraindications to being evaluated and listed for kidney transplantation except in some paraproteinemic conditions [66].

The risk of recurrence of MPGN after transplantation is variable depending on etiology. The current classification of MPGN has given better understanding of the disease and clinical course after transplantation. The overall recurrence rate of MPGN after transplant is up to 50% within the first 24 months post-transplant [85]. Immune complex-mediated GN has a lower recurrence risk, and progresses slowly [87]. Excluding Type II MPGN (which in current classification includes C3GN and DDD) and patients with fibrillary glomerulonephritis, Lorenz et al. from Mayo Clinic reported a recurrence of 41% [87]. Hence, this study included almost exclusively Type I or Immune complex-mediated MPGN. This rate of recurrence is the most accurate as they employed protocol biopsies in this study, thus identifying disease early and in asymptomatic stage. Median time to recurrence was 3.3 months with a range of 1 week to 14 months [87]. In contrast, C3 glomerulopathy has a very high risk of recurrence of up to 70% within a median of 28 months post-transplantation, and generally has a later recurrence than immune complex-mediated MPGN [88]. Risk factors for recurrence include living-related donation, low complement level at transplantation, and monoclonal IG-associated MPGN [87, 89]. Overall graft failure in MPGN is worse than in other etiologies (45% vs 38%), with a majority of these grafts failing due to recurrent disease [90]. Graft failure from recurrent disease is worse with C3 Glomerulopathy (Type II MPGN) and can be as high as 50% in those who experience recurrence [88, 89, 91]. Recurrence with paraproteinemic renal disease also has a more aggressive course [84].

As seen with other recurrent glomerular diseases, the potential donor and recipient should be educated and advised about recurrence of MPGN and its potential negative impact on the allograft kidney.

Diagnosis

Recurrent MPGN can present as proteinuria, hematuria, and/or deterioration of allograft function. It is important to note that in early stages, a slow allograft dysfunction may be the only presentation, particularly in complement -mediated MPGN [85]. Histological picture of recurrent MPGN is similar to the original disease. Interestingly, transplant glomerulopathy also has similar histological appearance, and needs to be differentiated from recurrence. Absence of IG deposits (in complement-mediated MPGN), absence of C4d staining on biopsy, and absence of donor-specific antibodies in the serum help to differentiate it from transplant glomerulopathy or chronic antibody -mediated rejection [84]. Because of a similar histological appearance between these conditions, some authors believe that true incidence of recurrence may be over-estimated particularly in the past when the pathogenesis of the conditions was not clearly known [84].

Management Post-Transplantation

As in the primary disease, treatment of recurrent MPGN is not well established. Just as in the primary disease, high-dose steroids, plasmapheresis, and rituximab have been tried with variable success. Most of these are case reports or small series with limited follow-up [92-94]. In relation to recurrent C3GN and DDD, eculizumab has shown some benefit, but this has not been definitively studied in clinical trials, and dose and duration of therapy not well established [92, 95]. In a retrospective cohort study of 60 patients with native kidney C3GN, those maintained on immunosuppressive corticosteroids and mycophenolate were more likely to achieve clinical remission compared to untreated patients or those on other immunosuppressive regimens [96]. Whether this strategy is beneficial in kidney transplantation is unknown. Thus, management of recurrent MPGN can be frustrating without definitive treatment strategies available so far.

LUPUS GLOMERULONEPHRITIS

Overview

Approximately 10% of patients with Lupus Nephritis (LN) progress to ESRD, and LN constitutes 2.6% of all transplants performed in the US [97]. It is ideal for the lupus activity to be quiescent at the time of transplantation. Preemptive transplantation can improve outcomes as opposed to patients whose transplantation is delayed until dialysis is initiated [98]. The incidence of acute rejection, graft, and patient outcomes after transplantation for patients with lupus nephritis are similar to those of non-lupus patients [97]. Recurrent LN is seen in 2 to 30% of patients with LN undergoing transplant with higher incidence reported from centers doing protocol biopsies [99-101]. In a large study using the UNOS database, Non-Hispanic black race, female gender, and age <33 years were independent risk factors for recurrent LN; median time to develop recurrence was 4.3 years after transplant [101]. The type of immunosuppression did not influence the rate of recurrence.

Presentation is similar to LN in native kidneys with proteinuria, hematuria, and kidney dysfunction. Transplant kidney biopsy will confirm the recurrence; serological parameters are of little help in the diagnosis of recurrent LN [99]. The same pathologic classification is followed for recurrent LN categories as for LN in native kidneys.

Management Post-Transplantation

Induction and maintenance immunosuppressive management could follow the same regimens as for non-lupus patients except that maintenance regimens should always include steroids to minimize the risk of recurrence. In a biopsy series evaluating the pathologic findings in 41 kidney transplant recipients with lupus erythematosus, 22 patients were found to have a recurrence of LN on their biopsy. However, the cases were subclinical and limited to LN classes 1 and 2 [102]. This suggests that transplant immunosuppressive regimens can modulate the immune system and minimize disease progression. In fact, graft failure in patients with SLE is predominantly due to rejection accounting for up to 86% of graft failures [101].

While no specific therapy guidelines exist for treatment of recurrent lupus, in class III, early class IV and Class V lesions, the dose of mycophenolate mofetil could be increased to 2 to 3 g/day [99], with increase of steroid dose, often starting with a pulse methylprednisolone. In more aggressive lesions of class IV with crescents and/or renal dysfunction, cyclophosphamide can be used as in LN of native kidneys. Anti-proliferative agents are to be withheld for the duration of treatment with cyclophosphamide [99]. In resistant recurrent LN, isolated case reports show the benefit of Rituximab.

Despite the risk of recurrence, patients with LN have equivalent allograft survival as that of the general transplant population [97].

Atypical Hemolytic Uremic Syndrome (aHUS)

Overview

Thrombotic microangiopathy (TMA) is a disease process caused by thrombotic occlusions of systemic microvasculature, leading to end-organ ischemia and infarction [103]. TMA is characterized by thrombocytopenia, microangiopathic hemolytic anemia, and organ damage such as acute renal failure. The major types of TMA consist of thrombocytopenic purpura (TTP), hemolytic-uremic syndrome (HUS), and atypical hemolytic uremic syndrome (aHUS), in which the latter is caused by the mutation of complement proteins which causes dysregulation of the balance of complement activation and regulation on endothelial cells. Such mutations can be either acquired or hereditary. It is thought that aHUS occurs as a result of a trigger event (disease, viral infection, medications, pregnancy, brain death, immunosuppressive agent s, etc.) in a person with a genetic susceptibility predisposing them to complement overactivation particularly affecting endothelial surfaces [104]. Therefore, the cornerstone of aHUS treatment is eculizumab, a humanized monoclonal antibody to complement C5 [105]. Treatment should be initiated early to offer renal recovery.

Pre-Transplantation

Patients with aHUS can be evaluated for kidney transplantation but should be cautioned about the risk of recurrence. aHUS is associated with a very high risk of recurrence and subsequent graft loss. Patients with a pathological variant of complement factor H (CFH), Complement Factor I, C3, Complement Factor B, or high titer anti-CFH autoantibodies have 80-90% risk of recurrence [66]. In a cohort of patient with aHUS transplanted before 2009, graft survival was only 51% at 5 years with graft loss being due to recurrence in all cases [106].

It is important to remember that aHUS is a disease due to complement dysfunction; therefore, when allocating a deceased donor organ to these patients, it is best to avoid transplant factors that may trigger the complement system. These include expanded criteria donors at high risk for delayed graft function, and donors with whom there are donor-specific antibodies or a positive cross-match.

Diagnosis

Diagnosis of recurrent aHUS should be suspected when there is allograft dysfunction, hemolytic anemia, and thrombocytopenia. However, not all transplant recipients with aHUS/TMA will have hemolysis and thrombocytopenia. Diagnosis is confirmed with transplant biopsy. The diagnosis of recurrent aHUS can be challenging as allografts can have *de novo* TMA from calcineurin inhibitor toxicity or from acute rejection [107]; however, with the right clinical context and high degree of suspicion, a diagnosis of recurrent aHUS can be made.

Management Post-Transplantation

As in the native kidney, Eculizumab is an effective treatment to prevent aHUS recurrence in the kidney transplant. Before the advent of Eculizumab, one strategy to prevent aHUS recurrence was through performing a combined liver -kidney transplant in an attempt to cure aHUS patients in whom mutations in genes encoding liver-produced circulating factors had been identified such as complement factor H and complement factor B [108]. While this is a suitable strategy to reduce recurrence, liver transplant ation is a high-risk procedure with significant associated risks, including mortality. Therefore, most centers today will add eculizumab on top of standard induction regimen in order to prevent aHUS recurrence. This strategy is successful with centers reporting no recurrences with median follow up of up to 25 months [109]. There is no consensus yet as to the duration of treatment with Eculizumab post-transplant ation.

KDIGO recommends that if a transplant candidate has an abnormality in complement regulation that places them at high risk, they should not proceed with transplantation unless a complement inhibitor can be administered or a combined liver -kidney transplant can be performed [66]. Maintenance immunosuppression with a combination of calcineurin inhibitor and mTOR inhibitor has been associated with higher risk of recurrence [110-112]. This data, however, predates eculizumab widespread use and it is unknown whether this combination is safe in patients on prophylactic eculizumab.

Dysproteinemias

Overview

Dysproteinemias encompass a group of diseases which are characterized by the overproduction of immunoglobulins. These immunoglobulins are monoclonal (MIg) as a result of clonal proliferation of immunoglobulin -producing cells (plasma cells or B cells).

Dysproteinemias can cause acute kidney injury secondary to various forms of injury in different locations in the kidney (Table 1). They can also lead to the progression of ESKD [113].

Table 1. Biopsy findings of different dysproteinemias that can recur in the allograft

	Glomerular Nodularity	Mesangial PAS	Proliferative Changes	Congo Red	Fibrils
Monoclonal immune deposition disease (MIDD) (includes Multiple Myeloma, light chain, and light and heavy chain deposition disease)	Yes	Strong	No	No	No
AL Amyloidosis	Yes	Weak	No	Yes	Yes
Immunotactoid GN	No	No	Yes	No	Yes
PGNMID	No	Weak	Yes	No	No
C3 glomerulopathy	Yes	Weak	Yes	No	No
Cast Nephropathy	No	No	No	No	No
Fibrillary GN	No	Strong	Yes	No	Yes

Most patients with dysproteinemias are asymptomatic on presentation but will have abnormal renal function and unexplained proteinuria. Work-up consists of hematological evaluation, serum and urine electrophoresis, serum immunofixation, serum free light chain analysis, bone marrow biopsy, and kidney biopsy.

In some cases, patients with dysproteinemias can be managed conservatively with ACEI/ARB and close monitoring of their renal function. However, when an active B-cell clone is recognized, treatment should be directed at treating the clone with bortezomib-based regimens, rituximab, and immunomodulators [114]. Treatments are continued until the patient achieves remission. Some diseases will require stem cell transplantation to achieve remission.

Pre-Transplantation

Patients with dysproteinemias are generally contraindicated from kidney transplantation unless they have received curative treatment and are in stable remission [66]. However, a carefully select group of patients may benefit from kidney transplantation. Risks of recurrence post-transplant ation should be discussed with the donor. Below, we briefly discuss the recurrences of specific dysproteinemias.

Monoclonal gammopathy of unknown significance (MGUS) is the most frequently encountered dysproteinemia. In one of the largest studies evaluating 3518 kidney transplant patients between 1963 through 2006, only 42 had a monoclonal protein. Of those, only 23 had MGUS pre-transplant, and 19 had MGUS post-transplant. Despite immunosuppression post-transplantation, only 2 patients progressed to smoldering multiple myeloma (MM) and none had symptomatic MM [115]. In another large study, only 1.6% of kidney transplant recipients had MGUS (30% pre-transplant and 70% post-transplant). None developed MM though 2 patients did develop another hematologic malignancy [116]. Similar findings of no progression to MM following transplantation was found in another large study as well [117].

In 35 patients with multiple myeloma who received a kidney transplant, median patient survival was 9.6 years. 17 patients died during follow-up and causes of death were varied with cardiac and infectious causes being the most common causes of death [118].

In a retrospective review of 923 patients with renal AL amyloidosis of which 221 required dialysis, 21 patients underwent kidney transplantation (unclear whether they were in full remission at the time) [119]. At 5 years post-transplant ation, there was scintigraphic evidence of recurrent amyloid in 6 renal allografts, of which 5 had proteinuria. Nevertheless, one- and 5-year patient survival rates were estimated to be as high as 95.2% and 71.4%, respectively. Two patients died from amyloid with functioning grafts [119].

One of the more challenging dysproteinemias to evaluate and treat is proliferative glomerulonephritis with monoclonal immunoglobulin deposits (PGNMID). This is due to its known very high risk of recurrence post-transplant ation [120, 121]. Approximately 70% of these patients have no detectable monoclonal proteins in serum or urine, making a kidney biopsy the main means of diagnosis. In a series of 20 patients with PGNMID transplanted at Mayo Clinic between 2003 and 2016, 90% had recurrence of their disease within a median of 7 months post-transplantation with 83% of recurrences occurring within the first year post-transplantation. Recurrence was associated with a decline in kidney function with proteinuria of >1.5g/day occurring in only 4 patients [120].

Diagnosis

Recurrence of dysproteinemia is suspected in the setting of allograft dysfunction and proteinuria; kidney biopsy will confirm the diagnosis [122]. Patients will need hematological evaluation as mentioned above.

Management Post-Transplantation

Kidney transplantation followed by autologous hematopoietic cell transplantation offers increased survival in patients with end stage renal disease due to dysproteinemias [123]. Alternatively, kidney transplantation can follow autologous hematopoietic stem cell transplantation [124-126]. These strategies offer survival benefit for the patient and the allograft. Immunosuppressive therapies are generally not targeted to the clone and include standard post-transplant immunosuppressive regimens. The management of dysproteinemia recurrence is challenging and is directed at the clone. Overall, the recurrence of dysproteinemia has been associated with poor outcomes for both patient and allograft [122, 127].

Conclusion

In conclusion, recurrent disease of the allograft represents a significant cause of allograft failure. Different diseases have different rates of recurrences, time to recurrence and associated risks of graft failure. Therefore, having a high suspicion of glomerulonephritis pre-transplant is imperative to allow for appropriate post-transplant management and active surveillance for disease recurrence.

References

[1] Wolfe RA, Ashby VB, Milford EL, Ojo AO, Ettenger RE, Agodoa LY, et al. Comparison of mortality in all patients on dialysis, patients on dialysis awaiting transplantation, and recipients of a first cadaveric transplant. *N Engl J Med.* 1999; 341:1725–30.

[2] Hariharan S, Johnson CP, Bresnahan BA, Taranto SE, McIntosh MJ, Stablein D. Improved graft survival after renal transplantation in the United States, 1988 to 1996. *N Engl J Med.* 2000;342(9):605-12.

[3] Lamb KE, Lodhi S, Meier-Kriesche HU. Long-term renal allograft survival in the United States: a critical reappraisal. *Am J Transplant.* 2011;11(3):450-62.

[4] Saran R, Robinson B, Abbott KC, Agodoa LYC, Bhave N, Bragg-Gresham J, et al. US Renal Data System 2017 Annual Data Report: Epidemiology of Kidney Disease in the United States. *Am J Kidney Dis.* 2018;71(3 Suppl 1):A7.

[5] Saran R, Robinson B, Abbott KC, Bragg-Gresham J, Chen X, Gipson D, et al. US Renal Data System 2019 Annual Data Report: Epidemiology of Kidney Disease in the United States. *Am J Kidney Dis.* 2020;75(1 Suppl 1):A6-a7.

[6] El-Zoghby ZM, Stegall MD, Lager DJ, Kremers WK, Amer H, Gloor JM, et al. Identifying specific causes of kidney allograft loss. *Am J Transplant.* 2009;9(3):527-35.

[7] Briganti EM, Russ GR, McNeil JJ, Atkins RC, Chadban SJ. Risk of renal allograft loss from recurrent glomerulonephritis. *N Engl J Med.* 2002;347(2):103-9.

[8] Cosio FG, Cattran DC. Recent advances in our understanding of recurrent primary glomerulonephritis after kidney transplantation. *Kidney Int.* 2017;91(2):304-14.

[9] Allen PJ, Chadban SJ, Craig JC, Lim WH, Allen RDM, Clayton PA, et al. Recurrent glomerulonephritis after kidney transplantation: risk factors and allograft outcomes. *Kidney Int.* 2017;92(2):461-9.

[10] Regunathan-Shenk R, Avasare RS, Ahn W, Canetta PA, Cohen DJ, Appel GB, et al. Kidney Transplantation in C3 Glomerulopathy: A Case Series. *Am J Kidney Dis.* 2019;73(3):316-23.

[11] Grupper A, Cornell LD, Fervenza FC, Beck LH, Jr., Lorenz E, Cosio FG. Recurrent Membranous Nephropathy After Kidney Transplantation: Treatment and Long-Term Implications. *Transplantation.* 2016;100(12):2710-6.

[12] Uffing A, Pérez-Sáez MJ, Mazzali M, Manfro RC, Bauer AC, de Sottomaior Drumond F, et al. Recurrence of FSGS after Kidney Transplantation in Adults. *Clin J Am Soc Nephrol.* 2020;15(2):247-56.

[13] Rodrigues JC, Haas M, Reich HN. IgA Nephropathy. *Clin J Am Soc Nephrol.* 2017;12(4):677-86.

[14] Levy M, Berger J. Worldwide perspective of IgA nephropathy. *Am J Kidney Dis.* 1988;12(5):340-7.

[15] O'Shaughnessy MM, Hogan SL, Thompson BD, Coppo R, Fogo AB, Jennette JC. Glomerular disease frequencies by race, sex and region: results from the International Kidney Biopsy Survey. *Nephrol Dial Transplant.* 2018;33(4):661-9.

[16] Magistroni R, D'Agati VD, Appel GB, Kiryluk K. New developments in the genetics, pathogenesis, and therapy of IgA nephropathy. *Kidney Int.* 2015; 88(5): 974-89.

[17] Praga M, Gutiérrez E, González E, Morales E, Hernández E. Treatment of IgA nephropathy with ACE inhibitors: a randomized and controlled trial. *J Am Soc Nephrol.* 2003;14(6):1578-83.

[18] Manno C, Torres DD, Rossini M, Pesce F, Schena FP. Randomized controlled clinical trial of corticosteroids plus ACE-inhibitors with long-term follow-up in proteinuric IgA nephropathy. *Nephrol Dial Transplant.* 2009;24(12):3694-701.

[19] Odum J, Peh CA, Clarkson AR, Bannister KM, Seymour AE, Gillis D, et al. Recurrent mesangial IgA nephritis following renal transplantation. *Nephrol Dial Transplant.* 1994;9(3):309-12.

[20] Ortiz F, Gelpi R, Koskinen P, Manonelles A, Räisänen-Sokolowski A, Carrera M, et al. IgA nephropathy recurs early in the graft when assessed by protocol biopsy. *Nephrol Dial Transplant.* 2012;27(6):2553-8.

[21] Avasare RS, Rosenstiel PE, Zaky ZS, Tsapepas DS, Appel GB, Markowitz GS, et al. Predicting Post-Transplant Recurrence of IgA Nephropathy: The Importance of Crescents. *Am J Nephrol.* 2017;45(2):99-106.

[22] Berthoux F, Suzuki H, Mohey H, Maillard N, Mariat C, Novak J, et al. Prognostic Value of Serum Biomarkers of Autoimmunity for Recurrence of IgA Nephropathy after Kidney Transplantation. *J Am Soc Nephrol.* 2017;28(6):1943-50.

[23] Berthelot L, Robert T, Vuiblet V, Tabary T, Braconnier A, Dramé M, et al. Recurrent IgA nephropathy is predicted by altered glycosylated IgA, autoantibodies and soluble CD89 complexes. *Kidney Int.* 2015;88(4):815-22.

[24] Han SS, Huh W, Park SK, Ahn C, Han JS, Kim S, et al. Impact of recurrent disease and chronic allograft nephropathy on the long-term allograft outcome in patients with IgA nephropathy. *Transpl Int.* 2010;23(2):169-75.

[25] Andresdottir MB, Hoitsma AJ, Assmann KJ, Wetzels JF. Favorable outcome of renal transplantation in patients with IgA nephropathy. *Clin Nephrol.* 2001; 56(4): 279-88.

[26] McDonald SP, Russ GR. Recurrence of IgA nephropathy among renal allograft recipients from living donors is greater among those with zero HLA mismatches. *Transplantation.* 2006;82(6):759-62.

[27] Andresdottir MB, Haasnoot GW, Doxiadis, II, Persijn GG, Claas FH. Exclusive characteristics of graft survival and risk factors in recipients with immunoglobulin A nephropathy: a retrospective analysis of registry data. *Transplantation.* 2005;80(8):1012-8.

[28] Blosser CD, Bloom RD. Recurrent glomerular disease after kidney transplantation. *Curr Opin Nephrol Hypertens.* 2017;26(6):501-8.

[29] Wyld ML, Chadban SJ. Recurrent IgA Nephropathy After Kidney Transplantation. *Transplantation.* 2016;100(9):1827-32.

[30] Clayton P, McDonald S, Chadban S. Steroids and recurrent IgA nephropathy after kidney transplantation. *Am J Transplant.* 2011;11(8):1645-9.

[31] Berthoux F, El Deeb S, Mariat C, Diconne E, Laurent B, Thibaudin L. Antithymocyte globulin (ATG) induction therapy and disease recurrence in renal transplant recipients with primary IgA nephropathy. *Transplantation.* 2008;85(10): 1505-7.

[32] Tomas NM, Beck LH, Jr., Meyer-Schwesinger C, Seitz-Polski B, Ma H, Zahner G, et al. Thrombospondin type-1 domain-containing 7A in idiopathic membranous nephropathy. *N Engl J Med.* 2014;371(24):2277-87.

[33] Ronco P, Debiec H. Membranous nephropathy: A fairy tale for immunopathologists, nephrologists and patients. *Mol Immunol.* 2015;68(1):57-62.

[34] Couser WG. Primary Membranous Nephropathy. *Clin J Am Soc Nephrol.* 2017; 12(6):983-97.

[35] Alsharhan L, Beck LH, Jr. Membranous Nephropathy: Core Curriculum 2021. *Am J Kidney Dis.* 2021;77(3):440-53.

[36] Glassock RJ. Diagnosis and natural course of membranous nephropathy. *Semin Nephrol.* 2003;23(4):324-32.

[37] Beck LH, Jr., Bonegio RG, Lambeau G, Beck DM, Powell DW, Cummins TD, et al. M-type phospholipase A2 receptor as target antigen in idiopathic membranous nephropathy. *N Engl J Med.* 2009;361(1):11-21.

[38] Beck LH, Jr., Fervenza FC, Beck DM, Bonegio RG, Malik FA, Erickson SB, et al. Rituximab -induced depletion of anti-PLA2R autoantibodies predicts response in membranous nephropathy. *J Am Soc Nephrol.* 2011;22(8):1543-50.

[39] Sprangers B, Lefkowitz GI, Cohen SD, Stokes MB, Valeri A, Appel GB, et al. Beneficial effect of rituximab in the treatment of recurrent idiopathic membranous nephropathy after kidney transplantation. *Clin J Am Soc Nephrol.* 2010;5(5):790-7.

[40] Rodriguez EF, Cosio FG, Nasr SH, Sethi S, Fidler ME, Stegall MD, et al. The pathology and clinical features of early recurrent membranous glomerulonephritis. *Am J Transplant.* 2012;12(4):1029-38.

[41] Leon J, Pérez-Sáez MJ, Batal I, Beck LH, Jr., Rennke HG, Canaud G, et al. Membranous Nephropathy Posttransplantation: An Update of the Pathophysiology and Management. *Transplantation.* 2019;103(10):1990-2002.

[42] Ward HJ, Koyle MA. Immunopathologic features of de novo membranous nephropathy in renal allografts. *Transplantation.* 1988;45(3):524-9.

[43] Debiec H, Martin L, Jouanneau C, Dautin G, Mesnard L, Rondeau E, et al. Autoantibodies specific for the phospholipase A2 receptor in recurrent and De Novo membranous nephropathy. *Am J Transplant.* 2011;11(10):2144-52.

[44] Blosser CD, Ayalon R, Nair R, Thomas C, Beck LH, Jr. Very early recurrence of anti-Phospholipase A2 receptor -positive membranous nephropathy after transplantation. *Am J Transplant.* 2012;12(6):1637-42.

[45] Leon J, Perez-Saez MJ, Batal I, Beck LH, Jr., Rennke HG, Canaud G, et al. Membranous Nephropathy Posttransplantation: An Update of the Pathophysiology and Management. *Transplantation.* 2019;103(10):1990-2002.

[46] Cosyns JP, Couchoud C, Pouteil-Noble C, Squifflet JP, Pirson Y. Recurrence of membranous nephropathy after renal transplantation: probability, outcome and risk factors. *Clin Nephrol.* 1998;50(3):144-53.

[47] Batal I, Vasilescu ER, Dadhania DM, Adel AA, Husain SA, Avasare R, et al. Association of HLA Typing and Alloimmunity With Posttransplantation Membranous Nephropathy: A Multicenter Case Series. *Am J Kidney Dis.* 2020;76: 374–83.

[48] Stahl R, Hoxha E, Fechner K. PLA2R autoantibodies and recurrent membranous nephropathy after transplantation. *N Engl J Med.* 2010;363(5):496-8.

[49] Quintana LF, Blasco M, Seras M, Pérez NS, López-Hoyos M, Villarroel P, et al. Antiphospholipase A2 Receptor Antibody Levels Predict the Risk of Posttransplantation Recurrence of Membranous Nephropathy. *Transplantation.* 2015;99(8):1709-14.

[50] Couchoud C, Pouteil-Noble C, Colon S, Touraine JL. Recurrence of membranous nephropathy after renal transplantation. Incidence and risk factors in 1614 patients. *Transplantation.* 1995;59(9):1275-9.

[51] Berchtold L, Letouzé E, Alexander MP, Canaud G, Logt AV, Hamilton P, et al. HLA -D and PLA2R1 risk alleles associate with recurrent primary membranous nephropathy in kidney transplant recipients. *Kidney Int.* 2021;99(3):671-85.

[52] Seitz-Polski B, Payré C, Ambrosetti D, Albano L, Cassuto-Viguier E, Berguignat M, et al. Prediction of membranous nephropathy recurrence after transplantation by monitoring of anti-PLA2R1 (M-type phospholipase A2 receptor) autoantibodies: a case series of 15 patients. *Nephrol Dial Transplant.* 2014;29(12):2334-42.

[53] Andrésdóttir MB, Wetzels JF. Increased risk of recurrence of membranous nephropathy after related donor kidney transplantation. *Am J Transplant.* 2012; 12(1):265-6.

[54] Josephson MA, Spargo B, Hollandsworth D, Thistlethwaite JR. The recurrence of recurrent membranous glomerulopathy in a renal transplant recipient: case report and literature review. *Am J Kidney Dis.* 1994;24(5):873-8.

[55] Dabade TS, Grande JP, Norby SM, Fervenza FC, Cosio FG. Recurrent idiopathic membranous nephropathy after kidney transplantation: a surveillance biopsy study. *Am J Transplant.* 2008;8(6):1318-22.

[56] Honda K, Horita S, Toki D, Taneda S, Nitta K, Hattori M, et al. De novo membranous nephropathy and antibody -mediated rejection in transplanted kidney. *Clin Transplant.* 2011;25(2):191-200.

[57] Larsen CP, Walker PD. Phospholipase A2 receptor (PLA2R) staining is useful in the determination of de novo versus recurrent membranous glomerulopathy. *Transplantation.* 2013;95(10):1259-62.

[58] Kearney N, Podolak J, Matsumura L, Houghton D, Troxell M. Patterns of IgG subclass deposits in membranous glomerulonephritis in renal allografts. *Transplant Proc.* 2011;43(10):3743-6.

[59] Bose B, Cattran D. Glomerular diseases: FSGS. *Clin J Am Soc Nephrol.* 2014;9(3): 626-32.

[60] D'Agati VD, Kaskel FJ, Falk RJ. Focal segmental glomerulosclerosis. *N Engl J Med.* 2011;365(25):2398-411.

[61] De Vriese AS, Sethi S, Nath KA, Glassock RJ, Fervenza FC. Differentiating Primary, Genetic, and Secondary FSGS in Adults: A Clinicopathologic Approach. *J Am Soc Nephrol.* 2018;29(3):759-74.

[62] Hommos MS, De Vriese AS, Alexander MP, Sethi S, Vaughan L, Zand L, et al. The Incidence of Primary vs Secondary Focal Segmental Glomerulosclerosis: A Clinicopathologic Study. *Mayo Clin Proc.* 2017;92(12):1772-81.

[63] Sethi S, Zand L, Nasr SH, Glassock RJ, Fervenza FC. Focal and segmental glomerulosclerosis: clinical and kidney biopsy correlations. *Clin Kidney J.* 2014;7(6):531-7.

[64] Laurinavicius A, Hurwitz S, Rennke HG. Collapsing glomerulopathy in HIV and non-HIV patients: a clinicopathological and follow-up study. *Kidney Int.* 1999;56(6):2203-13.

[65] Rovin BH, Caster DJ, Cattran DC, Gibson KL, Hogan JJ, Moeller MJ, et al. Management and treatment of glomerular diseases (part 2): conclusions from a Kidney Disease: Improving Global Outcomes (KDIGO) Controversies Conference. *Kidney Int.* 2019;95(2):281-95.

[66] Chadban SJ, Ahn C, Axelrod DA, Foster BJ, Kasiske BL, Kher V, et al. Summary of the Kidney Disease: Improving Global Outcomes (KDIGO) Clinical Practice Guideline on the Evaluation and Management of Candidates for Kidney Transplantation. *Transplantation.* 2020;104(4):708-14.

[67] Abbott KC, Sawyers ES, Oliver JD, 3rd, Ko CW, Kirk AD, Welch PG, et al. Graft loss due to recurrent focal segmental glomerulosclerosis in renal transplant recipients in the United States. *Am J Kidney Dis.* 2001;37(2):366-73.

[68] Francis A, Trnka P, McTaggart SJ. Long-Term Outcome of Kidney Transplantation in Recipients with Focal Segmental Glomerulosclerosis. *Clin J Am Soc Nephrol.* 2016;11(11):2041-6.

[69] Sener A, Bella AJ, Nguan C, Luke PP, House AA. Focal segmental glomerular sclerosis in renal transplant recipients: predicting early disease recurrence may prolong allograft function. *Clin Transplant.* 2009;23(1):96-100.

[70] Hickson LJ, Gera M, Amer H, Iqbal CW, Moore TB, Milliner DS, et al. Kidney transplantation for primary focal segmental glomerulosclerosis: outcomes and response to therapy for recurrence. *Transplantation.* 2009;87(8):1232-9.

[71] Newstead CG. Recurrent disease in renal transplants. *Nephrol Dial Transplant.* 2003;18 Suppl 6:vi68-74.

[72] Fujisawa M, Iijima K, Ishimura T, Higuchi A, Isotani S, Yoshiya K, et al. Long-term outcome of focal segmental glomerulosclerosis after Japanese pediatric renal transplantation. *Pediatr Nephrol.* 2002;17(3):165-8.

[73] Delville M, Sigdel TK, Wei C, Li J, Hsieh SC, Fornoni A, et al. A circulating antibody panel for pretransplant prediction of FSGS recurrence after kidney transplantation. *Sci Transl Med.* 2014;6(256):256ra136.

[74] Shoji J, Mii A, Terasaki M, Shimizu A. Update on Recurrent Focal Segmental Glomerulosclerosis in Kidney Transplantation. *Nephron.* 2020;144 Suppl 1:65-70.

[75] Santín S, Bullich G, Tazón-Vega B, García-Maset R, Giménez I, Silva I, et al. Clinical utility of genetic testing in children and adults with steroid-resistant nephrotic syndrome. *Clin J Am Soc Nephrol.* 2011;6(5):1139-48.

[76] McCarthy HJ, Bierzynska A, Wherlock M, Ognjanovic M, Kerecuk L, Hegde S, et al. Simultaneous sequencing of 24 genes associated with steroid-resistant nephrotic syndrome. *Clin J Am Soc Nephrol.* 2013;8(4):637-48.

[77] Lipska BS, Iatropoulos P, Maranta R, Caridi G, Ozaltin F, Anarat A, et al. Genetic screening in adolescents with steroid-resistant nephrotic syndrome. *Kidney Int.* 2013;84(1):206-13.

[78] Canaud G, Dion D, Zuber J, Gubler MC, Sberro R, Thervet E, et al. Recurrence of nephrotic syndrome after transplantation in a mixed population of children and adults: course of glomerular lesions and value of the Columbia classification of histological variants of focal and segmental glomerulosclerosis (FSGS). *Nephrol Dial Transplant.* 2010;25(4):1321-8.

[79] Ponticelli C. Recurrence of focal segmental glomerular sclerosis (FSGS) after renal transplantation. *Nephrol Dial Transplant.* 2010;25(1):25-31.

[80] Raina R, Wang J, Sharma A, Chakraborty R. Extracorporeal Therapies in the Treatment of Focal Segmental Glomerulosclerosis. *Blood Purif.* 2020;49(5):513-23.

[81] Colucci M, Labbadia R, Vivarelli M, Camassei FD, Emma F, Dello Strologo L. Ofatumumab rescue treatment in post-transplant recurrence of focal segmental glomerulosclerosis. *Pediatr Nephrol.* 2020;35(2):341-5.

[82] Solomon S, Zolotnitskaya A, Del Rio M. Ofatumumab in post-transplant ation recurrence of focal segmental glomerulosclerosis in a child. *Pediatr Transplant.* 2019;23(4):e13413.

[83] Bernard J, Bruel A, Allain-Launay E, Dantal J, Roussey G. Ofatumumab in post-transplant ation recurrence of a pediatric steroid-resistant idiopathic nephrotic syndrome. *Pediatr Transplant.* 2018;22(4):e13175.

[84] Masani N, Jhaveri KD, Fishbane S. Update on membranoproliferative GN. *Clin J Am Soc Nephrol.* 2014;9(3):600-8.

[85] Lim WH, Shingde M, Wong G. Recurrent and de novo Glomerulonephritis After Kidney Transplantation. *Front Immunol.* 2019;10:1944.

[86] Faedda R, Satta A, Tanda F, Pirisi M, Bartoli E. Immunosuppressive treatment of membranoproliferative glomerulonephritis. *Nephron.* 1994;67(1):59-65.

[87] Lorenz EC, Sethi S, Leung N, Dispenzieri A, Fervenza FC, Cosio FG. Recurrent membranoproliferative glomerulonephritis after kidney transplantation. *Kidney Int.* 2010;77(8):721-8.

[88] Zand L, Lorenz EC, Cosio FG, Fervenza FC, Nasr SH, Gandhi MJ, et al. Clinical findings, pathology, and outcomes of C3GN after kidney transplantation. *J Am Soc Nephrol.* 2014;25(5):1110-7.

[89] Alasfar S, Carter-Monroe N, Rosenberg AZ, Montgomery RA, Alachkar N. Membranoproliferative glomerulonephritis recurrence after kidney transplantation: using the new classification. *BMC Nephrol.* 2016;17:7.

[90] Angelo JR, Bell CS, Braun MC. Allograft failure in kidney transplant recipients with membranoproliferative glomerulonephritis. *Am J Kidney Dis.* 2011;57(2):291-9.

[91] Medjeral-Thomas NR, O'Shaughnessy MM, O'Regan JA, Traynor C, Flanagan M, Wong L, et al. C3 glomerulopathy: clinicopathologic features and predictors of outcome. *Clin J Am Soc Nephrol.* 2014;9(1):46-53.

[92] Muczynski KA. Plasmapheresis maintained renal function in an allograft with recurrent membranoproliferative glomerulonephritis type I. *Am J Nephrol.* 1995;15(5):446-9.

[93] Farooqui M, Alsaad K, Aloudah N, Alhamdan H. Treatment-resistant recurrent membranoproliferative glomerulonephritis in renal allograft responding to rituximab: case report. *Transplant Proc.* 2015;47(3):823-6.

[94] Pérez-Sáez MJ, Toledo K, Navarro MD, Lopez-Andreu M, Redondo MD, Ortega R, et al. Recurrent membranoproliferative glomerulonephritis after second renal graft treated with plasmapheresis and rituximab. *Transplant Proc.* 2011;43(10):4005-9.

[95] Welte T, Arnold F, Kappes J, Seidl M, Häffner K, Bergmann C, et al. Treating C3 glomerulopathy with eculizumab. *BMC Nephrol.* 2018;19(1):7.

[96] Rabasco C, Cavero T, Román E, Rojas-Rivera J, Olea T, Espinosa M, et al. Effectiveness of mycophenolate mofetil in C3 glomerulonephritis. *Kidney Int.* 2015;88(5):1153-60.

[97] Bunnapradist S, Chung P, Peng A, Hong A, Chung P, Lee B, et al. Outcomes of renal transplantation for recipients with lupus nephritis: analysis of the Organ Procurement and Transplantation Network database. *Transplantation.* 2006;82(5): 612-8.

[98] Naveed A, Nilubol C, Melancon JK, Girlanda R, Johnson L, Javaid B. Preemptive kidney transplantation in systemic lupus erythematosus. *Transplant Proc.* 2011;43(10):3713-4.

[99] Lionaki S, Skalioti C, Boletis JN. Kidney transplantation in patients with systemic lupus erythematosus. *World J Transplant.* 2014;4(3):176-82.

[100] Goral S, Ynares C, Shappell SB, Snyder S, Feurer ID, Kazancioglu R, et al. Recurrent lupus nephritis in renal transplant recipients revisited: it is not rare. *Transplantation.* 2003;75(5):651-6.

[101] Contreras G, Mattiazzi A, Guerra G, Ortega LM, Tozman EC, Li H, et al. Recurrence of lupus nephritis after kidney transplantation. *J Am Soc Nephrol.* 2010;21(7):1200-7.

[102] Norby GE, Strøm EH, Midtvedt K, Hartmann A, Gilboe IM, Leivestad T, et al. Recurrent lupus nephritis after kidney transplantation: a surveillance biopsy study. *Ann Rheum Dis.* 2010;69(8):1484-7.

[103] Brocklebank V, Wood KM, Kavanagh D. Thrombotic Microangiopathy and the Kidney. *Clin J Am Soc Nephrol.* 2018;13(2):300-17.

[104] Zuber J, Le Quintrec M, Morris H, Frémeaux-Bacchi V, Loirat C, Legendre C. Targeted strategies in the prevention and management of atypical HUS recurrence after kidney transplantation. *Transplant Rev* (Orlando). 2013;27(4):117-25.

[105] Legendre CM, Licht C, Muus P, Greenbaum LA, Babu S, Bedrosian C, et al. Terminal complement inhibitor eculizumab in atypical hemolytic-uremic syndrome. *N Engl J Med.* 2013;368(23):2169-81.

[106] Le Quintrec M, Zuber J, Moulin B, Kamar N, Jablonski M, Lionet A, et al. Complement genes strongly predict recurrence and graft outcome in adult renal transplant recipients with atypical hemolytic and uremic syndrome. *Am J Transplant.* 2013;13(3):663-75.

[107] Mundra VRR, Mannon RB. Thrombotic Microangiopathy in a Transplant Recipient. *Clin J Am Soc Nephrol.* 2018;13(8):1251-3.

[108] Saland JM, Ruggenenti P, Remuzzi G. Liver-kidney transplantation to cure atypical hemolytic uremic syndrome. *J Am Soc Nephrol.* 2009;20(5):940-9.

[109] Alpay N, Ozçelik U. Renal Transplantation in Patients With Atypical Hemolytic Uremic Syndrome: A Single Center Experience. *Transplant Proc.* 2019;51(7):2295-7.

[110] Fortin MC, Raymond MA, Madore F, Fugère JA, Pâquet M, St-Louis G, et al. Increased risk of thrombotic microangiopathy in patients receiving a cyclosporin-sirolimus combination. *Am J Transplant.* 2004;4(6):946-52.

[111] Robson M, Côte I, Abbs I, Koffman G, Goldsmith D. Thrombotic micro-angiopathy with sirolimus -based immunosuppression: potentiation of calcineurin -inhibitor -induced endothelial damage? *Am J Transplant.* 2003;3(3):324-7.

[112] Lovric S, Kielstein JT, Kayser D, Bröcker V, Becker JU, Hiss M, et al. Combination of everolimus with calcineurin inhibitor medication resulted in post-transplant haemolytic uraemic syndrome in lung transplant recipients --a case series. *Nephrol Dial Transplant.* 2011;26(9):3032-8.

[113] Hogan JJ, Weiss BM. Bridging the Divide: An Onco-Nephrologic Approach to the Monoclonal Gammopathies of Renal Significance. *Clin J Am Soc Nephrol.* 2016;11(9):1681-91.

[114] Varga C, Titus SE, Toskic D, Comenzo RL. Use of novel therapies in the treatment of light chain amyloidosis. *Blood Rev.* 2019;37:100581.

[115] Naina HV, Harris S, Dispenzieri A, Cosio FG, Habermann TM, Stegall MD, et al. Long-term follow-up of patients with monoclonal gammopathy of undetermined significance after kidney transplantation. *Am J Nephrol.* 2012;35(4):365-71.

[116] Cuéllar-García C, Sevillano Ruiz-Mateos C, Mazuecos Blanca MA, Narvaez Mejia C, Fernandez Valle MC, Martin Reina V, et al. Follow-up monoclonal gammopathy of undetermined significance in kidney transplant. *Transplant Proc.* 2015;47(1):78-80.

[117] Soltero L, Carbajal H, Xu J, McCarthy J, Suki WN, Gaber AO, et al. Initial survival data of kidney transplant patients with pre-transplant monoclonal gammopathy. *Clin Transplant.* 2012;26(2):300-4.

[118] Tsakiris DJ, Stel VS, Finne P, Fraser E, Heaf J, de Meester J, et al. Incidence and outcome of patients starting renal replacement therapy for end-stage renal disease due to multiple myeloma or light -chain deposit disease: an ERA -EDTA Registry study. *Nephrol Dial Transplant.* 2010;25(4):1200-6.

[119] Pinney JH, Lachmann HJ, Bansi L, Wechalekar AD, Gilbertson JA, Rowczenio D, et al. Outcome in renal Al amyloidosis after chemotherapy. *J Clin Oncol.* 2011;29(6):674-81.

[120] Buxeda A, Said SM, Nasr SH, Leung N, El Ters M, Cosio FG. Recurrent Proliferative Glomerulonephritis With Monoclonal Immunoglobulin Deposits in Kidney Allografts Treated With Anti-CD20 Antibodies. *Transplantation.* 2019;103(7):1477-85.

[121] Said SM, Cosio FG, Valeri AM, Leung N, Sethi S, Salameh H, et al. Proliferative glomerulonephritis with monoclonal immunoglobulin G deposits is associated with high rate of early recurrence in the allograft. *Kidney Int.* 2018;94(1):159-69.

[122] Kamal J, Khairallah P, Crew RJ, Ye X, Swanson SJ, Kudose S, et al. Clinicopathologic Assessment of Monoclonal Immunoglobulin-associated Renal Disease in the Kidney Allograft: A Retrospective Study and Review of the Literature. *Transplantation.* 2020;104(7):1341-9.

[123] Sánchez Quintana A, Rull PR, Atienza JB, McDonnell CN. Renal transplant in plasma cell dyscrasias with lenalidomide treatment after autologous stem cell transplantation. *Nephrology* (Carlton, Vic). 2013;18(9):641-3.

[124] Badros A, Barlogie B, Siegel E, Roberts J, Langmaid C, Zangari M, et al. Results of autologous stem cell transplant in multiple myeloma patients with renal failure. *Br J Haematol.* 2001;114(4):822-9.

[125] Barraclough KA, Dowling JP, Schwarer AP, Perry GJ. Sequential autologous peripheral blood stem cell transplantation and kidney transplantaion of light chain deposition disease. *Nephrol Dial Transplant.* 2007;22(4):1268-9.

[126] Beitinjaneh A, Burns LJ, Majhail NS. Solid organ transplantation in survivors of hematopoietic cell transplantation: a single institution case series and literature review. *Clin Transplant.* 2010;24(4):E94-102.

[127] Nambirajan A, Bhowmik D, Singh G, Agarwal SK, Dinda AK. Monoclonal gammopathy of renal significance with light -chain deposition disease diagnosed postrenal transplant: a diagnostic and therapeutic challenge. *Transpl Int.* 2015;28(3):375-9.

In: Issues in Kidney Disease – Transplantation
Editors: B. V. R. Murthy and S. Z. Fadem

ISBN: 978-1-53619-960-4

Chapter 12

LONG-TERM CARE OF THE KIDNEY TRANSPLANT RECIPIENT

Joseph Alge*[1]*, MD and Jenny S. Pan*[2,*]*, MD
[1]Division of Nephrology, Department of Pediatrics,
Baylor College of Medicine, Houston, TX, USA
[2]Selzman Institute for Kidney Health, Section of Nephrology,
and Michael E. DeBakey Veterans Affairs Medical Center,
Baylor College of Medicine, Houston, TX, USA

ABSTRACT

Transplantation has become the treatment of choice for patients with end-stage kidney disease (ESKD). Significant improvements in short-term outcomes have translated into a growing number of kidney transplant recipients (KTRs) with long-functioning allografts. In addition to transplant-related care, those providing long-term care to KTRs must be cognizant of the complex medical issues that commonly affect these patients. Early recognition of these comorbidities after transplantation and appropriate management can improve patient and allograft survival. Topics including overview of the long-term care of KTRs, monitoring for allograft dysfunction and transplant failure, immunosuppression and common medical issues that affect the kidney transplant recipient (e.g., cardiovascular disease, hypertension, diabetes, obesity, infectious complications, bone disease, malignancy, vaccination and pregnancy) are discussed in this chapter. Although some aspects of kidney transplantation are similar in adults and children, pediatric KTRs are a unique population with issues that warrant special consideration. Key differences in long-term care of pediatric kidney transplant recipients versus adults are also addressed in this section.

* Corresponding Author's Email: jenny.pan@bcm.edu.

Keywords: kidney transplantation, immunosuppression, allograft dysfunction, cardiovascular health, mineral bone disease, anemia, opportunistic infection, vaccination, family planning and pregnancy, pediatric transplant recipient

INTRODUCTION

The first successful kidney transplant was performed in 1954. Since then, transplantation has become the treatment of choice for patients with end-stage kidney disease (ESKD). Due to significant advances in immunosuppression, transplantation practices, and management of comorbid conditions, short-term outcomes after kidney transplantation have steadily improved. This has resulted in a large number of patients with long functioning allografts who have unique and complex long-term medical care needs. In the early post-transplant period, the focus was on optimization of graft function, prevention of perioperative complications, acute rejection, and opportunistic infection. The aims for long-term care of the kidney transplant recipient are to preserve good allograft function, ensure adherence to medication, follow-up and recommended general health maintenance, and prevent the long-term consequences of immunosuppression.

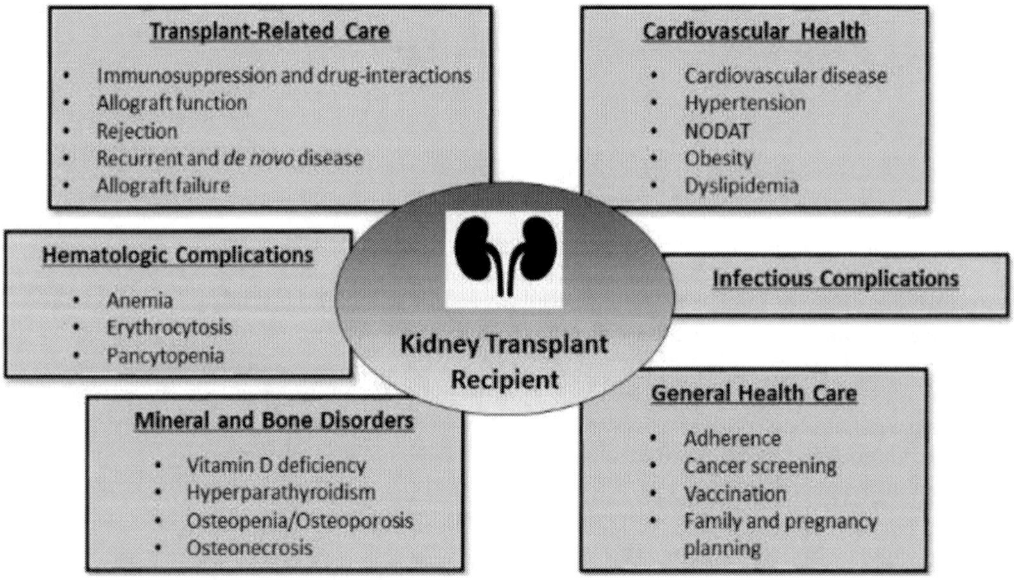

Figure 1. Long-term care of the kidney transplant recipient key components.

Due to the high prevalence of pre-transplant cardiovascular disease (CVD) and cardiovascular risk factors, as well as exacerbation of these risk factors by immunosuppressive agents post-transplant, CVD remains a leading cause of long-term morbidity and mortality in kidney transplant recipients. Aggressive cardiovascular risk factor identification and modification are important components of post-transplant care. Due to the need to remain on chronic immunosuppression, kidney transplant recipients (KTRs) will always remain at higher risk for infections including opportunistic pathogens. Care of the kidney transplant recipient requires remaining diligent for potential infections, having knowledge of antimicrobial therapy needed, and developing a vaccination plan. With the successes of kidney transplantation, post-transplant pregnancies have become more common [1]. Thus, all KTRs with childbearing potential must receive counseling about contraception and pregnancy planning. These (cardiovascular health, infectious complications, family planning and pregnancy) and other key components of the long-term medical care of KTRs (Figure 1) are discussed in this section.

Nearly half of all kidney transplant recipients will be alive with functioning transplants 10 years after transplantation. The total number of kidney transplant recipients alive with a functioning graft is on track to pass 250,000 in the next 1-2 years [2]. Due to a limited number of transplant nephrologists, constraints of transplant centers and other factors, many KTRs will receive most of their long-term care from providers in the community. It is important for general nephrologists and internists to be familiar with the unique medical issues and care requirements that these patients need, which includes effective care coordination and communication between transplant centers and community providers. Optimization of long-term care can significantly improve patient and allograft outcomes.

TRANSPLANT-RELATED CARE

Immunosuppression

A detailed review of the classes of immunosuppressive agents and immunosuppression strategies in kidney transplantation is presented elsewhere in this book. An overview of immunosuppression monitoring in the long-term care of kidney transplant recipients is discussed in this section. With a functioning allograft, KTRs require maintenance immunosuppressive medication indefinitely. One essential purpose of the follow-up visits over the long term is monitoring and reinforcing the importance of continued adherence to the immunosuppression regimen. Non-adherence is a major risk for late rejection and kidney allograft failure [3]. Thus, issues hindering compliance such as financial constraints, medication side effects, and lack of understanding of the importance of the medications prescribed need to be promptly addressed.

Most patients are prescribed triple therapy as maintenance, consisting of a calcineurin -inhibitor (CNI), an antiproliferative agent, and corticosteroids [4]. The combination of tacrolimus (TAC), mycophenolate mofetil (MMF) and corticosteroids are associated with the lowest rates of acute rejection, superior graft function, and patient survival [5]. In some patients, other immunosuppressive agents may be used for specific indications. For example, mycophenolate may be switched to sirolimus in patients with post-transplant malignancy or switched to azathioprine during pregnancy. As recipients are further from transplantation, target levels for the immunosuppressive agents are lower. However, many immunosuppressive agents have a narrow therapeutic window. Thus, it is imperative to continue close monitoring of drug levels in the long-term recipients. Typically, tacrolimus, cyclosporine or sirolimus levels are monitored at each clinic visit. Levels should also be checked when any medication with possible interactions is prescribed or when there is unexplained graft dysfunction [4]. There are numerous classes of drugs, foods and supplements that interact with immunosuppressive medications, particularly CNIs. It is important for healthcare providers caring for KTRs to be familiar with the most common drug interaction s, and consider consulting a transplant pharmacist before introducing new medications. Patients should be educated on the potential for drug interactions and advised to consult with their transplant provider before starting or stopping medications and supplements. Lastly, in the long-term care of KTRs, the use of generic medication can substantially reduce cost. However, generic medications may not be identical in strength or bioavailability as the brand-name drug or other generic formulations. It is important that the patient and prescriber are made aware of any change in a prescribed immunosuppressive medication, including a change to a generic drug. Kidney Disease Improving Global Outcomes (KDIGO) recommends that after switching to a generic medication it is monitored using blood levels. In addition, obtain levels and adjust the dose as often as necessary until a stable therapeutic target is achieved [6].

Monitoring Allograft Function and Transplant Failure

Regular monitoring of kidney function is required throughout the life of the transplanted kidney, even in stable patients. Most transplant centers report patient visits at least every 3 to 6 months after the first year [7]. Allograft function is monitored through the measurement of serum creatinine values and urinalyses; rise in serum creatinine or proteinuria both warrant further evaluation. In the late post-transplant period, allograft dysfunction may present with either acute kidney injury (AKI) or a slow decline in graft function. The major causes of AKI post-transplant include decreased kidney perfusion (e.g., volume depletion, transplant renal artery stenosis, CNI toxicity), obstruction from ureteral stricture, neurogenic bladder or prostatic hypertrophy, drug toxicity, and infection (e.g., transplant pyelonephritis, BK virus). Acute rejection (antibody -mediated or cellular) is uncommon in the late post-transplant period but should be suspected if immunosuppression was recently reduced or if there is concern for medication non-adherence. Rejection can also manifest as chronic antibody-mediated rejection (CAMR), which is typically characterized by a slow, progressive decline in graft function, increasing proteinuria, and worsening hypertension. CAMR is the most common cause of transplant failure after the first year [8]. The topic of kidney transplant rejection is reviewed in detail elsewhere in this book.

Another major cause of kidney allograft dysfunction and transplant failure is glomerulonephritis, either recurrent or *de novo*. The cumulative incidence of allograft glomerulonephritis is reported to be 5% at 1-year, 22% at 5-years, and 42% at 10-years post-transplant [8]. The most common glomerulonephritis to recur post-transplant are focal segmental glomerulosclerosis (FSGS), membranous nephropathy, membranoproliferative glomerulonephritis (MPGN), hemolytic uremic syndromes (HUS), and IgA nephropathy. A detailed review of recurrent disease after kidney transplantation is presented elsewhere in this book. The most common *de novo* glomerulonephritis post-transplant are FSGS and IgA nephropathy. Risk factors for development of *de novo* FSGS include conditions that lead to reduction in nephron mass with compensatory hyperfiltration (e.g., diabetes, BK nephropathy, CNI therapy, rejection) and sirolimus -associated podocyte injury [9]. *De novo* membranous nephropathy and MPGN primarily related to secondary causes including viral infection s, rejection, CNI and thrombotic microangiopathy can also occur, but are much less common. An allograft biopsy is indicated in any patient presenting with proteinuria, hematuria, and a decline in kidney function to evaluate for acute or chronic rejection and allograft glomerulonephritis.

Lastly, despite significant improvement in short-term outcomes after kidney transplant, long-term allograft survival remains a challenge. Thus, an important component of the long-term care of KTRs is providing guidance when the transplant stops working. The physician must provide psychosocial support as the patient may have difficulty accepting the loss of his/her transplant and develop depression [10]. Other issues to address include: 1) planning for return to dialysis; 2) the decision to maintain, taper or withdraw immunosuppression; 3) need for transplant nephrectomy; and 4) planning for re-transplantation if appropriate. These issues are discussed in detail elsewhere in this book.

INFECTIOUS COMPLICATIONS

Infections are common in kidney transplant recipients predominantly due to the use of immunosuppressive medications. An individual patient's risk of infection is determined by the intensity of immunosuppression and epidemiologic exposures, including donor-derived infections, recipient-derived infections present at the time of transplantation, nosocomial infections, and community -acquired infections. Generally, the incidence and type of common infectious complications can be divided into 3 distinct time periods after transplantation: 1) the first month; 2) the second through the sixth months; and 3) the late post-transplant period beyond 6 months.

Infections during the first month after transplantation are typically post-surgical infections similar to those observed in non-immunosuppressed patients. These include urinary tract infections (UTIs), wound infection s, pneumonia, and line-associated infections. Allograft-related surgical complications such as lymphocele, perigraft hematoma or urine leak increase the risk of early post-transplant infections [11]. Infections in the donor can also be transmitted to the recipient, including viral infections (e.g., viral hepatitis, West Nile virus), bacteria from a donor with bacteremia or bacteriuria, and fungal infections (e.g., histoplasma, cryptococcus). Other early infectious complications may result from undetected pre-existing infections in the recipient that are exacerbated by immunosuppression. Opportunistic infections are uncommon in this early post-transplant period.

Opportunistic infections are most likely to occur during the second to sixth month post-transplant period. Cytomegalovirus (CMV), BK virus, *Pneumocystis jiroveci pneumonia* (PJP), *Nocardia*, and *Listeria monocytogenes* are some of the common pathogens. KTRs are routinely administered prophylactic antimicrobial therapy against CMV, PJP and oral candidiasis soon after transplant surgery. Duration of prophylaxis is determined by the CMV status of the donor and recipient, as well as the intensity of immunosuppression administered to the patient. In the long-term transplant recipient, prophylactic therapy may need to be restarted in the setting of treatment for acute rejection.

In recipients with well-functioning allografts, the risk of infection diminishes after six months due to reduction in overall immunosuppression. The most common infections in this time period are community -acquired respiratory illnesses, UTIs, and other infections that affect the general population. However, opportunistic infections must also be considered. As an example, while CMV reactivation/disease typically occurs 1 to 4 months post-transplant, it may manifest later especially within a few months after prophylaxis is discontinued [12]. Those who provide care for kidney transplant recipients must always be aware of their increased susceptibility to infection. Furthermore, it is important to recognize that due to the use of immunosuppressive medication, patients may not present with the usual signs and symptoms of infection, such as fever and leukocytosis. Infectious complications after kidney transplantation are reviewed in detail elsewhere in this book.

Cardiovascular Health

Although successful kidney transplantation improves long-term survival in patients with ESKD compared to dialysis therapy, recipients remain at higher risk for cardiovascular disease (CVD)-related morbidity and mortality when compared with the general population [13]. In addition to the high prevalence of pre-existing cardiovascular risk factors and CVD in patients receiving kidney transplants, recipients encounter additional risk factors post-transplant that result in the development of CVD. These include adverse effects of immunosuppression on blood pressure, diabetes and lipid metabolism, as well as obesity, chronic inflammation, proteinuria, and chronic anemia [14]. Several of these risk factors are described in further detail below. CVD is the leading cause of death with a functioning graft in kidney transplant recipients (KTRs). Thus, it is important to optimize CVD care post-transplant. Aggressive risk factor identification and modification have the potential to significantly impact long-term patient and allograft survival .

Hypertension

Hypertension is the most common CVD risk factor in KTRs, occurring in up to 80% of patients. In addition to essential hypertension, transplant -related factors such as allograft dysfunction, use of immunosuppressive medication (calcineurin inhibitors and corticosteroids), and transplant renal artery stenosis contribute to the pathogenesis of *de novo* hypertension post-transplant [15]. Aggressive management of blood pressure in the long-term care of KTRs is imperative, as hypertension is associated with adverse cardiovascular outcomes, CVD-related mortality, and allograft dysfunction [16]. A retrospective cohort analysis of KTRs found that every 10mmHg increase in systolic blood pressure was associated with a 5% increased risk of allograft failure and death [15].

Although there are no trials examining optimal blood pressure targets in KTRs, published guidelines recommend a treatment goal of <130/80 mmHg [6, 17]. Patients should be counseled on lifestyle modifications, including dietary sodium restriction, weight loss, smoking cessation, and physical exercise. In addition, the majority of KTRs will require antihypertensive medication to achieve target blood pressure. Most classes of antihypertensive medications can be used and are effective in treating KTRs, but it is important to be familiar with potential drug interactions and side effects in this population. The American College of Cardiology Foundation/American Heart Association 2017 Guidelines on Blood Pressure Management recommended calcium channel blockers (CCBs) as the initial drug of choice. The vasodilatory properties of CCBs may counteract the vasoconstrictive and nephrotoxic effects of calcineurin inhibitors (CNIs), leading to improved glomerular filtration rate and allograft survival [18]. However, verapamil and diltiazem both increase CNI levels with potential for overimmunosuppression and nephrotoxicity; CNI blood levels must be monitored closely if therapy with these CCBs is initiated or the dose is adjusted. ACE-inhibitors or ARBs are recommended in KTRs with significant proteinuria (≥1 g/day) and/or diabetes due to their potential protective effects against hyperfiltration -mediated injury and CNI-induced fibrosis [6, 12]; potential side effects include hyperkalemia, allograft dysfunction, and anemia. β-blockers are recommended in patients with CVD. Diuretics can be useful as CNI- and corticosteroid-related hypertension can be sodium dependent. Patients on diuretic therapy should be monitored closely for volume depletion and electrolyte abnormalities.

New-Onset Diabetes after Transplantation (NODAT)

The prevalence of pre-existing diabetes is high in patients receiving kidney transplants, as diabetes is the most common cause of ESKD. In addition, several risk factors post-transplant lead to worsening of pre-existing diabetes and the development of new-onset diabetes after transplantation (NODAT), which affects up to 40% of transplant recipients [8]. Risk factors for the development of NODAT include weight gain, hepatitis C virus (HCV) infection, and immunosuppressive medications (CNIs, steroids, mTOR-inhibitors). CNIs are known to affect pancreatic beta cell function, with tacrolimus being more diabetogenic compared to cyclosporine [19]. mTOR-inhibitors may also increase the risk of NODAT by reducing pancreatic beta cell proliferation and decreasing insulin sensitivity [14]. All KTRs should be screened periodically for diabetes, and management of diabetic patients should follow the American Diabetes Association treatment guidelines. Weight loss, dietary modification, and exercise should be encouraged, and referral to an endocrinologist and/or dietician may be of benefit. In addition, consider modifying the immunosuppressive regimen including withdrawing or reducing the dose of steroids, CNIs, and mTOR-inhibitors. However, the benefits must be carefully weighed against the increased risk of rejection, especially with steroid withdrawal .

Obesity

Weight gain is common post-kidney transplant with most patients gaining an average of 5-10% in the first year [14]. The etiology of weight gain is multifactorial, including improved appetite with restoration of kidney function, increased caloric intake, and lack of physical activity. Corticosteroid use may also increase appetite; however, weight gain in patients on steroid-withdrawal immunosuppressive regimens appears similar to those on steroid therapy [20]. Obesity is an independent risk factor for CVD, and exacerbates other CVD risk factors, including hypertension, NODAT, dyslipidemia, metabolic syndrome, and inflammation. Thus, BMI should be assessed at each clinic visit, and kidney transplant patients need to be counseled early and routinely on lifestyle measures to maintain a healthy weight or to achieve weight loss targets.

Dyslipidemia

The prevalence of dyslipidemia is high post-kidney transplant due to effects of immunosuppressive medications and common comorbid conditions such as obesity, NODAT, and proteinuria. The Assessment of Lescol in Renal Transplantation (ALERT) study showed a significant reduction in LDL cholesterol, risk of myocardial infarction, and

CVD -related mortality in recipients treated with fluvastatin [21]. KDIGO guidelines recommend measuring fasting lipids on an annual basis and treating all KTRs with a statin regardless of LDL concentration [6, 22]. Fenofibrates can be used in patients with significant hypertriglyceridemia. However, note that statins and fibrates can interact with CNIs, increasing the risk of hepatitis, myositis, and rhabdomyolysis [23]. Ezetimibe has been shown to be well-tolerated when used alone or in combination with statin therapy in KTRs. Immunosuppressive agents that have been associated with dyslipidemia include corticosteroids, mTOR-inhibitors, and cyclosporine [6]. Dose reduction or a switch to alternative immunosuppressive agents (e.g., cyclosporine to tacrolimus) may improve dyslipidemia.

Mineral and Bone Disorders

Disorders of bone and mineral metabolism are common after kidney transplantation. KTRs have unique risk factors for bone disease, including pre-existing renal osteodystrophy, persistent alterations in mineral and bone disease (MBD) parameters, hypogonadism, age -related bone loss, and deleterious effects of immunosuppressive agents on osteoblast/osteoclast activity [24]. The spectrum of bone and mineral metabolism abnormalities commonly encountered post-transplant includes hypophosphatemia, hypercalcemia, vitamin D deficiency, secondary and tertiary hyperparathyroidism, osteoporosis, and osteonecrosis. Bone fracture rates are high – between 6 to 45% have been reported after kidney transplantation [23]. Osteonecrosis, a pathological condition characterized by bone death strongly associated with steroid use, has been reported to occur in up to 40% of patients post-transplant [24]. These bone disorders are associated with significant morbidity in KTRs, and in the case of osteonecrosis, there is no proven therapy once it develops. Thus, monitoring of bone and mineral metabolism parameters and institution of preventive and therapeutic measures are essential in all KTRs, and should begin early after transplantation and continue over the long-term. Biochemical assessment should include routine measurement of serum calcium, phosphorus, 25-hydroxyvitamin D, and intact parathyroid hormone levels (iPTH) [25]. It is recommended that dual X-ray absorptiometry (DXA) scans be obtained at regular intervals after transplantation, although significant limitations remain in using DXA to predict fracture risk in this patient population. After the immediate post-kidney transplant period, the frequency of monitoring should be based on the rate of progression of CKD, the presence and magnitude of abnormalities, and whether the patient is receiving treatments for CKD-MBD.

Treatment of MBD post-transplant requires a multifactorial approach with ultimate focus on bone health, instead of focusing on individual lab abnormalities. General measures such as regular exercise, weight resistance training, and avoidance of alcohol and smoking should be encouraged to prevent bone loss. In patients at high risk of fractures, consider use of a steroid avoidance protocol or rapid taper of prednisone to below 7.5 mg/day. It is important to recognize that other medications commonly used post-transplant can contribute to bone loss, including tacrolimus, sirolimus, and proton pump inhibitors [26, 27]. Reversal of MBD abnormalities (e.g., hypophosphatemia, hypo- or hypercalcemia) and vitamin D deficiency is the focus of initial management. With successful transplantation, iPTH levels may slowly decline over the first year as spontaneous regression of the hyperplastic parathyroid gland occurs. Cinacalcet is used for the management of severe hypercalcemia associated with tertiary hyperparathyroidism, and parathyroidectomy is reserved for patients who fail medical therapy [24]. Consider employing antiresorptive agents (e.g., bisphosphonates, denosumab, teriparatide) in patients with substantially reduced bone mineral density (BMD) and elevated markers of bone turnover. However, while these agents improve BMD, no evidence exists for changes in fracture risk in KTRs. Furthermore, bisphosphonate use and oversuppression of PTH can lead to adynamic bone disease.

Hematologic Complications

Hematologic disorders after kidney transplantation are frequently observed. In the long-term follow-up of KTRs, a complete blood count should be performed at regular intervals, and after any change in medication that may cause leukopenia, anemia, or thrombocytopenia [6]. The most common post-transplant hematologic complications are peripheral blood cytopenias and post-transplant erythrocytosis. While other hematologic disorders are observed, including thrombotic microangiopathy, post-transplant lymphoproliferative disorder, and the hemophagocytic syndrome, they are not discussed in this section.

Leukopenia and thrombocytopenia in either isolation or involving all three cell lines (pancytopenia) occur most frequently in the first six months after kidney transplantation. The predominant cause is myelosuppression due to immunosuppressive agents (e.g., mycophenolate, sirolimus, lymphocyte depleting drugs), prophylactic antimicrobial drugs (e.g., bactrim, valcyte), and CMV infection. Treatment typically consists of dose reduction or discontinuation of causative medications. However, this may increase the risk of acute rejection or CMV reactivation/disease, and recipients need to be monitored closely for the development of these complications .

Post-transplant erythrocytosis, defined as hemoglobin > 17 g/dL or hematocrit > 51%, is commonly observed in patients with excellent graft function. The pathophysiological mechanism is thought to be due to excess erythropoietin production by the remaining native kidneys, which is not affected by negative feedback mechanisms [28]. Erythrocytosis increases plasma viscosity and may cause thrombotic events. ACE-inhibitors and ARBs are associated with a drop in hemoglobin in KTRs, and may be used to manage post-transplant erythrocytosis. In rare cases, phlebotomy is used in patients who do not respond to treatment with ACE-inhibitors or ARBs and in those who present with a hemoglobin > 18.5 mg/dL.

Anemia is the most common hematologic disorder encountered in long-term care of the kidney transplant recipient. Contributory factors include reduced allograft function, effects of commonly prescribed medications (e.g., mycophenolate, azathioprine, sirolimus, ACE-inhibitors), iron deficiency, infections (e.g., parvovirus B19), and an increased inflammatory state. Underlying causes of anemia should be identified and treated. Chronic anemia in KTRs should be managed in the same way as other patients with CKD [6].

General Health Maintenance and Preventive Care

Cancer Screening

It is important to recognize that malignancies are more common in kidney transplant recipients (KTRs) than in the general population due to chronic use of immunosuppressive medications. Non-melanomatous cancers of the skin and lip are the most common malignancies in KTRs. Other cancers that have a higher incidence after transplantation include Kaposi's sarcoma, non-Hodgkin's lymphoma, renal cell carcinoma (RCC), post-transplant lymphoproliferative disorders (PTLD), and cervical cancer [12, 23]. Patients should be counseled regarding sun protection measures and undergo skin surveillance by a healthcare professional annually. Age appropriate screening for cervical, breast, colon, and prostate cancer as recommended for the general population should be performed. Although RCCs are seen more frequently post-transplant, there are no established screening guidelines; hematuria in KTRs warrants evaluation for urologic malignancies in both the native and transplanted kidneys [8]. In patients diagnosed with cancer after transplantation, reduction in immunosuppression may be required, especially for cancers that are virally related (e.g., Kaposi's sarcoma, PTLD). Studies have suggested that a switch from calcineurin -inhibitor to mTOR-inhibitor may be beneficial in certain cancers due to its anti-proliferative properties [29]. The chapter on "Malignancies After Transplantation" in this book provides a detailed review of this topic.

Vaccination

Kidney transplant recipients are at increased risk for more severe clinical illness caused by infections, thus vaccination is a critical component of preventing infection -related morbidity and mortality. Vaccination status should be reviewed in all transplant recipients and a vaccination plan should be developed during the first post-transplant visit. Due to their immunosuppressed condition, the efficacy of vaccines may be lower in KTRs than in the general population [12]. Although the optimal timing of vaccination after transplantation has not been fully evaluated, most centers restart vaccination 3-6 months post-transplant when immunosuppression is generally reduced to maintenance levels; vaccination during active treatment of rejection should also be avoided. The 2009 KDIGO transplant work group recommended avoiding vaccinations in the first 6 months post-transplant. An exception is the influenza vaccine, which can be given as early as one-month post-transplant prior to the onset of the annual influenza season, regardless of status of immunosuppression [6].

All KTRs are encouraged to receive inactivated vaccines unless contraindicated. These include the diphtheria-pertussis -tetanus, haemophilus influenza B, hepatitis A and B, streptococcus pneumonia conjugated and polysaccharide (PCV13 and PPSV23), inactivated polio, influenza, meningococcus, and recombinant herpes zoster (Shingrix) vaccines [6]. In general, the guidelines for administration of these vaccines should follow that of the general population. Some vaccine -specific recommendations include: 1) annual influenza vaccination; 2) pneumococcal vaccination every 5 years after initial vaccination; and 3) annual hepatitis B surface antibody (HBsAb) titers and revaccination if the titer falls below 10 mIU/mL. KTRs need to be educated about avoiding live vaccines, such as the intranasal influenza, MMR (measles, mumps, and rubella), smallpox, live oral polio, yellow fever, and shingles (Zostavax) vaccines given the increased risk of infection. However, there is accumulating data that certain live-attenuated vaccines may be given to select post-transplant patients safely (e.g., pediatric population); appropriate counseling and close follow-up should be provided in these specific cases. The 2019 American Society of Transplantation updated guidelines on vaccination of solid organ transplant candidates and recipients can be referred to for more detailed recommendations [30].

Family Planning and Pregnancy

Chronic kidney disease is associated with decreased fertility; pregnancies are uncommon in patients with advanced CKD [31]. However, fertility is improved and often restored to normal in both male and female recipients soon after successful kidney transplantation [32]. Thus, it is important for physicians caring for recipients to counsel those with childbearing potential about contraception and pregnancy planning early and frequently after transplantation. Male fertility may be affected by immunosuppressive medications. For example, sirolimus is associated with low sperm count and reduced testosterone; male KTRs who wish to maintain fertility may consider avoiding sirolimus or banking sperm prior to sirolimus use [6]. Pregnancies fathered by KTRs appear to have similar outcomes compared to the general population.

Although successful pregnancies within the first year post-transplant have been reported, it is recommended that female KTRs wait for at least 1 year after transplantation without acute rejection before pregnancy [6, 33]. In fact, pregnancy within the first 2 years post-transplant may increase the risk of graft loss [34]. It is also recommended that women who wish to become pregnant meet these additional criteria before conception: 1) stable estimated GFR with serum creatinine < 1.5 mg/dL; 2) proteinuria < 1 g/day; 3) no recent episodes of acute rejection; 4) well-controlled blood pressure; and 5) discontinued/replaced teratogenic medications (e.g., mycophenolate, ACE-inhibitor, ARB) [8]. Mycophenolate has been reported to cause severe fetal malformations, including cleft lip and palate, microtia, and absence of external auditory canals [35, 36]. Thus, mycophenolate should be discontinued or changed to azathioprine at least 6-weeks, ideally 3-months, before conception. There is limited safety data on the use of mTOR-inhibitors and pregnancy. However, the FDA -approved package labeling for sirolimus notes that the drug was embryo/fetotoxic in animal studies when given in doses approximately 0.2 to 0.5 times the human doses adjusted for body surface area. Thus, the 2009 KDIGO transplant work group recommended that mTOR-inhibitors be discontinued or replaced before pregnancy is attempted [6]. Prednisone, azathioprine, cyclosporine and tacrolimus are generally considered safe in pregnancy when used at standard doses.

Table 1. Special considerations in pediatric kidney transplant recipients

- **Cause of End-Stage Kidney Disease (ESKD)**
  - *Congenital anomalies of the kidneys and urinary tract (CAKUT)*
  - *Genetic diseases*
- **Immunosuppression**
  - *Corticosteroid avoidance due to adverse effects on growth*
  - *Differences in immunobiology and drug metabolism*
- **Detection of Rejection**
  - *Low baseline serum creatinine and minimal change with mild rejection due to small body size*
- **Infectious Complications**
  - *Naïve to common infections pre-transplant (e.g., CMV, EBV)*
  - *Incomplete vaccination status pre-transplant*
- **Psychosocial Determinants of Health**
  - *Dependence on adult caregivers*
  - *Impact of ESKD and transplantation on physical, emotional, and sexual growth*
  - *Risk of non-adherence during adolescence*
- **Transitional Care to Adult Nephrology**

Pregnant transplant recipients should be managed in close conjunction by a transplant nephrologist and a high-risk obstetrician. It is important to monitor closely for the development of medical complications such as worsening hypertension, preeclampsia, urinary tract infection, worsening anemia, intrauterine growth retardation and preterm delivery, which are more common for pregnancies in KTRs. Blood levels of certain immunosuppressive drugs need to be monitored more frequently due to increase in the volume of distribution and metabolism by the placenta. For example, a 20-25% dose elevation of CNIs from pre-pregnancy levels is typically required [37]. Vaginal delivery is safe and is neither affected by, nor does it affect, the transplant kidney; cesarean sections should only be performed for obstetrical indications. Breastfeeding is not contraindicated for transplant recipients taking prednisone, azathioprine, cyclosporine, tacrolimus or sirolimus [38]; the amount of these immunosuppressive drugs in breastmilk is minimal. Data is lacking for mycophenolate and belatacept, and breastfeeding should be avoided in transplant recipients taking these immunosuppressive drugs.

Table 2. Clinical pearls

- Significant improvements in short-term outcomes after kidney transplantation has resulted in a large number of patients with long functioning allografts who have unique and complex long-term medical care needs.
- Major causes of allograft dysfunction in the late post-transplant period include decreased kidney perfusion (e.g., volume depletion, transplant renal artery stenosis, CNI toxicity), obstruction, drug toxicity, infections (e.g., transplant pyelonephritis, BK virus), rejection (acute or CAMR), and recurrent or *de novo* glomerulonephritis .
- Immunosuppressive medications contribute to the development of many medical issues after kidney transplantation, including hypertension, obesity, new-onset diabetes, anemia, and bone disorders.
- Cardiovascular disease (CVD) remains a leading cause of death with a functioning graft in kidney transplant recipients, so optimizing CVD care post-transplant is imperative.
- The spectrum of bone and mineral metabolism abnormalities commonly encountered post-transplant includes hypophosphatemia, hypercalcemia, vitamin D deficiency, secondary and tertiary hyperparathyroidism, osteoporosis, and osteonecrosis.
- Transplant recipients are at increased risk for certain malignancies (e.g., non-melanomatous skin cancer s, Kaposi's sarcoma, RCC, leukemia) as compared to the general population, primarily due to chronic use of immunosuppressive medications.
- In general, kidney transplant recipients are encouraged to receive inactivated vaccines as per the general population, but should avoid live vaccines.
- It is important to counsel recipients with childbearing potential about contraception and pregnancy planning early and frequently after transplantation. Several commonly used post-transplant medications are teratogenic.
- "Children are not little adults " and long-term care of the pediatric kidney transplant recipient requires consideration of distinct issues including: 1) the impact of CAKUT and genetic diseases post-transplant; 2) the effects of immunosuppression on growth; 3) a unique infection risk profile; and 4) the transition to adult nephrology care.

Long-Term Care of the Pediatric Kidney Transplant Recipient

"Children are not little adults ." The pediatrician 's mantra applies to kidney transplantation, and in this section we give special consideration to the key features that distinguish pediatric kidney transplant recipients from their adult counterparts. Long-term care of this special population requires a nuanced understanding of several key issues including: 1) the most common of causes of end-stage kidney disease in children and the impact of congenital anomalies on the patient's post-transplant care; 2) immunosuppression and detection of allograft rejection; 3) unique infection risk profile of children; and 4) the unique psychosocial challenges that impact the care of children with kidney disease (Table 1). While volumes have been written on these topics, the following is intended to be a primer for the physician tasked with caring for a member of this unique patient population.

Causes of End-Stage Kidney Disease in Children

Causes of ESKD in children differ dramatically from that of adults. Congenital anomalies of the kidneys and urinary tract (CAKUT) are the most common underlying etiology of ESKD in children, accounting for approximately 30% of all cases and with disproportionate representation in younger age groups [39, 40]. CAKUT is a catch-all term for structural kidney diseases that includes conditions as varied as renal aplasia /dysplasia /hypoplasia, obstructive uropathies, such as posterior urethral valves, and reflux nephropathy secondary to vesicoureteral reflux (VUR). Focal segmental glomerulosclerosis is the second most common cause of ESKD in children, but tends to present at a later age, and is more common among black children [39, 40]. Other important causes of pediatric ESKD include genetic conditions such as Alport syndrome, cystic kidney diseases (autosomal recessive polycystic kidney disease and nephronophthisis), cystinosis, and primary hyperoxaluria. Causes of primary and secondary glomerulonephritis, such as lupus nephritis also merit mention. Lastly, it is noteworthy that many children with ESKD develop kidney disease in the setting of the management of other clinical conditions such as malignancy, cardiac disease, or liver disease .

The clinical heterogeneity of pediatric ESKD is a stark contrast with adult ESKD and each disease requires a specialized approach to post-transplant care. In particular, children with ESKD due to CAKUT often have comorbid urologic issues that impact their care in the pre- and post-transplant period. These children generally continue to make a significant amount of urine output after progression to end-stage, and they will frequently have persistent VUR and recurrent urinary tract infections (UTI). While native urine output diminishes post-transplant, native nephrectomy is sometimes performed before transplant to reduce the risk of UTI after transplant. Children with certain genitourinary anomalies need surgical intervention such as creation of an open vesicostomy or a catheterizable appendico-vesicostomy, and bladder augmentation, in which bladder volume is expanded using a segment of the ileum in order to reduce intravesical pressure or increase capacity. Success of kidney transplantation in these children depends upon appropriate management of their underlying urologic issues after transplant.

As previously mentioned, many children with ESKD have a primary genetic cause, and it is critical to understand the non-renal manifestations of the conditions and to recognize the limitations of kidney transplantation for these patients. For instance, patients with X-linked Alport syndrome suffer from sensorineural hearing loss in addition to kidney failure, and while kidney transplantation addresses their kidney disease, hearing impairment has a significant negative impact on quality of life. In more dramatic fashion, kidney transplant alone is not curative for some conditions, such as autosomal recessive polycystic kidney disease, primary hyperoxaluria, and methylmalonic acidemia, and patients with these conditions require dual liver -kidney transplantation. Finally, it is important to remember that if kidney transplant is successful, children with genetic kidney diseases will grow up into adults with heritable genetic kidney diseases, and so genetic counseling for the purposes of family planning is prudent.

Immunosuppression and Allograft Rejection

Like adults, pediatric kidney transplant recipients require careful long-term management of immunosuppression to prevent rejection, and outcomes are generally excellent with a 5-year allograft survival of 95% for living donors and 90% for deceased donors [40]. Following induction of immunosuppression at the time of transplant, children typically receive a combination of a calcineurin inhibitor (CNI) and mycophenolate for maintenance immunosuppression. Corticosteroids are generally avoided due to their adverse effects, including impaired growth, although they may be used for children who are on a steroid-based immunosuppression regimen pre-transplant. Tacrolimus is the preferred CNI due to its lower risk of rejection and chronic allograft nephropathy compared to cyclosporine [41, 42]. Tacrolimus trough levels must be closely monitored, and many factors including drug interaction s, certain foods, and gastrointestinal illness can affect its absorption and metabolism. As in adult KTRs, higher drug levels are targeted in the early post-transplant period to maximize immunosuppression, and the target level is slowly decreased over the first several months after transplant. Goals may be adjusted if there is an episode of rejection or opportunistic infection. An important component of management includes monitoring for adverse effects of immunosuppressive medications, including acute kidney injury (tacrolimus), diabetes (tacrolimus and corticosteroids) and cytopenias (mycophenolate).

Allograft rejection is the chief concern for the pediatric nephrologist, although the rate of acute rejection has declined in recent years following improvements in immunosuppression [40]. The diagnosis, staging, and treatment of rejection is similar to that of adults, and three general types of acute rejection are observed cellular, antibody - mediated, and vascular rejection. Detection of early or mild rejection is more challenging in children. Pediatric kidney transplant recipients typically have a low baseline creatinine due to their comparatively small body size relative to a high glomerular filtration rate, and therefore a large reduction in kidney function is necessary to cause a significant change in the patient's serum creatinine. For this reason, many pediatric transplant centers perform surveillance biopsies at set time points after transplant, although this practice is somewhat controversial [43].

Immunity and Infection

Immunosuppressed children, like adults, are at increased risk of infection, and pediatric kidney transplant recipients should receive prophylactic antimicrobial therapy against candidal infection, *Pneumocystis jiroveci* pneumonia (PJP), and CMV infection for the first six months after transplantation. Nystatin or fluconazole are appropriate for antifungal prophylaxis; the former is preferred because fluconazole inhibits metabolism of tacrolimus [44]. Thus, patients on fluconazole prophylaxis require significantly lower doses of tacrolimus to achieve therapeutic drug levels and, conversely, missing doses of fluconazole can precipitously decrease the tacrolimus level and increase the risk of rejection. Trimethoprim-sulfamethoxazole is typically used for PJP prophylaxis. However, if patients have delayed graft function, prolonged renal insufficiency, or cytopenias, then inhaled pentamidine may be substituted. For prevention of reactivation of latent CMV infection, patients are treated with prophylactic ganciclovir or valganciclovir. Pediatric kidney recipients have a significantly higher rate of CMV negativity at the time of transplantation and a higher risk of post-transplant primary CMV infection. High-risk patients, that is these recipients who are CMV seronegative and receive an organ from a seropositive donor, may also receive anti-CMV immunoglobulin and should undergo regular surveillance testing for CMV reactivation with plasma viral load measurement. In addition to these infections, pediatric kidney transplant recipients are at risk of reactivation of latent Epstein-Barr virus (EBV) and BK polyomavirus infections, particularly if the recipient is naive to these infections. Patients who are EBV seronegative and receive a kidney from an EBV positive donor are at increased risk of post-transplant lymphoproliferative disorder (PTLD), which occurs in about 1-3.5% of pediatric kidney transplant recipients, and these patients should undergo routine evaluation for EBV reactivation using quantitative PCR blood testing [40, 45]. While CMV and EBV serology are routinely ascertained for both the donor and recipient prior to transplantation, BK virus testing is not done. However, the incidence of BK nephropathy in pediatric kidney transplant recipients is 4-5% in the first 2 years after transplant, and one-fourth of patients with BK nephropathy develop graft failure within the next 2 years [46]. The diagnosis of BK nephropathy should be suspected whenever there is significant allograft dysfunction. *BK viruria* and *BK viremia* can be detected by PCR in urine and blood, respectively, and the diagnosis is confirmed histologically on biopsy. In addition to the allograft injury caused by BK virus infection, there is a heightened risk of rejection because the mainstay of management of BK nephropathy (and reactivation of other viruses) is reduction in immunosuppression. In summary, the long-term care of the pediatric kidney transplant recipient involves a variety of measures to prevent infectious complications from immunosuppression and vigilant monitoring for early signs of serious infections.

In addition to the previously discussed infections, children who undergo kidney transplantation have a unique infection risk profile compared to adults. While there are important differences between the immune system of a child, compared to that of an adult, a detailed analysis of the nuances of pediatric immunobiology is beyond the scope of this discussion. Suffice to say, the immune system continues to develop throughout childhood and children are often naive to common pathogens. Therefore, children with ESKD should be protected from infection by updating their immunizations prior to transplantation, and it is also important to verify immunity with serological titers and provide boosters as needed before transplant because patients with advanced or end-stage kidney disease may not respond appropriately to vaccination. Like adults, pediatric transplant recipients generally should not receive live vaccinations, but certain live-attenuated vaccines (MMR and varicella) might be given to carefully selected post-transplant patients safely [30]. Maintaining an up-to-date vaccination status, including annual influenza vaccination, is a critically important component of preventive medicine for pediatric kidney transplant patients.

Psychosocial Determinants of Health in Pediatric Kidney Transplant Recipients

Children are uniquely impacted by psychosocial determinants of health, and the kidney transplant recipient is no exception. Pediatric kidney transplant recipients are entirely dependent on their adult caregivers for their medications and transportation to follow up appointments, and caregivers must undergo rigorous education in the peri-transplant period to ensure that the child receives adequate care after transplant. In the post-transplant period, special attention is required to identify psychosocial stress ors that could negatively impact the transplant recipient and increase the risk of medical non-adherence, such as divorce, parental unemployment, the birth of a sibling, etc. Additionally, children with end-stage kidney disease have high rates of depression and neurocognitive impairment, and many of these psychological comorbidities persist and can negatively impact post-transplant outcomes [47, 48]. Finally, it is important to note that rates of rejection and graft loss increase dramatically during adolescence and young adulthood [49]. The end goal for the pediatric nephrologist is to assist the patient and their caregivers to navigate the obstacles that arise after transplant, especially during this challenging period and, ultimately, to help the patient become independent of their caregivers and successfully transition to adult nephrology care.

CONCLUSION

Significant improvements in short-term outcomes after kidney transplantation has resulted in a large number of patients with long functioning allografts. This unique patient population has complex long-term medical care needs, including transplant -related care and management of comorbidities that are often exacerbated by chronic use of immunosuppressive medications. The aims for long-term care of the kidney transplant recipient are to preserve good allograft function, ensure adherence to medication, follow-up and recommended general health maintenance, and prevent the long-term consequences of immunosuppression. Early recognition of these medical issues after transplantation and implementing the respective management strategies may improve long-term patient and allograft outcomes.

REFERENCES

[1] McKay DB, Josephson MA. Pregnancy after kidney transplantation. *Clin J Am Soc Nephrol.*, 2008, 3 Suppl 2, S117-25.

[2] Hart A, Smith JM, Skeans MA, Gustafson SK, Wilk AR, Castro S, et al. OPTN/SRTR 2018 Annual Data Report: Kidney. *Am J Transplant.*, 2020, 20 Suppl s1, 20-130.

[3] Scheel J, Reber S, Stoessel L, Waldmann E, Jank S, Eckardt KU, et al. Patient-reported non-adherence and immunosuppressant trough levels are associated with rejection after renal transplantation. *BMC Nephrol.*, 2017, 18(1), 107.

[4] Baker RJ, Mark PB, Patel RK, Stevens KK, Palmer N. Renal association clinical practice guideline in post-operative care in the kidney transplant recipient. *BMC Nephrol.*, 2017, 18(1), 174.

[5] Ekberg H, Tedesco-Silva H, Demirbas A, Vitko S, Nashan B, Gurkan A, et al. Reduced exposure to calcineurin inhibitors in renal transplantation. *N Engl J Med.*, 2007, 357(25), 2562-75.

[6] Kasiske BL, Zeier MG, Chapman JR, Craig JC, Ekberg H, Garvey CA, et al. KDIGO clinical practice guideline for the care of kidney transplant recipients: a summary. *Kidney Int.*, 2010, 77(4), 299-311.

[7] Kasiske BL, Vazquez MA, Harmon WE, Brown RS, Danovitch GM, Gaston RS, et al. Recommendations for the outpatient surveillance of renal transplant recipients. American Society of Transplantation. *J Am Soc Nephrol.*, 2000, 11 Suppl 15, S1-86.

[8] Voora S, Adey DB. Management of Kidney Transplant Recipients by General Nephrologists: Core Curriculum 2019. *Am J Kidney Dis.*, 2019, 73(6), 866-79.

[9] Lim WH, Shingde M, Wong G. Recurrent and de novo Glomerulonephritis After Kidney Transplantation. *Front Immunol.*, 2019, 10, 1944.

[10] Messa P, Ponticelli C, Berardinelli L. Coming back to dialysis after kidney transplant failure. *Nephrol Dial Transplant.*, 2008, 23(9), 2738-42.

[11] Khoury JA, Brennan DC. Infectious complications in kidney transplant recipients: review of the literature. *Saudi J Kidney Dis Transpl.*, 2005, 16(4), 453-97.

[12] Cohen D, Galbraith C. General health management and long-term care of the renal transplant recipient. *Am J Kidney Dis.*, 2001, 38(6 Suppl 6), S10-24.

[13] Ojo AO. Cardiovascular complications after renal transplantation and their prevention. *Transplantation.*, 2006, 82(5), 603-11.

[14] Rangaswami J, Mathew RO, Parasuraman R, Tantisattamo E, Lubetzky M, Rao S, et al. Cardiovascular disease in the kidney transplant recipient: epidemiology, diagnosis and management strategies. *Nephrol Dial Transplant.*, 2019, 34(5), 760-73.

[15] Kasiske BL, Anjum S, Shah R, Skogen J, Kandaswamy C, Danielson B, et al. Hypertension after kidney transplantation. *Am J Kidney Dis.*, 2004, 43(6), 1071-81.

[16] Opelz G, Dohler B. Collaborative Transplant, S. Improved long-term outcomes after renal transplantation associated with blood pressure control. *Am J Transplant.*, 2005, 5(11), 2725-31.

[17] Whelton PK, Carey RM, Aronow WS, Casey DE, Jr. Collins KJ, Dennison Himmelfarb C, et al. 2017 ACC/AHA/AAPA/ABC/ACPM/AGS/ APhA/ASH/ ASPC/NMA/PCNA Guideline for the Prevention; Detection; Evaluation; and Management of High Blood Pressure in Adults: A Report of the American College of Cardiology/American Heart Association Task Force on Clinical Practice Guidelines. *J Am Coll Cardiol.*, 2018, 71(19), e127-e248.

[18] Cross NB, Webster AC, Masson P, O'Connell PJ, Craig JC. Antihypertensive treatment for kidney transplant recipients. *Cochrane Database Syst Rev.*, 2009, (3), CD003598.

[19] Vincenti F, Friman S, Scheuermann E, Rostaing L, Jenssen T, Campistol JM, et al. Results of an international, randomized trial comparing glucose metabolism disorders and outcome with cyclosporine versus tacrolimus. *Am J Transplant.*, 2007, 7(6), 1506-14.

[20] de Oliveira CM, Moura AE, Goncalves L, Pinheiro LS, Pinheiro FM, Jr. Esmeraldo RM. Post-transplantation weight gain: prevalence and the impact of steroid-free therapy. *Transplant Proc.*, 2014, 46(6), 1735-40.

[21] Holdaas H, Fellstrom B, Cole E, Nyberg G, Olsson AG, Pedersen TR, et al. Long-term cardiac outcomes in renal transplant recipients receiving fluvastatin: the ALERT extension study. *Am J Transplant.*, 2005, 5(12), 2929-36.

[22] Wanner C, Tonelli M. Kidney Disease: Improving Global Outcomes Lipid Guideline Development Work Group M. KDIGO Clinical Practice Guideline for Lipid Management in CKD: summary of recommendation statements and clinical approach to the patient. *Kidney Int.*, 2014, 85(6), 1303-9.

[23] Schaefer HM. Long-term management of the kidney transplant recipient. *Blood Purif.*, 2012, 33(1-3), 205-11.

[24] Vangala C, Pan J, Cotton RT, Ramanathan V. Mineral and Bone Disorders After Kidney Transplantation. *Front Med* (Lausanne)., 2018, 5, 211.

[25] Isakova T, Nickolas TL, Denburg M, Yarlagadda S, Weiner DE, Gutierrez OM, et al. KDOQI US Commentary on the 2017 KDIGO Clinical Practice Guideline Update for the Diagnosis, Evaluation, Prevention, and Treatment of Chronic Kidney Disease-Mineral and Bone Disorder (CKD -MBD). *Am J Kidney Dis.*, 2017, 70(6), 737-51.

[26] Martin-Fernandez M, Rubert M, Montero M, de la Piedra C. Effects of Cyclosporine, Tacrolimus, and Rapamycin on Osteoblasts. *Transplant Proc.*, 2017, 49(9), 2219-24.

[27] Lenihan CR, Sukumaran Nair S, Vangala C, Ramanathan V, Montez-Rath ME, Winkelmayer WC. Proton Pump Inhibitor Use and Risk of Hip Fracture in Kidney Transplant Recipients. *Am J Kidney Dis.*, 2017, 69(5), 595-601.

[28] Reindl-Schwaighofer R, Oberbauer R. Blood disorders after kidney transplantation. *Transplant Rev* (Orlando)., 2014, 28(2), 63-75.

[29] Mathew T, Kreis H, Friend P. Two-year incidence of malignancy in sirolimus - treated renal transplant recipients: results from five multicenter studies. *Clin Transplant.*, 2004, 18(4), 446-9.

[30] Danziger-Isakov L, Kumar D, Practice AICo. Vaccination of solid organ transplant candidates and recipients: Guidelines from the American society of transplantation infectious diseases community of practice. *Clin Transplant.*, 2019, 33(9), e13563.

[31] Reddy SS, Holley JL. Management of the pregnant chronic dialysis patient. *Adv Chronic Kidney Dis.*, 2007, 14(2), 146-55.

[32] Kim HW, Seok HJ, Kim TH, Han DJ, Yang WS, Park SK. The experience of pregnancy after renal transplantation: pregnancies even within postoperative 1 year may be tolerable. *Transplantation.*, 2008, 85(10), 1412-9.

[33] Sarkar M, Bramham K, Moritz MJ, Coscia L. Reproductive health in women following abdominal organ transplant. *Am J Transplant.*, 2018, 18(5), 1068-76.

[34] Rose C, Gill J, Zalunardo N, Johnston O, Mehrotra A, Gill JS. Timing of Pregnancy After Kidney Transplantation and Risk of Allograft Failure. *Am J Transplant.*, 2016, 16(8), 2360-7.

[35] Le Ray C, Coulomb A, Elefant E, Frydman R, Audibert F. Mycophenolate mofetil in pregnancy after renal transplantation: a case of major fetal malformations. *Obstet Gynecol.*, 2004, 103(5 Pt 2), 1091-4.

[36] Sifontis NM, Coscia LA, Constantinescu S, Lavelanet AF, Moritz MJ, Armenti VT. Pregnancy outcomes in solid organ transplant recipients with exposure to mycophenolate mofetil or sirolimus. *Transplantation.*, 2006, 82(12), 1698-702.

[37] Shah S, Verma P. Overview of Pregnancy in Renal Transplant Patients. *Int J Nephrol.*, 2016, 2016, 4539342.

[38] Constantinescu S, Pai A, Coscia LA, Davison JM, Moritz MJ, Armenti VT. Breast-feeding after transplantation. *Best Pract Res Clin Obstet Gynaecol.*, 2014, 28(8), 1163-73.

[39] Saran R, Robinson B, Abbott KC, Bragg-Gresham J, Chen X, Gipson D, et al. US Renal Data System 2019 Annual Data Report: Epidemiology of Kidney Disease in the United States. *Am J Kidney Dis.*, 2020, 75(1 Suppl 1), A6-A7.

[40] Chua A, Cramer C, Moudgil A, Martz K, Smith J, Blydt-Hansen T, et al. Kidney transplant practice patterns and outcome benchmarks over 30 years: The 2018 report of the NAPRTCS. *Pediatr Transplant.*, 2019, 23(8), e13597.

[41] Trompeter R, Filler G, Webb NJ, Watson AR, Milford DV, Tyden G, et al. Randomized trial of tacrolimus versus cyclosporin microemulsion in renal transplantation. *Pediatr Nephrol.*, 2002, 17(3), 141-9.

[42] Meier M, Nitschke M, Weidtmann B, Jabs WJ, Wong W, Suefke S, et al. Slowing the progression of chronic allograft nephropathy by conversion from cyclosporine to tacrolimus: a randomized controlled trial. *Transplantation.*, 2006, 81(7), 1035-40.

[43] Rose EM, Kennedy SE, Mackie FE. Surveillance biopsies after paediatric kidney transplantation: A review. *Pediatr Transplant.*, 2016, 20(6), 748-55.

[44] Mahnke CB, Sutton RM, Venkataramanan R, Michaels M, Kurland G, Boyle GJ, et al. Tacrolimus dosage requirements after initiation of azole antifungal therapy in pediatric thoracic organ transplantation. *Pediatr Transplant.*, 2003, 7(6), 474-8.

[45] Francis A, Johnson DW, Teixeira-Pinto A, Craig JC, Wong G. Incidence and predictors of post-transplant lymphoproliferative disease after kidney transplantation during adulthood and childhood: a registry study. *Nephrol Dial Transplant.*, 2018, 33(5), 881-9.

[46] Smith JM, Dharnidharka VR, Talley L, Martz K, McDonald RA. BK virus nephropathy in pediatric renal transplant recipients: an analysis of the North America n Pediatric Renal Trials and Collaborative Studies (NAPRTCS) registry. *Clin J Am Soc Nephrol.*, 2007, 2(5), 1037-42.

[47] Kogon AJ, Matheson MB, Flynn JT, Gerson AC, Warady BA, Furth SL, et al. Depressive Symptoms in Children with Chronic Kidney Disease. *J Pediatr.*, 2016, 168, 164-70 e1.

[48] Ruebner RL, Laney N, Kim JY, Hartung EA, Hooper SR, Radcliffe J, et al. Neurocognitive Dysfunction in Children, Adolescents, and Young Adults With CKD. *Am J Kidney Dis.*, 2016, 67(4), 567-75.

[49] Van Arendonk KJ, James NT, Boyarsky BJ, Garonzik-Wang JM, Orandi BJ, Magee JC, et al. Age at graft loss after pediatric kidney transplantation: exploring the high-risk age window. *Clin J Am Soc Nephrol.*, 2013, 8(6), 1019-26.

In: Issues in Kidney Disease – Transplantation
Editors: B. V. R. Murthy and S. Z. Fadem
ISBN: 978-1-53619-960-4

Chapter 13

SHORT AND LONG-TERM OUTCOMES AFTER KIDNEY TRANSPLANTATION

Elizabeth Godfrey*, MD and Abbas Rana, MD
Division of Abdominal Transplantation, Department of Surgery,
Baylor College of Medicine, Houston, TX, USA

ABSTRACT

Short-term outcomes of kidney transplantation – those pertaining to the first year – are excellent across the US and peer nations. Patient survival is over 95%, and graft survival well over 90%. The traditional challenges of the perioperative period and early post-transplant period have included hyperacute and acute rejection, now sharply curtailed by pre-transplant matching and highly effective induction protocols. The switch to the relatively well-tolerated tacrolimus and mycophenolate mofetil regimen used in the majority of transplant recipients has provided stable and effective immunosuppression and reduced infection rates, presumably by providing stable coverage that requires fewer high-intensity pulses of immunosuppression. Delayed graft function (DGF) remains a challenge which cannot easily be resolved, particularly given its frequency in deceased donor and extended criteria allografts, with both a high material and personal cost for transplant recipients. However, with assiduous rejection prevention and medical management, its impact on long-term function can be attenuated. Post-transplant hospitalizations are particularly impressive areas of improvement, likely in large part due to excellent pre-transplant optimization practices.

Long-term outcomes of kidney transplantation are also good, and have improved in recent years, although they have been far outpaced by the improvements in short-term outcomes. Graft half-life is now between 10 and 13 years for a deceased donor allograft, and despite increasing medical complexity and waiting times, recipients are doing better, and surviving longer. Some of this is due to improvements in medication options and immunosuppression and some due to improved dialysis outcomes, among other strides. Long-term therapy remains a tight rope walk between rejection and infection, with lifelong

* Corresponding Author's Emails: Elizabeth.Godfrey@yale.edu or ElizabethLGodfrey@gmail.com.

immunosuppression carrying risks of diabetes, other metabolic disorder s, and ultimately both cardiovascular and malignant disease. Multidisciplinary management including lifestyle and medication-based management of comorbidities, robust surveillance for malignancy, and a high index of suspicion for infection – whether typical or atypical – remain the cornerstones of long-term care.

Keywords: renal transplantation, graft survival, patient survival

Introduction

Short-term outcomes – those within the first year after transplantation – and long-term outcomes – those after the first year – have significantly improved over the years in the US and across the world. These successes have been made possible by the development of effective and safe immunosuppressive drugs, highly effective induction protocols, and significant advances in management of acute rejection aided by the discovery of highly effective drugs targeting the crucial steps of the immune reaction. While significant advances have been made in long-term outcomes after kidney transplantation, these were also limited because of several complications. Some of these complications are a consequence of immunosuppression such as infections or malignancy, some because of adverse effects of medications such as new onset diabetes and hypertension, and others because of complications of original disease causing end-stage renal disease such as diabetes and hypertension. But what is creditable is that these outcomes have been achieved despite increasing complexity of comorbidities. This chapter discusses these aspects in detail and attempts to bring out the continuing challenges and opportunities in further improving these outcomes.

Short-Term Outcomes of Kidney Transplantation

Short-term outcomes – that is, within the first year after transplantation – are excellent in the United States, encouraged ever-upward in part by close regulatory scrutiny. First-year outcomes, in fact, are comparable to or better than much of the western world, including Australia, New Zealand, the UK, the European continent, and Canada [1, 2].

Short-Term Patient and Graft Survival

Patient and graft survival in the first year after transplantation has been trending slowly upward most years since 2000, according to the US Renal Data System's recent annual reports [3–5]. The most up-to-date 1-year patient survival rate is 95.4% for recipients of deceased donor transplants, and 98.8% for recipients of living donor transplants. Graft survival is just slightly lower, at 93% and 96.9% for deceased and living donor recipients, respectively. This is up from the 94% one-year patient survival and 97% graft survival reported for patients who received deceased donor transplants back in 1999 [4].

These improvements occur despite an increasing age and medical complexity at the time of both listing and transplantation. It has been noted that the proportion of older recipients rose from 3.4% in 1990 to 18.4% by 2011, with an increase in the proportion of female and African American recipients, dialysis vintage, obesity, and prevalence of hypertension and diabetes – yet one-year survival after transplantation even among recipients 75 years and older improved from 79% to 89% in the same period [6]. Beyond merely survival, graft function as assessed by estimated glomerular filtration rate (eGFR) at one year after transplant has been demonstrated to be largely stable since the early 2000s despite increasingly unfavorable donor and recipient demographics [7]. Even the small but growing population of human immunodeficiency virus (HIV) positive kidney transplant recipients have experienced improved patient and graft survival, with or without HIV-specific center experience [8].

These improvements are due in part to immunologic factors like optimized cross-matching and immunosuppression, particularly the transition to tacrolimus and mycophenolate as the most common maintenance regimen, and various induction protocols [7, 9, 10]. Technical refinement and excellence, of course, has a role in the most immediate post-operative outcomes. Finally, comorbidity management and pre- and perioperative optimization strongly contribute to the excellent outcomes observed in the short term. This is supported by the relatively greater patient and graft survival gains among patients with diabetes, and a recent meta-analysis by Foroutan et al. who demonstrated that comorbidities such as obesity, diabetes, and hypertension are no longer independently associated with graft loss [10–12]. Although more directly associated with waiting list survival gains, dialysis technology and practice have improved and, logically, such improvements are likely also protective in the post-operative period relative to older techniques [13].

Short-Term Complications

Among the most immediate negative outcomes in renal transplantation is hyperacute rejection, a form of rejection that begins intraoperatively once perfusion is restored to the allograft, as the recipient's pre-formed antibodies, usually against ABO- or HLA -antigens, immediately bind to the graft and initiate destruction of graft tissues. Hyperacute rejection is generally irreversible and necessitates transplant nephrectomy. Fortunately, pre-transplant ABO typing and HLA cross-matching have made hyperacute rejection an extremely rare and almost completely preventable event in modern transplantation. While not recently studied among adult recipients in the United States, the rate in pediatric recipients is now less than 1% [14]. Hyperacute rejection has also been nearly eliminated among even ABO-incompatible transplants, as antibody -targeted regimens including plasmapheresis, IVIG, rituximab, and other immunoadsorption methods have been implemented in renal transplantation worldwide [15, 16].

Delayed hyperacute rejection or accelerated acute rejection (AAR) also involves preformed antibodies and prior sensitization but, rather than occurring immediately due to a high titer of antibodies, it occurs days after transplantation when alloresponse from memory B- and plasma cells triggers increasing donor-specific antibodies (DSA) titers [17]. Pre-transplantation crossmatching may be negative even if patients are sensitized. No recent studies have reported on the overall incidence of AAR, but it has been reported periodically particularly in multiparous women, although alloimmunization, particularly to HLA, may also be observed in individuals with prior transplants or blood transfusion s. While not always reversible, immunosuppressive treatments including a combination of intensified dosing, plasmapheresis, anti-thymocyte globulin, and switching to tacrolimus /mycophenolate, if another regimen was previously in use, have been successful in the past [18, 19]. In other words, as the name "accelerated acute rejection" would suggest, management is similar to management of acute antibody -mediated rejection in general.

Aside from hyperacute rejection, early graft loss (EGL) after kidney transplantation, generally defined as graft loss within 30 days of transplantation, remains an issue affecting short-term outcomes. Early graft loss may describe primary allograft non-function – the graft's failure to provide any appreciable renal function at any point – or secondary non-function when some initial function is detectable but then diminishes. Graft loss particularly in the first 30 days can be caused by donor kidney injury, vascular occlusion, preservation injury, ureteral or other post-renal injury, and rejection [20, 21]. Early graft loss is relatively rare and continuing to decrease; the United States data as represented in the OPTN STAR kidney file suggests a rate of only 0.6% of early death-censored graft failure in the recent 2011-2017 era, down from 7.1% in 1984-1990 [22]. Rates were demonstrated to follow a similar trend in Ireland [23]. An older study from 2002 to 2012 in Great Britain of a prospectively maintained database returned a rate of 6.2% of EGL, slightly higher than contemporaneous estimates of 5%, and demonstrated that 2.5% of grafts, or just under half of EGL cases, experience primary non-function, while the second biggest contributor to EGL is vascular occlusion [21]. Early graft loss is more common among extended criteria donors, as well as donation after circulatory death donors. However, even when early graft loss occurs, long-term outcomes for patients are still superior to remaining on the waitlist, emphasizing the value of expanding donor graft utilization [21].

Delayed graft function (DGF) is the other side of the early graft loss coin: acute kidney injury of the graft in the peri-transplantation period that is typically defined by requiring dialysis support in the first postoperative week. This may continue for weeks to months, carrying a significant financial and quality of life burden. In contrast with EGL, rates of DGF have risen in recent years, with a particularly notable increase after the 2014 Kidney Allocation System (KAS) was implemented. Delayed graft function occurred in approximately 24.5% of transplants nationwide prior to KAS implementation while it was reported to occur in 29.2% of transplants 12 months after implementation, although rates vary widely from center-to-center [24, 25]. This increase after KAS implementation was not completely unexpected, as highly sensitized patients, among other high-risk groups, are more relatively prioritized but it does highlight the increasingly broad impact of DGF on the field of kidney transplantation .

The response -to-injury hypothesis describes the pathophysiology of delayed graft function: ischemia and reperfusion cause a cycle of tissue injury and inflammatory response, which can be exacerbated by microangiopathy, coagulopathy, or nephrotoxic immunosuppressants [25]. Warm and cold ischemic time are known to impact DGF, with something of a dose-dependent response demonstrated between cold ischemic time and DGF in particular [26]. Largely because of this relationship between ischemia and tissue injury, DGF, like EGL, occurs primarily in deceased donor grafts (somewhere between 2 and 10% of living donor transplants suffer DGF), and more commonly in donation after circulatory death grafts. Donor factors like age, female sex, elevated creatinine at procurement, and recipient factors like male sex, diabetes, and previous transplant, as well as BMI in both donor and recipient, increase the rate of DGF [25, 27, 28]. While many of these factors are not modifiable, hypothermic machine perfusion reduces the impact of cold ischemic time and significantly improves rates of delayed graft function [29]. While DGF has a wide-reaching impact on numerous short- and long-term outcomes after kidney transplantation, no magic bullet for prevention has been identified other than general medical optimization and minimization of ischemic time, and effective treatments have been elusive. Supportive care and dialysis when necessary remain the standard of care.

One of the outcomes to which DGF predisposes recipients is rejection, which is a major factor impacting first-year graft and patient survival. Acute rejection can be T-cell mediated, antibody mediated, or a mixture thereof, with the antibody-mediated component being much more associated with graft failure. Presence of donor-specific antibodies (DSA) at or after transplantation, higher panel-reactive antibody levels, and greater HLA mismatch (often leading to DSAs) contribute to antibody-mediated rejection (AbMR), but not all sensitized patients develop AbMR [30]. Acute rejection is fortunately decreasing in the modern era. It was estimated in 2012 to occur in about 10% of deceased donor kidney transplant recipients in the first year after transplantation, an improvement from the 15-25% observed back in 2000; in a study of recipients from 2003 – 2013 undergoing T-cell depletion, the rate was even lower, around 5% [31, 32].

Numerous induction regimens and a variety of maintenance regimens have developed to address rejection. The dominant maintenance regimen, tacrolimus and mycophenolate, appears to have a durable effect on reducing rejection episodes and graft failure in the first year and beyond [7, 9]. While a meta-analysis of the topic was not able to support that any particular induction regimen decreases incidence of rejection, a retrospective study found that for deceased donor kidney recipients on maintenance tacrolimus and mycophenolate with initial steroids, additional induction with anti-thymocyte globulin (ATG) reduces incidence of rejection; without steroids, ATG does not have a statistically significant impact on rejection but does reduce graft failure rates [32]. Anti-IL-2 induction has been used as well, and has been shown to reduce anti-HLA antibodies, although evidence that it improves graft outcomes is unclear. A widely used and seemingly effective protocol for sensitized patients has become IVIG and plasmapheresis, with IL-2 or ATG added for T-cell depletion [33]. Numerous other drugs have been tested and are used in some instances, including bortezomib and berinert. Eculizumab, in particular, is increasingly used either in induction or for rejection that is not responding to other therapies, and has shown promising results in at least one randomized controlled trial [17, 34]. A more detailed discussion of these therapies is discussed elsewhere in this book.

A surprising and positive trend, or lack thereof, has been that despite a reduction in acute rejection events, studies of Medicare -enrolled transplant recipients have shown that post-transplant ation hospitalizations for infection have been stable, with about 1 in 5 recipients requiring hospitalization for infection in the first three years after transplantation, and a median time to hospitalization of 0.93 years (indicating that at least 10% of patients in this population are generally hospitalized for infection in the first year). Lenihan et al. suggest that this may be due to the reduced need for pulsed or escalated immunosuppression in the post-transplant period as well as a trend towards steroid withdrawal [10]. However, given that the vast majority of transplant recipients are managed on tacrolimus and mycophenolate, which has been suggested to be the reason for improved rejection rates, there may be minimal room for further population-wide improvements in either infection or rejection rates until another superior regimen is identified. It is worth noting that while there may be limited opportunities for population-wide improvement at present, studies have demonstrated center-level disparities in short-term infectious complications, specifically urinary tract and surgical site infections, that represent gaps that should be addressed. Incidence of postoperative UTIs ranges from 0 to 14% between centers, and for surgical site infections, from 0 to 17% [35].

The first year after transplantation is the most perilous for infectious complications; beyond the Lenihan study, others reported over 20% of patients are hospitalized for infection in the first year [36]. For this reason, a complete and appropriate vaccination regimen is critical for any preventable bacterial and viral infections during transplant evaluation; live attenuated vaccinations can only be given prior to transplant as they are not safe in the post-transplant immunosuppressed patient. Fungal and antiviral prophylaxis is also key in the first post-transplant year. Diagnosing infection is challenging in transplant recipients because immunosuppression and altered anatomy mean that classic signs of infection such as fever, leukocytosis, or even pain may not be present, so early and comprehensive workup should be initiated whenever there is an unexplained decrement in kidney function, any typically infectious sign like dysuria or fever, or nonspecific systemic signs. While a high index of suspicion for infection should always be the case when caring for a transplant patient, even greater attention should be given to the older recipient; patients over 65 years of age have been demonstrated to have more cytomegalovirus (CMV) viremia and late UTIs than younger recipients [37]. Treatment should also be quickly initiated to avoid further graft damage or escalation to sepsis. Urinary tract infections should always be treated as complicated because of the altered anatomy of the allograft and its ureter, including the short distance to the renal pelvis [38].

One area of impressive gains in short- and long-term renal transplantation outcomes, conversely, has been a reduction of non-infection -related post-transplant ation hospitalizations, especially for cardiovascular events. A study of Medicare -enrolled patients who received renal transplants between 1998 and 2011 demonstrated, in every year of transplantation beginning with 2003, a significantly decreased rate of having an initial hospitalization for a cardiovascular event by the third year after transplantation. By 2011, the unadjusted sub-distribution hazard ratio of a first cardiovascular hospitalization, relative to 1998, was 0.7, and the event rate was 3.0 hospitalizations/100 patient years, compared to 4.5 in 1998 – a 67% decrease [10]. This is not due to a healthier or younger population of transplant candidates – as previously mentioned, recipients are increasing in age and more likely to have a longer dialysis vintage, diabetes, and/or hypertension [6, 39]. A Canadian study had similar findings from 1994 to 2009, although in their case, rates of cardiovascular events in recipients were overall stable rather than decreasing – until adjustment for age and comorbidities, which demonstrated decreasing risk over time [40]. Given the increasingly high-risk profile of transplant candidates and recipients, cardiac optimization, revascularization when necessary, and medical management are likely key to these improved outcomes. Short-term cardiac outcomes for transplant patients are mostly determined before the patient ever rolls back to surgery.

LONG-TERM OUTCOMES OF KIDNEY TRANSPLANTATION

It has been a point of concern for American regulatory bodies, transplant institutions, and researchers that long-term outcomes of kidney transplantation have not gained as much ground as short-term outcomes in recent decades, particularly because long-term outcomes in the US are not on par with nations with similarly resourced and long-running renal transplant programs. Canada, Australia and New Zealand, the UK, and Europe all have higher 5-year contemporary graft and patient survival rates than the US [1, 2]. A 2016 study reported 5-year patient and graft survival rates of 86.1% and 72.4%, respectively for deceased donor transplants in the US; the same rates in Australia and New Zealand's registry were 90 and 81%; and in Europe, 87.1 and 77.8%. Canadian graft survival at five years was 81.4% [1]. There have been gains in long-term graft and patient survival across all regions, including the US; the long-term graft failure decreased about 3% every year between 1988 and 2014 [2].

Long-Term Patient and Graft Survival

The most recent US Renal Data System report from 2020 reported a five- and ten-year graft survival rate of 76.7 and 49.2% for deceased donor grafts [3]. On the other hand, living donor graft recipients have five- and ten-year graft survival of 85.0 and 65.2%. Currently, five- and ten-year patient survival for deceased donor graft recipients are 79.7 and 49.2%. Patient survival rates for living donor graft recipients are 88.0 and 61.5%. Another mode of assessing long-term outcomes of renal transplantation is graft half-life, i.e., the time it takes for half of grafts to fail, either by failing in a recipient who remains alive, or by the recipient's death. A 2011 study of the Scientific Registry of Transplant Recipients (SRTR) data estimated an unadjusted half-life of 8.8 years for deceased donor grafts transplanted as recently as 2005, and 12 years for living donor grafts; a previous study using the similar UNOS data files up to 2000 provided a more optimistic estimate of 13.8 years for deceased donor grafts transplanted in 1995, and 21.6 years for living donor grafts [41, 42].

The US Renal Data System reports, particularly the 2018 report, highlighted the improvement in long-term outcomes over time; while not in parallel and with a less consistent trend, significant gains have still been identified. From 1999 to 2015, one-year survival rates improved from 94 to 96% for deceased donor kidney transplant (DDKT), and five-year survival improved from 1999 to 2011 by a greater margin of 81 to 85% [4]. The studies on renal allograft half-life, although producing somewhat different results in terms of projected outcome, also highlight considerable improvement: the 2000 study reported a 75% increase in graft half-life for cadaveric grafts, and 70% increase for living donor grafts. The more conservative 2011 study reported a 33% increase in graft half-life for cadaveric grafts and a relatively flat graft half-life for living donor grafts. Both emphasized that while long-term graft survival has been increasing at a greater rate among black recipients than nonblack recipients, half-life is still demonstrably lower among black recipients [41, 42].

The increase in graft survival is impressive in the context of both increasingly high-risk recipients, and increasing utilization of "marginal" grafts, including donation after cardiac death, those with prolonged ischemic time, and grafts that met criteria for donor AKI. Likely the same factors that are responsible for improved short-term outcomes also drive the gains in long-term outcomes, although to differing magnitudes, with a few exceptions. In particular, more stable and effective maintenance immunosuppression and better induction therapies that reduce incidence and lengthen time to first rejection episodes no doubt have improved graft and patient outcomes. An example of factors that are less impactful in the long term than in the short term are cold ischemic time (CIT) and DGF: while CIT is a driver of the important short-term outcome of DGF, and DGF itself has significant impact on post-transplant experience and quality of life, it has less of an independent impact on long-term outcomes than previously feared. An analysis of paired kidney transplants with different total ischemic times revealed that longer CIT and related DGF were not strongly associated with reduced long-term graft failure, hence justifying national sharing when warranted [26]. Another study demonstrated that DGF only appears to be related to long-term failure when the kidney donor profile index (KDPI) is also high (>85%) [27].

Long-Term Complications

Major long-term complications in kidney transplant recipients largely arise from chronic allograft dysfunction, long-term effects of immunosuppression, and the effects of pre-existing and de novo comorbidities, such as hypertension and heart disease. Long-term complications are more difficult and more complex to manage, as they represent a composite of the patient's comorbidities, disease prior to transplant, health of the donor prior to procurement, and long-term effects of immunosuppression, all of which are contributors to the three primary causes of morbidity and mortality in renal transplant recipients: infection, malignancy, and cardiovascular complications.

Chronic allograft dysfunction or chronic allograft nephropathy (CAN) describes a decline in allograft function over time, usually defined clinically as reduced filtration rate and creatinine clearance, from a multifactorial combination of immune and non-immune etiologies. It was estimated in the 1990s that CAN accounted for between 50 and 80% of long-term death-censored graft losses [43]. Chronic antibody -mediated rejection (c-ABMR), an immune-mediated cause of CAN, is characterized histopathologically, as the name would suggest, by humoral immunity against the allograft, with an interrelationship between cytokine production by Th2-cells and donor-specific antibody (mostly anti-HLA) production by B-cells. Complement is deposited into peritubular capillaries; vasculopathy, interstitial fibrosis, and glomerulosclerosis occur, with a corresponding decline in kidney function [44].

Discrete episodes of injury, both before and after transplant, contribute to the chronic injury of CAN. Pre-transplant factors including older donor age, deceased-donor graft, and increased ischemic time, which have all been associated with greater risk of CAN [45]. However, these cannot all be alleviated, given the limited supply and high demand for kidneys. Factors that are more able to be mitigated by the transplant physician are those that arise after transplantation. Acute rejection episodes are a major risk factor for CAN and can occur at any time in the post-transplant period; more than one episode is a particularly negative predictor. A seven-year, single-center study of individuals who experienced at least one acute rejection episode found that individuals with a single episode have five-year graft survival rates of 85.1%, but individuals with more than one have an overall five-year graft survival rate of 52.5%, a difference almost entirely attributable to chronic rejection [46]. Hypertension, diabetes, and the general spectrum of renal diseases are other contributory non-immune factors, whether merely recurring or arising *de novo* [45, 47]. Infections, whether causing a more generalized inflammatory response or causing direct renal damage, also contribute [48, 49]. All these factors are crucial points of focus to preserve long-term graft function, beginning with pre-transplantation matching and optimization, and continuing with post-transplantation management .

Unfortunately, while strides have been made in medical management of everything from acute rejection episodes to hypertension itself, the immune component of CAN, or c-ABMR, remains as-yet insurmountable. Nephrotoxicity from immunosuppressive medications, especially calcineurin inhibitors, is an outstanding issue that limits a physician's ability to provide adequate immunosuppression [50]. No immunosuppressive regimen has proven highly effective in stopping CAN, although multimodal regimens with minimization of calcineurin inhibitors are favored at this point when possible. It is important to note that while appropriate minimization is helpful, replacement of tacrolimus with the less nephrotoxic sirolimus has not been a successful strategy in randomized trials [51]. When new-onset loss of kidney function is detected that is consistent with CAN, biopsy is often wise to assess whether rejection or nephrotoxicity is the predominant issue. If the latter occurs, switching to a less nephrotoxic regimen is indicated, even with the greater risk of rejection. If the former occurs, doses should be increased and steroids and/or IVIG considered. Adjuncts like eculizumab, rituximab, and bortezomib all have weak evidence suggesting they might be useful in refractory cases; studies continue to investigate these therapies along with numerous emerging therapies [52–54].

While prolonged graft survival is a key goal of renal transplantation, patient survival remains the most important focus. The most important cause of post-transplant morbidity and mortality in the US transplant population is believed to be cardiovascular disease; according to the 2020 USRDS report, 35.4% of deaths with a reported cause of death among transplant recipients are due to cardiovascular causes. Of those, the majority is due to arrhythmia or cardiac arrest, at 20.9%; 4.7% due to stroke, 5.1% to chronic heart failure, and 4.4% to acute infarction or other atherosclerotic disease [3]. Unfortunately, cause of death data is often incomplete, particularly beyond the first-year post-transplant, with 64% of causes of death unrecorded and 16.4% recorded as "unknown"; but it is undeniable that cardiovascular disease is a significant concern for the transplant physician and recipient.

Cardiovascular disease and, more broadly, metabolic disease, is intertwined with outcomes of ESRD and transplantation at every level; i.e., hypertension and diabetes, which are the most common etiologies of renal disease, are also common comorbidities in other forms of renal disease. Immunosuppression itself has metabolic effects that can cause or exacerbate hypertension, dyslipidemia, and diabetes, leading to worsening of existing and *de novo* cardiovascular complications. While incidence of post-transplant hypertension and dyslipidemia is hard to assess, post-transplantation diabetes (PTDM) occurs in approximately 30% of renal transplant recipients in one large US study, although incidence estimates range widely (from 10 to 74%); higher prednisone dosage over time is one modifiable risk factor [55, 56]. A small US study of 100 patients in the azathioprine /cyclosporine era demonstrated at least half had developed hypercholesterolemia by the end of 12 months but, fortunately, tacrolimus is less dyslipidemic. In another study, patients receiving tacrolimus were only a third as likely to be on cholesterol -lowering drugs as patients receiving cyclosporine [57, 58]. Importantly, as might be expected, PTDM confers a higher risk of post-transplant mortality with a relative risk of 1.38 [59]. In contrast to lipid dysregulation, tacrolimus is a more diabetogenic drug than its predecessors but still preferable due to its overall favorable outcomes [60]. Hypertension also contributes to higher risk of post-transplant death, but to a lesser degree with a relative risk of 1.18 [61].

While the short-term cardiovascular health of a transplant recipient is largely dependent on patient selection and pre-operative optimization, providing a long, healthy post-transplant life for a recipient is, as these numbers would suggest, dependent on more variables. Lifestyle factors; i.e., exercise, a healthy weight, and abstinence from tobacco are all instrumental in providing health advantages in the renal transplant recipient population just as they are in the general population. The clinician's role, in addition to encouraging healthy behavior, chiefly entails appropriate medical therapies to manage cardiovascular risk factors and comorbidities. Adequate blood pressure control is recommended. While calcium -channel blockers decrease blood pressure less efficiently than ACE-inhibitors, they also cause less decrement in kidney function [62]. Managing blood glucose and lipid levels is crucial, as well, with statins generally recommended for dyslipidemia in this population. No evidence conclusively demonstrates that statins reduce mortality in this population, but the ALERT randomized controlled trial did demonstrate that incidence of myocardial infarction is reduced by statin use [63]. Finally, given the role that immunosuppression plays as a driver of increasing cardiac risk, maintaining a stable but appropriately minimized regimen is perhaps the single best intervention for cardiovascular health in a transplant recipient and for almost every outcome.

Infection in the immunosuppressed patient is the second of the three major causes of post-transplant mortality and morbidity. It accounts for 17.2% of known post-transplant causes of death; while it is already a serious threat to non-diabetics, mortality incidence from infectious causes is twice as high in diabetics [3, 64]. In the long-term post-transplant period, the infections to which recipients are most susceptible are urinary tract infections (UTIs) and community respiratory and other viral infection s, including the dreaded BK virus that is particularly prone to reactivation in the renal transplant recipient, but also any number of common infections, from flu to hepatitis to the herpes family of viruses [65, 66]. BK virus, unfortunately, is still without a truly effective targeted antiviral therapy, so annual surveillance for replication, and reduction of immunosuppression if persistent viremia is detected, remains the clinician's main arsenal against progression to BK virus nephropathy. Some protocols have been found to be reasonably successful, with only a 9% incidence of rejection, but as a caution, only half of grafts lost to BK virus nephropathy are lost to the viral infection itself; half have historically been lost to rejection from reduced immunosuppression [49, 67, 68].

Fungal infections including pneumocystis pneumonia should also remain on the clinician's radar. By ten years after transplant, incidence of invasive fungal infection among kidney recipients is 5.0%, a relatively small group, but significant because mortality once it occurs is high, with a cumulative probability of 30.4% in the year after an invasive fungal infection [69]. Infection is tied not only to mortality, but in the long-term to graft failure. For example, CMV recurrence can directly attack the graft. UTIs cause pyelonephritis and graft injury and even septicemia at a higher rate in transplant recipients [38]. A more detailed review of this topic is covered elsewhere in this book.

As in the short-term post-transplant period, early recognition and treatment of infection is crucial to preserving graft and patient function, which requires consistent, reliable follow-up and a good relationship between the patient and his or her physician. In contrast to the short-term, however, long-term management is simply less proscriptive. Immunosuppression is typically decreased in the first few years, and anti-fungal and anti-viral prophylaxis are only prescribed short-term. Physicians caring for a transplant recipient need to be aware of the potentially atypical presentation of infection and should maintain a low threshold for treatment and for modification of the immunosuppressive regimen or referral to a more specialized provider as necessary.

Finally, in the long term, renal transplant patients are at higher risk for malignancy than either the general population or the population on dialysis, which is the third of the three major causes of morbidity and mortality among renal transplant recipients [70, 71]. According to the USRDS reports, 15.9% of deaths of renal transplant recipients in 2018, for example, were due to malignancy; 17.2% were due to malignancy in 2015 [3, 4]. Rates of long-term post-transplant death from malignancy have remained steady or increased consistently year-by-year since the 1990s [72]. Somewhat surprisingly, a relatively high proportion of these cancer deaths are among younger recipients, as cardiovascular events are a more common, competing cause of death in older recipients with more comorbidities [73]. While a variety of cancers have been shown to occur at a higher rate in renal transplant recipients, the cancers with the greatest increase in risk have been identified in a meta-analysis as lip and non-melanoma skin cancers (standardized infection ratio, or SIR of 29.5 and 12.1, respectively), renal cell carcinoma (SIR of 10.77), non-Hodgkin lymphoma (SIR of 10.66), and thyroid cancer (SIR of 5.04), with Hodgkin lymphoma following close behind [70]. Kaposi's sarcoma, while not included in that meta-analysis, also poses a vastly greater risk in transplant recipients [74, 75]. Post-transplant lymphoproliferative disorder (PTLD) may also occur.

Immunosuppression is known to be the major driver of malignancy in this population, which is supported by the association between dose, number, and duration of immunosuppressive medications in a patient's regimen, and the incidence of cancer [76–79]. Transmission of malignancy from a donor with known or unknown malignancy at the time of transplant can also occur but is rare. Unfortunately, not only is cancer more common among transplant recipients, but also is more likely to be aggressive and be associated with a poor outcome [80]. As in the general population, there is no magic bullet to address this issue: pre- and post-transplant screening is critically important, particularly since individuals on dialysis typically have elevated cancer risk. At present, a two- to five-year period of remission is recommended as a prerequisite to transplant in patients who have a history of malignancy [81]. Unlike in the general population, immunomodulation is a significant part of the transplant physician's arsenal. Reducing dosage is often a next step if a cancer diagnosed in the post-transplant period has a viral or immunosuppression - related etiology, and changing the patient's immunosuppressant regimen may be indicated. For example, mTOR inhibitors like sirolimus and everolimus were anticipated to have significant anti-malignant impact when they entered widespread use, although studies since have reported a more modest reduction in risk most strongly tied to non-melanoma skin cancers [82, 83]. A more detailed discussion on the incidence, management, and outcomes is provided in a separate chapter on "Malignancies after Transplantation."

One long-standing goal in solid-organ transplantation is inducing durable tolerance, i.e., clinical operational tolerance (COT) with minimal or no immunosuppression, given the pervasive risks inherent to long-term immunosuppression. It has remained particularly elusive in renal transplantation, as attempts to wean immunosuppression most often led to rejection episodes. However, an exceedingly small number of individuals have discontinued immunosuppression without rejection, a group characterized as attaining "operational tolerance." Genetic and immunologic changes of T-cells that have been suggested to be associated with tolerance include stronger alteration of the length distribution of the CDR3 hypervariable region, i.e., increased transcript accumulation for that region in T-cells of tolerant individuals and an abnormally high relative transcription of Vβ receptor families [84]. Some clinical factors that have been identified as contributors to operational tolerance include younger donor age, as well as progressive cessation of immunosuppression over years, with no particular association with disease etiology identified among the small group of individuals in which tolerance has occurred [85]. While it is impossible to estimate how many renal transplant recipients would be able to achieve tolerance, genetic studies based on known tolerance profiles predict that the incidence of operational tolerance could approach 7.3% [86]. Validating a prediction methodology, and one day being able to apply it clinically would revolutionize care for those patients able to achieve tolerance.

Despite the rarity of true operational tolerance, the optimization, as well as relative minimization, of immunosuppression remains a complex case-by-case decision for each individual patient based on their renal function, rejection likelihood and history, and side effects and comorbidities. Reduction of immunosuppression remains the only line of defense in some situations, like BK nephropathy. Reducing or eliminating steroid dosages is particularly desirable; a Cochrane review of the numerous studies on steroid withdrawal determined that doing so remains a risk for acute rejection – but this appears to be largely reversible with resumption of steroids, as the risk of graft failure or death within five years does not appear to be increased [87]. An earlier meta-analysis had similar findings and also concluded that cardiovascular metrics improve with steroid avoidance or withdrawal [88]. However, long-term studies on this topic are yet uncommon, so it is impossible to rule out long-term effects. In short, carefully monitored minimization of steroid therapy should be a part of long-term immunosuppressive management when clinically appropriate.

Conclusion

Short-term outcomes of renal transplantation are plateaued at an all-time high in the US, comparing favorably to nations with similar populations and programs around the globe. Rejection and infection are the primary challenges of the first-year post-transplant, with infections somewhat able to be mitigated by prophylaxis regimens in the short-term. Contrary to conventional wisdom, there actually have been considerable gains over the past few decades in long-term outcomes but gains in peer nations have outstripped those in the US. Cardiovascular, infections, and malignant complications are the major causes of long-term morbidity and mortality among renal transplant recipients, and walking the clinical line between over- and under-immunosuppression remains the transplant physician's greatest challenge.

References

[1] Wang JH, Skeans MA, Israni AK. Current Status of Kidney Transplant Outcomes: Dying to Survive. *Adv Chronic Kidney Dis*. 2016;23(5):281–6.
[2] Merion RM, Goodrich NP, Johnson RJ, McDonald SP, Russ GR, Gillespie BW, et al. Kidney transplant graft outcomes in 379 257 recipients on 3 continents. *Am J Transplant.* 2018;18(8):1914–23.
[3] United States Renal Data System. 2020 USRDS *Annual Data Report: Epidemiology of kidney disease in the United States.* Bethesda, MD: National Institutes of Health, National Institute of Diabetes and Digestive and Kidney Diseases; 2020. https://www.usrds.org/annual-data-report/.
[4] United States Renal Data System. 2018 USRDS *Annual Data Report: Epidemiology of kidney disease in the United States.* Bethesda, MD: National Institutes of Health,

National Institute of Diabetes and Digestive and Kidney Diseases; 2018. https://www.usrds.org/annual-data-report/previous-adrs/.

[5] United States Renal Data System. 2017 *USRDS Annual Data Report: Epidemiology of kidney disease in the United States.* Bethesda, MD: National Institutes of Health, National Institute of Diabetes and Digestive and Kidney Diseases; 2017. https://www.usrds.org/annual-data-report/previous-adrs/.

[6] McAdams-Demarco MA, James N, Salter ML, Walston J, Segev DL. Trends in kidney transplant outcomes in older adults. *J Am Geriatr Soc*. 2014;62(12):2235–42.

[7] Huang Y, Tilea A, Gillespie B, Shahinian V, Banerjee T, Grubbs V, et al. Understanding trends in kidney function 1 year after kidney transplant in the United States. *J Am Soc Nephrol*. 2017;28(8):2498–510.

[8] Locke JE, Reed RD, Mehta SG, Durand C, Mannon RB, Maclennan P, et al. Center-Level Experience and Kidney Transplant Outcomes in HIV -Infected Recipients. *Am J Transplant*. 2015;15(8):2096–104.

[9] Keith DS, Vranic G, Nishio-Lucar A. Graft Function and Intermediate-Term Outcomes of Kidney Transplants Improved in the Last Decade. *Transplant Direct*. 2017;3(6):e166.

[10] Lenihan CR, Liu S, Montez-Rath ME, Winkelmayer WC. Trends in the Medical Complexity and Outcomes of Medicare -insured Patients Undergoing Kidney Transplant in the Years 1998–2014. *Transplantation*. 2019;103(11):2413–22.

[11] Schold JD, Buccini LD, Poggio ED, Flechner SM, Goldfarb DA. Association of Candidate Removals from the Kidney Transplant Waiting List and Center Performance Oversight. *Am J Transplant*. 2016;16(4):1276–84.

[12] Foroutan F, Friesen EL, Clark KE, Motaghi S, Zyla R, Lee Y, et al. Risk factors for 1-year graft loss after kidney transplantation; systematic review and meta-analysis. *Clin J Am Soc Nephrol*. 2019;14(11):1642–50.

[13] Foster BJ, Mitsnefes MM, Dahhou M, Zhang X, Laskin BL. Changes in Excess Mortality from End Stage Renal Disease in the United States from 1995 to 2013. *Clin J Am Soc Nephrol*. 2018;13(1):91–9.

[14] Dharnidharka VR. 43 - Pediatric Renal Transplantation [Internet]. Fourth Edi. Vol. 661, *Chronic Kidney Disease, Dialysis, and Transplantation*. Elsevier Inc.; 2020. 661-675.e7 p.

[15] Opelz G, Morath C, Süsal C, Tran TH, Zeier M, Döhler B. Three-Year Outcomes Following 1420 ABO-Incompatible Living-Donor Kidney Transplants Performed After ABO Antibody Reduction. *Transplantation*. 2015; 99(2):400–4.

[16] Takahashi K, Saito K, Takahara S, Okuyama A, Tanabe K, Toma H, et al. Excellent long-term outcome of ABO-incompatible living donor kidney transplantation in Japan. *Am J Transplant*. 2004;4(7):1089–96.

[17] Zhang R. Donor-specific antibodies in kidney transplant recipients. *Clin J Am Soc Nephrol*. 2018;13(1):182–92.

[18] Chen SC, Kuo MC, Hung CC, Huang CH, Chen HC. Delayed recovery of accelerated acute rejection. *Dial Transplant*. 2009;38(8):332–4.

[19] Loss GE, Grewal HP, Siegel CT, Peace D, Mead J, Bruce DS, et al. Reversal of delayed hyperacute renal allograft rejection with a tacrolimus -based therapeutic regimen. *Transplant Proc*. 1998;30(4):1249–50.

[20] Foster K, Cohen DJ, D'Agati VD, Markowitz GS. Primary renal allograft dysfunction. *Am J Kidney Dis*. 2004;44(2):376–81.

[21] Hamed MO, Chen Y, Pasea L, Watson CJ, Torpey N, Bradley JA, et al. Early graft loss after kidney transplantation: Risk factors and consequences. *Am J Transplant*. 2015;15(6):1632–43.

[22] *Organ Procurement and Transplantation Network.* OPTN STAR file, Kidney-Pancreas. United Network for Organ Sharing; 2017.

[23] Phelan PJ, O'Kelly P, Tarazi M, Tarazi N, Salehmohamed MR, Little DM, et al. Renal allograft loss in the first post-operative month: Causes and consequences. *Clin Transplant*. 2012;26(4):544–9.

[24] Wang CJ, Wetmore JB, Israni AK. Old versus new: Progress in reaching the goals of the new kidney allocation system. *Hum Immunol*. 2017;78(1):9–15.

[25] Mannon RB. Delayed graft function: The AKI of kidney transplantation. *Nephron*. 2018;140(2):94–8.

[26] Kayler LK, Srinivas TR, Schold JD. Influence of CIT-induced DGF on kidney transplant outcomes. *Am J Transplant*. 2011;11(12):2657–64.

[27] Arias-Cabrales CE, Pérez-Sáez MJ, Redondo-Pachón D, Buxeda A, Burballa C, Duran X, et al. Relevance of KDPI value and acute rejection on kidney transplant outcomes in recipients with delayed graft function – a retrospective study. *Transpl Int*. 2020;33(9):1071–7.

[28] Mogulla MR, Bhattacharjya S, Clayton PA. Risk factors for and outcomes of delayed graft function in live donor kidney transplantation – a retrospective study. *Transpl Int*. 2019;32(11):1151–60.

[29] O'Callaghan JM, Morgan RD, Knight SR, Morris PJ. Systematic review and meta-analysis of hypothermic machine perfusion versus static cold storage of kidney allografts on transplant outcomes. *Br J Surg*. 2013;100(8):991–1001.

[30] Sampaio MS, Chopra B, Sureshkumar KK. Depleting Antibody Induction and Kidney Transplant Outcomes: A Paired Kidney Analysis. *Transplantation*. 2017;101(10):2527–35.

[31] Dunn TB, Noreen H, Gillingham K, Maurer D, Ozturk OG, Pruett TL, et al. Revisiting Traditional Risk Factors for Rejection and Graft Loss After Kidney Transplantation. *Am J Transplant*. 2011;11(10):2132–43.

[32] Tanriover B, Jaikaransingh V, MacConmara MP, Parekh JR, Levea SL, Ariyamuthu VK, et al. Acute rejection rates and graft outcomes according to induction regimen

among recipients of kidneys from deceased donors treated with tacrolimus and mycophenolate. *Clin J Am Soc Nephrol*. 2016;11(9):1650–61.

[33] Djamali A, Kaufman DB, Ellis TM, Zhong W, Matas A, Samaniego M. Diagnosis and management of antibody -mediated rejection: Current status and novel approaches. *Am J Transplant*. 2014;14(2):255–71.

[34] Marks WH, Mamode N, Montgomery RA, Stegall MD, Ratner LE, Cornell LD, et al. Safety and efficacy of eculizumab in the prevention of antibody -mediated rejection in living-donor kidney transplant recipients requiring desensitization therapy: A randomized trial. *Am J Transplant*. 2019 Oct 19;19(10):2876–88.

[35] Parekh JR, Hirose R, Foley DP, Grieco A, Cohen ME, Hall BL, et al. Beyond death and graft survival —Variation in outcomes after kidney transplantation. Results from the NSQIP Transplant beta phase. *Am J Transplant*. 2019;19(9):2622–30.

[36] Cowan J, Bennett A, Fergusson N, McLean C, Mallick R, Cameron DW, et al. Incidence Rate of Post-Kidney Transplant Infection: A Retrospective Cohort Study Examining Infection Rates at a Large Canadian Multicenter Tertiary-Care Facility. *Can J Kidney Heal Dis*. 2018; 12;5:205435811879969.

[37] Hemmersbach-Miller M, Alexander BD, Sudan DL, Pieper C, Schmader KE. Infections after kidney transplantation. Does age matter ? *Clin Transplant*. 2019 Apr 28;33(4):e13516.

[38] Rice JC, Safdar N. Urinary Tract Infections in Solid Organ Transplant Recipients. *Am J Transplant*. 2009; 9:S267–72.

[39] Pippias M, Jager KJ, Caskey F, Casula A, Erlandsson H, Finne P, et al. Kidney transplant outcomes from older deceased donors: a paired kidney analysis by the European Renal Association–European Dialysis and Transplant Association Registry. *Transpl Int*. 2018;31(7):708–19.

[40] Lam NN, Kim SJ, Knoll GA, McArthur E, Lentine KL, Naylor KL, et al. The risk of cardiovascular disease is not increasing over time despite aging and higher comorbidity burden of kidney transplant recipients. *Transplantation*. 2017;101 (3):588–96.

[41] Hariharan S, Johnson CP, Bresnahan BA, Taranto SE, McIntosh MJ, Stablein D. Improved Graft Survival after Renal Transplantation in the United States, 1988 to 1996. *N Engl J Med*. 2000;342(9):605–12.

[42] Lamb KE, Lodhi S, Meier-Kriesche HU. Long-term renal allograft survival in the United States: A critical reappraisal. *Am J Transplant*. 2011;11(3):450–62.

[43] Paul LC. Chronic renal transplant loss. *Kidney Int*. 1995;47(6):1491–9.

[44] Bhatti AB, Usman M. Chronic Renal Transplant Rejection and Possible Anti-Proliferative Drug Targets. *Cureus*. 2015; 7(11):e376.

[45] Baluja P, Haragsim L, Laszik Z. Chronic Allograft Nephropathy. *Adv Chronic Kidney Dis*. 2006;13(1):56–61.

[46] Humar A, Payne WD, Sutherland DER, Matas AJ. Clinical Determinants of Multiple Acute Rejection Episodes in Kidney Transplant Recipients. *Transplantation*. 2000;69(11):2357–60.

[47] Lin J, Valeri AM, Markowitz GS, D???Agati VD, Cohen DJ, Radhakrishnan J. Angiotensin converting enzyme inhibition in chronic allograft nephropathy. *Transplantation*. 2002;73(5):783–8.

[48] Martin-Gandul C, Mueller NJ, Pascual M, Manuel O. The Impact of Infection on Chronic Allograft Dysfunction and Allograft Survival after Solid Organ Transplantation. *Am J Transplant*. 2015;15(12):3024–40.

[49] Mengel M. BK Virus Nephropathy Revisited. *Am J Transplant*. 2017;17(8):1972–3.

[50] Chapman JR. What are the key challenges we face in kidney transplantation today? *Transplant Res*. 2013; 2(S1):S1.

[51] Campath, calcineurin inhibitor reduction, and chronic allograft nephropathy (the 3C Study) - results of a randomized controlled clinical trial. *Am J Transplant*. 2018;18(6):1424–34.

[52] Riella LV, Djamali A, Pascual J. Chronic allograft injury: Mechanisms and potential treatment targets. *Transplant Rev*. 2017;31(1):1–9.

[53] Stegall MD, Diwan T, Raghavaiah S, Cornell LD, Burns J, Dean PG, et al. Terminal Complement Inhibition Decreases Antibody-Mediated Rejection in Sensitized Renal Transplant Recipients. *Am J Transplant*. 2011;11(11):2405–13.

[54] Aubert O, Suberbielle C, Gauthe R, Francois H, Obada EN, Durrbach A. Effect of a Proteasome Inhibitor Plus Steroids on HLA Antibodies in Sensitized Patients Awaiting a Renal Transplant. *Transplantation*. 2014;97(9):946–52.

[55] Bayer ND, Cochetti PT, Anil Kumar MS, Teal V, Huan Y, Doria C, et al. Association of Metabolic Syndrome With Development of New-Onset Diabetes After Transplantation. *Transplantation*. 2010;90(8):861–6.

[56] Shivaswamy V, Boerner B, Larsen J. Post-Transplant Diabetes Mellitus: Causes, Treatment, and Impact on Outcomes. *Endocr Rev*. 2016;37(1):37–61.

[57] Gonyea JE, Anderson CF. Weight Change and Serum Lipoproteins in Recipients of Renal Allografts. *Mayo Clin Proc*. 1992;67(7):653–7.

[58] Vincenti F, Jensik SC, Filo RS, Miller J, Pirsch J. A long-term comparison of tacrolimus (FK506) and cyclosporine in kidney transplantation: evidence for improved allograft survival at five years1. *Transplantation*. 2002;73(5):775–82.

[59] Cole EH, Johnston O, Rose CL, Gill JS. Impact of Acute Rejection and New-Onset Diabetes on Long-Term Transplant Graft and Patient Survival. *Clin J Am Soc Nephrol*. 2008;3(3):814–21.

[60] Webster AC, Taylor RR, Chapman JR, Craig JC. Tacrolimus versus cyclosporin as primary immunosuppression for kidney transplant recipients. *Cochrane Database Syst Rev*. 2005; http://doi.wiley.com/10.1002/14651858. CD003961.pub2.

[61] Kasiske BL, Anjum S, Shah R, Skogen J, Kandaswamy C, Danielson B, et al. Hypertension after kidney transplantation. *Am J Kidney Dis.* 2004;43(6):1071–81.

[62] Cross NB, Webster AC, Masson P, O'Connell PJ, Craig JC. Antihypertensives for Kidney Transplant Recipients: Systematic Review and Meta-Analysis of Randomized Controlled Trials. *Transplantation.* 2009;88(1):7–18.

[63] Holdaas H, Fellström B, Jardine AG, Holme I, Nyberg G, Fauchald P, et al. Effect of fluvastatin on cardiac outcomes in renal transplant recipients: a multicentre, randomised, placebo -controlled trial. *Lancet.* 2003;361(9374):2024–31.

[64] Weinrauch LA, D'Elia JA, Weir MR, Bunnapradist S, Finn P V., Liu J, et al. Infection and Malignancy Outweigh Cardiovascular Mortality in Kidney Transplant Recipients: Post Hoc Analysis of the FAVORIT Trial. *Am J Med.* 2018;131(2):165–72.

[65] Ramaswamy K, Madariaga HM, Thomas BS, Lerma E V. Kidney transplantation for the primary care provider. *Disease-a-Month.* 2020;66(3):100869.

[66] Greendyke WG, Pereira MR. Infectious Complications and Vaccinations in the Posttransplant Population. *Med Clin North Am.* 2016;100(3):587–98.

[67] Schaub S, Hirsch HH, Dickenmann M, Steiger J, Mihatsch MJ, Hopfer H, et al. Reducing Immunosuppression Preserves Allograft Function in Presumptive and Definitive Polyomavirus-Associated Nephropathy. *Am J Transplant.* 2010; 10(12): 2615–23.

[68] Hirsch HH, Randhawa P. BK Polyomavirus in Solid Organ Transplantation. *Am J Transplant.* 2013;13(s4):179–88.

[69] Hosseini-Moghaddam SM, Ouédraogo A, Naylor KL, Bota SE, Husain S, Nash DM, et al. Incidence and outcomes of invasive fungal infection among solid organ transplant recipients: A population -based cohort study. *Transpl Infect Dis.* 2020 5;22(2).

[70] Wang Y, Lan G Bin, Peng FH, Xie XB. Cancer risks in recipients of renal transplants: A meta-analysis of cohort studies. *Oncotarget.* 2018;9(20):15375–85.

[71] Campistol JM. Minimizing the Risk of Posttransplant Malignancy. *Transplant Proc.* 2008;40(10 SUPPL.):S40–3.

[72] Awan AA, Niu J, Pan JS, Erickson KF, Mandayam S, Winkelmayer WC, et al. Trends in the Causes of Death among Kidney Transplant Recipients in the United States (1996–2014). *Am J Nephrol* 2018;48(6):472–81.

[73] Kiberd BA, Rose C, Gill JS. Cancer Mortality in Kidney Transplantation. *Am J Transplant.* 2009;9(8):1868–75.

[74] Woodle ES, Hanaway M, Buell J, Gross T, First MR, Trofe J, et al. Kaposi sarcoma: an analysis of the US and international experiences from the Israel Penn international transplant tumor registry. *Transplant Proc.* 2001;33(7–8):3660–1.

[75] Euvrard S, Kanitakis J, Claudy A. Skin Cancers after Organ Transplantation. *N Engl J Med.* 2003; 348(17):1681–91.

[76] Ramsay HM, Fryer AA, Reece S, Smith AG, Harden PN. Clinical risk factors associated with nonmelanoma skin cancer in renal transplant recipients. *Am J Kidney Dis*. 2000;36(1):167–76.

[77] Dantal J, Hourmant M, Cantarovich D, Giral M, Blancho G, Dreno B, et al. Effect of long-term immunosuppression in kidney -graft recipients on cancer incidence: randomised comparison of two cyclosporin regimens. *Lancet*. 1998;351(9103):623–8.

[78] Opelz G, Döhler B. Lymphomas After Solid Organ Transplantation: A Collaborative Transplant Study Report. *Am J Transplant*. 2004;4(2):222–30.

[79] Rama I, Grinyó JM. Malignancy after renal transplantation: the role of immunosuppression. *Nat Rev Nephrol*. 2010;6(9):511–9.

[80] Miao Y, Everly JJ, Gross TG, Tevar AD, First MR, Alloway RR, et al. De Novo Cancers Arising in Organ Transplant Recipients are Associated with Adverse Outcomes Compared with the General Population. *Transplantation*. 2009;87(9): 1347–59.

[81] Au E, Wong G, Chapman JR. Cancer in kidney transplant recipients. *Nat Rev Nephrol*. 2018;14(8):508–20.

[82] Ying T, Wong G, Lim WH, Clayton P, Kanellis J, Pilmore H, et al. Everolimus and Long-Term Clinical Outcomes in Kidney Transplant Recipients: A Registry -based 10-year Follow-up of 5 Randomized Trials. *Transplantation*. 2019;103(8):1705–13.

[83] Alberú J, Pascoe MD, Campistol JM, Schena FP, Rial M del C, Polinsky M, et al. Lower Malignancy Rates in Renal Allograft Recipients Converted to Sirolimus-Based, Calcineurin Inhibitor-Free Immunotherapy: 24-Month Results From the CONVERT Trial. *Transplantation*. 2011;92(3):303–10.

[84] Brouard S, Dupont A, Giral M, Louis S, Lair D, Braudeau C, et al. Operationally tolerant and minimally immunosuppressed kidney recipients display strongly altered blood T-cell clonal regulation. *Am J Transplant*. 2005;5(2):330–40.

[85] Roussey-Kesler G, Giral M, Moreau A, Subra JF, Legendre C, Noël C, et al. Clinical operational tolerance after kidney transplantation. *Am J Transplant*. 2006;6(4):736–46.

[86] Roedder S, Li L, Alonso MN, Hsieh SC, Vu MT, Dai H, et al. A three-gene assay for monitoring immune quiescence in kidney transplantation. *J Am Soc Nephrol*. 2015;26(8):2042–53.

[87] Haller MC, Royuela A, Nagler E V., Pascual J, Webster AC. Steroid avoidance or withdrawal for kidney transplant recipients. *Cochrane Database Syst Rev*. 2016;2016(8).

[88] Knight SR, Morris PJ. Steroid avoidance or withdrawal after renal transplantation increases the risk of acute rejection but decreases cardiovascular risk. A Meta-analysis. *Transplantation*. 2010;89(1):1–14.

In: Issues in Kidney Disease – Transplantation
Editors: B. V. R. Murthy and S. Z. Fadem
ISBN: 978-1-53619-960-4

Chapter 14

MULTI-ORGAN TRANSPLANTATION INVOLVING THE KIDNEY: ELIGIBILITY AND CONTROVERSIES IN ALLOCATION

Angelina Edwards*, MD
Division of Kidney Diseases, Hypertension and Transplantation,
Department of Medicine, Houston Methodist Hospital, Houston, TX, USA

ABSTRACT

Both acute renal failure and chronic kidney disease are highly prevalent among non-renal organ transplant populations and contribute to increased morbidity and premature mortality in these patients. Criteria for kidney transplantation with simultaneous pancreas kidney (SPK), and simultaneous liver kidney (SLK) transplantation are well-defined by the United Network of Organ Sharing (UNOS), but criteria for simultaneous heart kidney transplantation (SHK) and combined lung-kidney transplantation (CLK) remain undefined, with most centers adopting their own criteria. While prioritization should continue to be given to those patients in urgent need in whom SHK and CLK are appropriate options, care must be taken to avoid kidney transplant in those candidates who have a chance of renal recovery and in those with poor-transplant survival. Future initiatives must focus on universally agreed upon guidelines for eligibility of SHK and CLK. A "safety net" policy that exists for SLK candidates is also needed for potential SKH and CLK candidates to optimize allocation of kidneys. As stewards of a limited resource, the governing organizations, as well as the transplant community, must continue to strive for fairness and beneficence in organ allocation, considering the obligation to the kidney alone recipient, particularly because the high-quality kidneys for multi-organ transplants are prioritized over pediatric and young adult kidney alone recipients who otherwise have a long expected post-transplant survival.

Keywords: multi-organ, transplantation, renal disease

---

* Corresponding Author's Email: aredwards@houstonmethodist.org.

Introduction

Kidney dysfunction is often seen in non-renal end organ failure. As heart, lung, and liver failure progress, incidence of acute kidney injury (AKI) and chronic kidney disease (CKD) increases. As patients with non-kidney organ failure are being considered for transplantation, those with renal insufficiency are considered for multi-organ transplant (MOT). Renal transplant is the preferred therapy for advanced kidney disease. Dialysis after non-renal transplant adds to the complexity of cost and care and contributes to morbidity and mortality. While the criteria for kidney transplant alone (KTA), simultaneous pancreas kidney (SPK), and simultaneous liver kidney (SLK) transplantation are well-defined by the United Network of Organ Sharing (UNOS), criteria for simultaneous heart kidney transplantation (SHK) and combined lung-kidney transplantation (CLK) remain undefined, with most centers adopting their own criteria. Given the disparity of supply and demand for kidney transplant alone, balancing equity along with utility in MOT remains a challenge. This chapter focuses on the rationale, current eligibility, and outcomes for MOT in the settings of SPK, SLK, SHK, and CLK transplantation, as well as considers the utility of each, in light of the current allocation policies.

Incidence and Pathophysiology of Renal Dysfunction in Non-Kidney Organ Failure

Chronic kidney disease is highly prevalent, affecting 30% to 50% of the non-renal organ transplant population. The annual end-stage renal disease risk is 1.5% to 2.0% with higher incidence mirroring the severity of the organ failure. Both acute renal failure and CKD contribute to increased morbidity and premature mortality [1].

The true incidence of CKD in the pre-transplant population is difficult to ascertain due to variation of definitions and means of assessment [2]. Therefore, its prevalence is often underestimated. Currently, the use of equations for estimated glomerular filtration (eGFR) fail to capture the extent of renal dysfunction that may be present. Patients with liver cirrhosis, heart failure, or hypoxemic lung disease often have diffuse muscle atrophy and poor nutrition, which make standard calculations of kidney dysfunction difficult to interpret. Serum creatinine and eGFR overestimate renal function in these patients. Use of a more sensitive marker, such as cystatin C, may prove beneficial in this population, as it is not dependent on muscle mass, its production is constant in every nucleated cell, and it does not vary with age, race, or sex. Use of the new Chronic Kidney Disease Epidemiology Collaboration (CKD-EPI) Equation with both creatinine and cystatin c more closely estimates renal function captured by the gold standard of inulin clearance [3]. While inulin clearance is not widely available, radionuclide markers (iohexol or iothalamate) for precise

GFR assessment are used; however, the increased cost, radiation exposure, and lack of accessibility limit their use [4].

Despite these limitations, the incidence of renal dysfunction in non-renal pre-transplant patients remains high. In pre-lung transplant patients with pulmonary hypertension, chronic kidney disease is a common comorbid condition that leads to increased mortality, often triggered by venous congestion, decreased cardiac output, and neurohormonal activation [5, 6]. End-stage heart failure patients are increasingly supported with a left ventricular assist device (LVAD) as a bridge to heart transplant or destination therapy. Patients with refractory heart failure and cardiorenal syndrome may see a benefit following LVAD placement but predicting reversibility of renal dysfunction remains challenging. Implantation of such device carries increased risk of AKI. AKI is usually observed in those with pre-existent CKD, prolonged cardiopulmonary bypass time, post-implant elevated central venous pressure, and post-implant right ventricular failure. These factors trigger prolonged ischemia and venous congestion to the kidneys. Patients with AKI after LVAD implantation have increased mortality in the first year of device therapy, are more likely to require dialysis, and less likely to receive a heart transplant [7].

Table 1. Universal risk factors for renal disease

<table>
<tr><td>• Age</td><td colspan="2">• Systemic Hypertension</td><td>• Diabetes mellitus</td></tr>
<tr><td colspan="2">• Nephrotoxic Agents
• (contrast, medications)</td><td colspan="2">• Acute Kidney Injury</td></tr>
<tr><td colspan="2">• Liver Failure</td><td colspan="2">• Heart Failure</td></tr>
<tr><td colspan="2">• NASH/Diabetic nephropathy</td><td colspan="2">• Decreased effective circulatory volume from diuretics</td></tr>
<tr><td colspan="2">• Hepatitis B and C Glomerulonephritis</td><td colspan="2">• Cardiorenal syndrome</td></tr>
<tr><td colspan="2">• Hepatorenal Syndrome</td><td colspan="2">• LVAD and advanced heart failure therapeutics</td></tr>
<tr><td colspan="2">• Hyperoxaluria</td><td colspan="2">• Renovascular atherosclerosis</td></tr>
<tr><td colspan="2">• Diuretic-induced hypovolemia</td><td colspan="2">• Hypertension</td></tr>
<tr><td colspan="2">• Lung Failure</td><td colspan="2">• Pancreas Failure</td></tr>
<tr><td colspan="2">• Chronic aminoglycoside use</td><td colspan="2">• Diabetic nephropathy</td></tr>
<tr><td colspan="2">• Cystic-fibrosis related diabetes</td><td colspan="2">• Autonomic dysfunction and chronic hypotension</td></tr>
<tr><td colspan="2">• Pulmonary hypertension</td><td colspan="2"></td></tr>
</table>

Patients with end-stage liver disease often manifest CKD related to the underlying liver disease, and the occurrence of AKI and Hepatorenal syndrome carries significant prognostic implications as severity of kidney disease mirrors liver disease. Hence, renal dysfunction is used in the liver transplant ation allocation priority through the Model for End-Stage Liver Disease (MELD) score [8, 9]. For patients with diabetes mellitus, renal dysfunction or nephropathy manifests following years of uncontrolled hyperglycemia, with other end-organ manifestations, including concomitant neuropathy, retinopathy, and gastroparesis [10]. Table 1 below highlights the common risk factors for impaired kidney function and renal disease in patients with end stage liver, heart, lung or pancreas failure [1, 7, 11, 12].

EVALUATION OF RENAL FUNCTION PRIOR TO NON-KIDNEY SOLID ORGAN TRANSPLANTATION

In an era of ever-increasing organ shortage and longer wait times, a robust assessment of kidney function in a candidate for a non-kidney organ transplant is mandatory. There are three areas to consider: 1) prior history of renal dysfunction or injury; 2) current stage of kidney disease; and 3) the likelihood of kidney injury and the rate of progression of kidney disease following solid organ transplantation. As previously discussed, despite some limitations, the first two areas can be quantified and assessed; however, the last one remains an area that is difficult to predict.

Prior history of renal dysfunction and current stage of kidney disease are key elements assessed in the pre-transplant evaluation; the initial evaluation is detailed in Table 2.

Table 2. Initial evaluation of renal function in a non-renal organ transplantation candidate

Laboratory Assessment	Urine Studies	Radiographic Studies
• Serum creatinine mg/dL	• Urine albumin/ creatinine ratio and/or protein/creatinine ratio	• Renal Ultrasonography with doppler
• Serum cystatin C mg/dL	• Urine electrolytes and osm	• CT Renal Stone Protocol
• Estimated GFR (mL/min)	• 24 Hour Urine for Creat Cl	• Nuclear medicine scan for GFR

Key caveats to remember when assessing current and future renal function include: 1) the limitations of estimating equations for GFR (discussed previously); 2) impact of medications, such as diuretics, on interpretation; 3) the unknown aspects of the peri-operative and post-operative period.

Urine assessment will reveal any underlying proteinuria or microscopic hematuria, concerning for glomerulonephritis. If an underlying glomerulonephritis is suspected, additional serology assessment with complement levels, immune markers, rheumatoid factor, cryoglobulins, Hepatitis B and C viral load, lactate dehydrogenase (LDH), and haptoglobin should be ordered. Urine sodium will assess urinary concentrating capability and effective circulating volume. Urine creatinine clearance from a 24-hour collection overestimates GFR in this subset of patients, due to enhanced tubular secretion of creatinine, and interpretation requires caution [13]. Renal imaging with Doppler ultrasound shows kidney anatomy, echogenicity, presence of stones, and renovascular disease. Findings of cortical thinning and small kidneys (less than 10 centimeters) with increased echogenicity are reflective of the presence of irreversible chronic kidney disease [14]. Normal sonographic appearance of the bladder rules out bladder outlet obstruction from enlarged prostate or neurogenic bladder. A kidney biopsy may be pursued if the common clinical workup is unrevealing and if the cause of renal dysfunction appears to be due to intrinsic kidney dysfunction rather than a low-flow state or chronic hypoperfusion. Transjugular native kidney biopsy carries a decreased risk of bleeding compared to percutaneous biopsy. Nevertheless, given underlying coagulopathy in these patients, post-biopsy bleeding risk is substantial and therefore a biopsy may not be feasible. When available, evaluation of kidney biopsy for underlying glomerulonephritis and assessing the degree of interstitial fibrosis, tubular atrophy, and glomerulosclerosis lends key prognostic information. Evidence of ≥ 30% interstitial fibrosis or ≥ 30% glomerulosclerosis on renal biopsy supports a diagnosis of advanced chronic kidney disease. Elevated parathyroid hormone and other metabolic derangements provide additional supportive evidence for chronic renal dysfunction [2].

Renal Outcomes in Non-Kidney Organ Transplantation

Recipients of nonrenal organ transplants including the liver, heart, and lung are at risk for developing acute kidney injury (AKI) and chronic kidney disease (CKD). Underlying hepatic or cardiopulmonary failure, prolonged intraoperative hemodynamic instability, and the use of calcineurin inhibitors and nephrotoxic medications have all been suggested to be contributory factors [15].

AKI and Renal Replacement Therapy

The incidence of perioperative AKI has been reported to occur in 17% to 95% of liver transplant recipients, 5% to 30% of heart transplant recipients, and 5% to 60% in recipients of lung transplants. Among those who develop AKI, renal replacement therapy is required in 5% to 35%, 5% to 15%, and 8% to 10% in liver, heart, and lung transplant recipients, respectively. The majority of patients are managed with continuous renal replacement therapy (CRRT) given less hemodynamic instability and more effective and efficient metabolic clearance and volume removal, with some centers advocating intraoperative CRRT at the time of transplant [15, 16].

Part of the wide range of reported AKI incidence is due to the varied criteria that have been used for the diagnosis of AKI. Acute kidney injury has been broadly defined as an abrupt decline in function, leading to retention of nitrogenous waste products, and a rise in blood urea nitrogen (BUN) and serum creatinine. Classification schemes initially established by the Acute Dialysis Quality Initiative (ADQI) included the Risk, Injury, Failure, Loss of kidney function, and End-stage kidney disease (RIFLE) staging criteria. The Acute Kidney Injury Network (AKIN) classification system modified the RIFLE Criteria and most recently the Kidney Disease Improving Global Outcomes (KDIGO) AKI Work-Group proposed criteria that incorporates both schemes [17]. The currently accepted definition of AKI is a rise in creatinine of > 0.3 mg/dL or 50% rise above baseline within 48 hours, with or without a reduction of urine output to less than 0.5 mL/kg/hour. Most publications of AKI have not followed this definition. Moving forward, use of established criteria should lessen the variability of AKI reporting and provide a more precise assessment of AKI incidence following non-renal solid organ transplantation.

Regardless of the incidence, AKI is strongly associated with increased morbidity, inferior allograft function, development of de-novo CKD and ESRD, and death. In addition to organ specific factors, sepsis, thrombotic microangiopathy, and calcineurin inhibitor nephrotoxicity may contribute to AKI. Acute kidney injury occurrence contributes to increased length of stay by nearly 3 weeks, as well as medical charges of more than $115,000 compared to those without AKI [18].

For liver transplant patients, AKI rates were highest in those with high pre-transplant MELD scores and a serum creatinine ≥ 2 mg/dL. Recent estimates show that 47% of liver transplant patients develop AKI with 7% requiring dialysis. For those patients with MELD scores > 30, the majority required renal replacement therapy post-transplant. Although serum creatinine is an important determinant of MELD, the actual severity of the liver disease, as demonstrated by pre-transplant international normalized ratio (INR), was associated with post-liver transplant AKI. Additional donor specific risk factors, such as donor age, cold and warm ischemic times, graft steatosis, and donation after circulatory death (DCD) all increase the occurrence of hepatic ischemia -reperfusion injury, graft dysfunction, and subsequent acute kidney injury [19].

A recent meta-analysis showed that almost 50% of all post-cardiac transplant patients develop AKI, with roughly 20% requiring renal replacement therapy. AKI proved an independent predictor of mortality post-transplant. Despite advances in cardiac transplant medicine and management, mortality rates in patients undergoing cardiac transplantation with AKI has not improved [20]. A recent meta-analysis showed that AKI post-cardiac transplant led to a 3.5-fold increased mortality in patients within 90 days of transplant and 2.3-fold increased mortality at one year. Pre-transplant factors that increase AKI incidence include previous cardiac operations, pre-existent diabetes, and older age. Common peri-operative and post-operative factors that predispose to AKI include older donor age, prolonged cardiopulmonary bypass time, surgery time, blood loss with transfusion dependence, high peripheral vascular resistance, and right ventricular failure with need for right ventricular assist device (RVAD) or veno-arterial extracorporeal membrane oxygenation (VA ECMO) [21, 22].

As with liver and heart transplant, AKI after lung transplantation is significantly associated with reduced short-term and long-term survival. Though survival following lung transplantation has improved over the past few decades, morbidity and mortality related to AKI after lung transplantation and resultant CKD remain high. Over 50% of lung transplant patients develop AKI and 10% of those require renal replacement therapy. Postoperative respiratory failure is as high as 55%. This degree of graft dysfunction and resultant hypoxia leads to reduced renal blood flow and AKI. Hypercapnia leads to peripheral vasodilation and decreased systemic vascular resistance with compensatory activation of the renin - angiotensin-aldosterone system (RAAS), leading to renal vasoconstriction and reduction in renal blood flow and GFR. Intraoperative hypotension, cardiopulmonary bypass time, and extracorporeal membrane oxygenation (ECMO) all lead to AKI [23].

Development of CKD and ESRD

With improved medical care, enhanced survival and increased longevity of solid organ transplant patients, CKD has become increasingly prevalent in these patients. Renal failure is common among recipients of non-renal solid organ transplants with rates of CKD of up to 16%; and in those with CKD, an ESRD incidence of up to 30% with most becoming dialysis -dependent within 3 years post-nonrenal organ transplantation [11, 18, 24]. The incidence of CKD often predates the transplant, is exacerbated by AKI events, and continues to deteriorate after transplantation. Risk factors for progression of kidney disease are summarized in Table 3.

Table 3. Risk Factors for CKD progression and ESRD following non-renal solid organ transplantation [25]

Pre-Transplant Conditions	• Pre-Existent Chronic kidney disease • Hypertension and Diabetes • Age • Hepatitis B- or C- related Glomerulonephritis • FSGS
Peri-Operative Conditions	• Ischemia-reperfusion injury • Prolonged Pump time • Hemodynamic instability and fluid shifts
Post-Transplant Factors	• Calcineurin Inhibitors • mTOR inhibitors and synergistic AKI • Progression of proteinuria • Development of Thrombotic Microangiopathy

The development of CKD and progression to ESRD results in a 4-fold increase in overall mortality [15]. According to Scientific Registry of Transplant Recipients (SRTR) data, kidney transplant for patients with prior non-renal organ transplant account for roughly 3% of transplants annually. Kidney transplant has a survival advantage for each type of non-renal transplant candidate, relative to maintenance dialysis. While most patients are placed on the deceased donor list preemptively, they suffer a significant and rapid decline, often not surviving the waiting time for kidney transplant. Given the high mortality while on the waiting list, targeted use of expanded criteria donor and/or living donor transplants may be particularly important in the non-renal transplant population [18].

MULTI-ORGAN TRANSPLANTATION

Multi-Organ Transplants (MOT) have been on the rise. Given the increased incidence of chronic kidney disease and the longevity of patients with non-renal organ failure managed with destination therapies, the need for MOT is increasing. In order to better utilize the pool of available kidney deceased donors, the Organ Procurement and Transplantation Network/United Network for Organ Sharing (OPTN/UNOS) restructured the Kidney Allocation System (KAS) in 2014. A key concept of the KAS is longevity matching, which aims to reduce the demand for subsequent kidney transplants and to increase the availability of kidneys for all prospective candidates [26]. However, the current allocation scheme places priority for MOT recipients above KTA, prioritizing urgency over longevity. Table 4 shows national trends of multi-organ transplants and the increasing incidence over the years [27].

Table 4. Combinations of organ involved in MOT and frequency (2013-2017)

	2013	2014	2015	2016	2017
Pancreas/Kidney (SPK)	762	709	719	798	789
Liver/Kidney (SLK)	494	558	627	730	739
Heart/Kidney (SHK)	85	104	141	140	187
Lung/Kidney (CLK)	7	5	1	4	7

The following discussion will highlight both the rationale for MOT involving a kidney transplant, as well as some of the ethical challenges of balancing equity and utility in MOT.

Simultaneous Pancreas Kidney (SPK) Transplant

Diabetes mellitus is a major health problem worldwide. In the United States, roughly 26 million adults are diabetic with 1.4 million being insulin -dependent type 1 diabetics and 2.9 million having type 2 diabetes managed with insulin [28]. Diabetes is reported as the cause for ESRD in nearly 40% of patients on the waitlist, with roughly 90,000 patients on the kidney transplant alone (KTA) list and 1,500 patients on the SPK waitlist [29]. Patients with diabetes and ESRD can choose one of the following options: dialysis, KTA, SPK, or Pancreas After Kidney (PAK), into a recipient with a function deceased- or living-donor kidney. This chapter will focus on the discussion of SPK. While the average waiting time for KTA under the new KAS policy remains 3-5 years, the average wait time for SPK is 2-4 years. Type 1 diabetics with ESRD have a 33% mortality rate in the first 5 years of dialysis initiation. Given the longer wait time for KTA, overall morbidity and mortality for wait-listed patients increases and diabetic KTA have worse kidney allograft function after transplant compared to other patients with non-diabetic ESRD [29]. Despite the surgical and immunosuppressive risks, SPK is the preferred treatment option for type 1 diabetics with ESRD. Pancreas transplant restores euglycemia, arrests further diabetic microvascular complications, and leads to improved patient and graft survival compared to KTA. This benefit is extended to select insulin-dependent type 2 diabetics who are increasingly being offered SPK and currently make up 18% of the waiting list for SPK [30].

Eligibility and Trends

The 2003 American Diabetes Association (ADA) criteria for simultaneous pancreas kidney transplant are as follows: 1) Patients with ESRD who meet criteria for renal transplant; 2) History of frequent, acute, severe metabolic complications (hypoglycemic unawareness, ketoacidosis), incapacitating clinical and emotional problems with exogenous insulin administration; and 3) Consistent failure of insulin therapy to prevent acute complications [31]. Given the survival advantage that a pancreas along with a kidney transplant confers, more SPK transplants should have been observed; however, numbers remained low. In 2014, UNOS changed the pancreas allocation system in order to increase the efficiency of allocation and availability of pancreas transplant. Prior to 2014, pancreas transplant alone and SPK transplants were not uniformly allocated. The revised policy established a separate waitlist and match run for these organs, separating these candidates from the kidney alone waitlist. It also established the following medical criteria for SPK: eligible for kidney transplant in a candidate who is on: 1) insulin with a C-peptide level < 2 ng/mL (i.e., true type 1 diabetic) or 2) insulin, with a C peptide > 2 ng/mL, with a BMI less than or equal to the maximum allowable cutoff (i.e., phenotypic type 2 diabetic). The UNOS mandated BMI cutoff was initially 28 in 2014, was modified to 30 in 2018, and was lifted completely in 2019. Currently, BMI cutoff for SPK in phenotypic type 2 diabetics is up to the discretion of transplant centers [32]. Critics point out that using C-peptide levels to differentiate between type 1 and type 2 diabetes can be misleading for the following reasons: 1) levels can be falsely elevated in patients with CKD /ESRD due to impaired excretion; 2) level can vary with patient's blood glucose levels; 3) level does not correlate with total daily insulin dose. Daily insulin requirements, as a surrogate of insulin resistance, seems to be a more reliable way to differentiate type 1 from type 2 diabetics [33]. Moreover, most centers establish set cutoffs for age and insulin requirement, with most pursuing SPK in those younger than 55 and insulin requirements not exceeding 1 unit/kg/day.

Outcomes, Controversies and Future Initiatives

Full assessment of the outcomes and benefits of SPK compared to living donor kidney transplantation alone (LD KTA) or deceased donor kidney transplantation alone (DD KTA) are difficult to quantify, as large registry data is lacking, and no randomized controlled trials have been performed. Retrospective reviews make up the bulk of observations, which are limited by patient, donor, and transplant center characteristics. Recent registry analysis has shown a slightly decreased survival and increased mortality in the first year with SPK compared to LD KTA and a survival difference that persists for nearly 5 years. This is attributed to the additional risk of the pancreas transplant and possibly additional dialysis time in SPK versus possible preemptive transplant or minimal dialysis vintage in LD KTA. However, mortality rate was two-fold lower in SPK recipients with functioning pancreas graft compared to DD KTA recipients [10]. Overall, the major benefits of SPK are reduced mortality and improved quality of life. The survival advantage is mainly attributed to a functional kidney transplant and freedom from dialysis, but a growing number of studies attribute improved survival to the pancreas allograft itself [34]. One study, in particular, showed that SPK recipients had improved patient survival, especially with a long-term functioning pancreas, compared with living-or deceased-donor kidney transplantation (LD KTA or DD KTA). Similar observations have been seen in retrospective reviews from individual transplant centers. Simultaneous pancreas kidney transplant in Type 2 diabetics show similar mortality benefit and non-inferior outcomes to those with Type 1 diabetes [33].

In addition to improved survival, SPK transplant also provides improved morbidity. Minimizing hyperglycemia and enhancing the counter-regulatory mechanisms that prevent hypoglycemia lead to restored euglycemia. Lipid parameters improve following SPK transplant, and progression of macrovascular atherosclerosis is slowed. Retinopathy and neuropathy are often stabilized and may even improve with restored euglycemia. Recipients reported enhanced quality of life and higher satisfaction. A substantial cost advantage was seen with SPK transplant compared to conventional medical therapy. One cost-effectiveness decision model analysis showed the estimated costs per quality adjusted year were $317, 746 for dialysis, but only $102,422 for SPK [35].

The following complications must be considered when discussing SPK outcomes. Most of these complications are observed in the first-year post-transplant and contribute to the increased morbidity and mortality observed in SPK compared to KTA. Table 4 outlines the most common complications post-transplant. Complications in the first 3 months are usually due to technical failure. Graft thrombosis remains the leading cause of early technical pancreas loss, with predisposing factors being prolonged cold ischemia time, graft pancreatitis, hypotension, reperfusion injury, and hypercoagulable states. From month 3-12, graft loss is due to death with a functioning graft, infections or acute/chronic rejection. One-year rates of immune-mediated pancreas graft loss are 1.5% in SPK compared to 4-5% in pancreas transplant alone. Pancreas graft failure has been difficult to define given lack of uniform definitions in the past. Only recently did UNOS outline the following definition for pancreas failure: 1) surgical removal of the pancreas; 2) the recipient dies; 3) the recipient is relisted for pancreas transplant; 4) recipient is listed for islet cell transplant after pancreas transplant; 5) insulin use of > 0.5 units/kg/day for ≥ 90 days [30].

Table 5. Common complications in simultaneous pancreas kidney transplant

Surgical Complications
• Graft thrombosis
• Peripancreatic abscess/fluid collection
• Anastomotic leaks
• Wound infection
Infectious Complications
• Bacterial, fungal, viral (CMV)
Metabolic Complications
• Chronic metabolic acidosis in patients with bladder-drained pancreata

Overall, SPK transplant is an attractive option for treatment of patients with diabetes and remains the primary treatment modality for diabetics with ESRD. Insulin-dependent patients on dialysis should be evaluated for SPK based on their predicted ability to tolerate the morbidity of the surgical procedure and the immunosuppression risks. The true benefit of pancreas transplant remains in question due to lack of prospective randomized trials; its full utility for Type 2 diabetics is still being evaluated. With the advent of closed loop insulin delivery systems, continuous glucose sensors, and future stem cell therapies, pancreas transplant outcomes will have to continue to improve to remain a clinically attractive therapy for insulin-dependent patients with diabetes [30].

APPROACH IN LIVER TRANSPLANT PATIENTS

Pre-existent CKD and AKI are common in patients with end-stage liver disease. By design, the MELD-based allocation for liver transplant ation prioritizes liver transplantation, particularly in those with renal insufficiency. Multiple studies have shown that liver transplant recipients with impaired renal function pre- and post-transplant experience increased morbidity and mortality. For those with end-stage liver disease awaiting liver transplant, the MELD score has not been able to predict which patients will have some degree of native kidney recovery and those who will need a concurrent renal transplant.

Rationale for SLK

In recent years, there has been a significant growth in the number of simultaneous liver kidney (SLK) transplants. Given the high mortality and morbidity associated with dialysis dependence post-liver transplant alone, a proposal was made and adopted by UNOS in 2016 to establish the SLK Allocation Policy. Table 6 outlines the current eligibility criteria that must be assessed by a Transplant Nephrologist, for wait-listing of a recipient for SLK, from the same deceased donor [36].

Table 6. Medical eligibility criteria for candidates under the liver -kidney allocation

If the Transplant Nephrologist confirms the diagnosis of:	Then the Transplant Program must report to the OPTN Contractor and document in the candidate's medical record:
• CKD with a measured or calculated GFR of ≤ 60 mL/min for greater than 90 days	At least one of the following: • Candidate has begun maintenance dialysis for ESRD, either in-center, in-hospital, or at home • At the time of registration on the kidney transplant waiting list, candidate GFR (calculated or measured) is ≤ 30 mL/min • On a date after the registration on the kidney transplant waiting list, the candidate's GFR (calculated or measured) is ≤ 30 mL/min
• Sustained acute kidney injury	At least one of the following or a combination of both of the following, for the last 6 weeks: • Candidate has been on dialysis at least once every 7 days • Candidate has a GFR (calculated or measured) of < 25 mL/min at least once every 7 days *if the candidates eligibility is not confirmed at least once every 7 days, for the last 6 weeks, the candidate is not eligible to receive a liver and kidney from the same donor
• Metabolic disease	A diagnosis of at least one of the following: • Hyperoxaluria • Atypical hemolytic uremic syndrome (aHUS) from mutations in factor H or factor I • Familial non-neuropathic systemic amyloidosis • Methylmalonic aciduria

Even with the current allocation guidelines, one of the challenges that many transplant nephrologists encounter is the difficulty to predict with full certainty whether a candidate's pre-existent kidney dysfunction is likely to recover after a liver transplant alone. Knowing the increased morbidity and mortality of dialysis dependence following liver transplant alone, the OPTN established a "safety - net" policy for those liver recipients with sustained kidney dysfunction. If a kidney candidate receives a liver transplant, but not a liver and kidney transplant from the same deceased donor, the candidate will be classified as a prior liver recipient. This liver recipient will be prioritized on the deceased donor kidney waiting list if they fulfill criteria outlined in Table 7 [36].

Table 7. Prioritization for liver recipients on the kidney alone waiting list

Both of the following must be met:
• Candidate is registered on the kidney transplant list prior to the one year anniversary of the liver transplant
• On a date that is at least 60 days but not more than 365 days after the liver transplant, the following are documented: • Candidate GFR (measured or calculated) < 20 mL/min • Candidate is on dialysis

Prioritization of "safety -net" candidates, using the new KAS, is outlined in Table 8 [36].

Table 8. Allocation sequence of safety -net liver transplant recipients with non-recovery of renal function

Sequence A	Sequence B	Sequence C	Sequence D
KDPI $\leq$ 20%	KDPI > 20% but < 35%	KDPI 35%-85%	KDPI> 85%
Highly Sensitized 0 ABDR MM Prior Living Donor Local Pediatrics	Highly Sensitized 0 ABDR MM Prior Living Donor Local Pediatrics	Highly Sensitized 0 ABDR MM Prior Living Donor Local Safety Net	Highly Sensitized 0 ABDR MM Local Safety Net
Local top 20% EPTS Local (all) Regional Pediatrics Regional EPTS<20% Regional (all) National Pediatrics National top 20% EPTS National (all)	Local Safety Net Local Adults Regional Pediatrics Regional Adults National Pediatrics National Adults	Local Adults Regional Adults National Adults	Local + Regional Adults National Adults

Of note, kidney after liver transplant allows allocation of kidneys to appropriate patients to maximize the longevity of the allograft and minimize mortality. An allocation system that maximizes the benefit of each organ balances utility, equity, and beneficence in a time when organ availability is limited [37].

Outcomes, Controversies and Future Initiatives

Based on single center and limited registry data, recipients of SLK have improved 1 year (86.2% vs 81.1%) and 5-year (70.1% vs 65.9%) survival compared to liver transplant alone [36]. In particular, SLK proves beneficial for patients with significant acute tubular necrosis (ATN) pre-transplant, as evidenced by dialysis dependence greater than 8 weeks and sustained creatinine ≥ 2.5 mg/dL. This observation characterizes those patients with low likelihood of native kidney recovery and true benefit from SLK.

However, when compared to KTA, SLK patients have increased morbidity and mortality. In a UNOS study of SLK versus kidney transplant patients who received the contralateral kidney, 5-year kidney graft survival (64% SLK vs. 75% KTA) and patient (66% SLK vs. 81% kidney-alone) survival were significantly lower in SLK [38]. These results highlight the challenge of balancing organ utility with equity. Since the new kidney allocation system in 2014, more kidneys are being allocated to SLK transplant recipients. Because multi-organ allocation occurs before kidney-alone allocation, highly sensitized ESRD patients, who are prioritized in the new KAS, lose the opportunity of these potential offers. Another concern is that kidneys used in SLK allocation tend to come from donors with lower kidney donor profile index (KDPI) and enhanced expected longevity. Unfortunately, these kidneys which would be prioritized to pediatric transplant candidates or young adults with the longest expected post-transplant survival, are allocated to SLK and MOTs in general. Of the total number of SLK transplants, 49% of donor kidneys had a KDPI < 35%. This diverts over 300 kidneys a year from pediatric and young adults, highly sensitized, and other high priority candidates on the kidney alone wait list. Data suggest that any of the kidney allografts that failed after SLK in the MELD era could have been used in a KTA and would have generated a median of 6 life-years [39]. Thus, care must be taken to avoid kidney transplant in those candidates who have a chance of renal recovery and in those with poor-transplant survival, where SLK would prove futile.

Care must also be given as to the timing of the transplant and considering delayed implant of the kidney until after the liver transplant has occurred. Using this model of maintaining the kidney on continuous hypothermic pulsatile machine perfusion and performing a two-surgery approach allows for decreased ATN and a more favorable environment for the kidney transplantation. It may allow re-allocation of the kidney transplant to the kidney alone waiting list, if the recipient is too unstable for transplant following the liver transplant [40, 41].

Future initiatives must focus on objective assessment of graft and patient outcomes under the new SLK Allocation criteria, observing the effectiveness of the "safety net" kidney allocation and exploring the use of higher KDPI donors in "safety net" candidates.

APPROACH IN HEART TRANSPLANT PATIENTS

Renal dysfunction is the most common comorbidity in patients with congestive heart failure (CHF), with roughly 50% of patients having eGFR< 60 mL/min. Increasing age and severity of heart failure correlate with increasing severity of renal dysfunction from cardiorenal syndrome and worse outcomes [42]. Concomitant diabetes, hypertension, renovascular disease, ongoing volume overload, low cardiac output, diuretic therapy, and intrinsic kidney disease all contribute to progression of end-stage renal failure [7]. In patients with advanced CHF refractory to medical therapy, LVAD as a bridge to orthotopic heart transplant (OHT) may initially improve renal function, but hemodynamic instability and right ventricular failure post-LVAD implantation can lead to AKI and further decline in GFR. Heart transplant remains the treatment of choice for end-stage heart disease. Unlike end-stage liver disease with the MELD scoring system, no prediction score exists in heart transplant to risk stratify candidates and determine pre-and post-transplant outcomes. The current heart allocation policy increases the likelihood of orthotopic heart transplantation (OHT) for the sickest patients, who have the greatest pre-transplant risk and post-transplant mortality [43].

Rationale for SHK

Analysis of the UNOS registry database shows a direct correlation between pre-OHT serum creatinine and 1-year post-OHT mortality, with a pre-OHT serum creatinine of > 2.5 mg/dl being associated with the highest risk of ESRD, need for kidney transplantation post-OHT, and almost double the mortality risk 1 year after OHT [44]. Patients requiring dialysis after transplant had a 41% mortality rate prior to discharge compared to just 3% for those not requiring dialysis. Therefore, there is a growing interest and demand for SHK transplant as a means of mortality risk mitigation in short- and long-term renal impairment in heart transplant recipients.

Eligibility and Trends

Unlike SLK transplantation, no UNOS mandated guideline exists to define the eligibility for SHK transplantation. Lack of consistent definitions of renal impairment limit objective candidacy assessment and listing for SHK. Given the lack of national eligibility criteria, individual transplant centers extrapolate GFR cutoffs and AKI duration from the SLK allocation policy to guide SHK transplant candidacy. General concepts of assessment of chronicity and reversibility guide the transplant nephrologist in assessing the degree of CKD. Predicting and considering future perioperative AKI events and the impact of calcineurin -inhibitor nephrotoxicity guides the decision for SHK versus OHT. Prolonged pre-transplant dialysis dependence and pre-existent CKD which appears irreversible are indications for SHK transplant. The SHK transplant occurs as a staged approach, with the heart transplant going first and the kidney transplant occurring 12-24 hours later, at the discretion of the medical team, once the recipient is hemodynamically stable.

Outcomes, Controversies, and Future Initiatives

UNOS data sets have shown improved survival of SHK compared to OHT alone. For patients with pre-transplant dialysis dependence, survival rates were 84% at 1-year and 73% at 5-year in SHK transplants compared to 69% at 1-year and 51% at 5-year in OHT alone. Similarly, for patients with pre-transplant non-dialysis dependent renal insufficiency, survival rates were 91% at 1-year and 80% at 5-year in SHK transplants compared to 81% at 1-year and 69% at 5-year in OHT alone [45]. Additional studies with multivariable adjustment of recipient and donor characteristics showed significant survival advantage in SHK transplants compared to OHT, with hazard ratios from 0.36-0.58 [46, 47]. Limitations to registry analysis include lack of reporting of post-transplant dialysis, particularly in the first month. A key observation has been that most SHK recipients are less critically ill, since only patients who are stable enough to undergo kidney transplantation after heart transplant undergo SHK. The selection bias may contribute to the overestimation of immediate improvement in survival of SHK recipients over OHT, which is unrelated to the kidney transplant. Therefore, questions arise regarding the comparability of the SHK and OHT groups and whether other differences contribute to the observed survival trends [48]. Kidney transplant at the time of heart transplant may be unnecessary in the setting of renal insufficiency from cardiorenal syndrome, where heart transplantation alone may lead to renal recovery .

When compared to KTA, SHK has inferior 1-year patient survival compared to DD KTA (84.0% vs 94.5%), higher relative risk of renal graft loss (HR of 1.41) with post-SHK dialysis dependence, and roughly 40% incidence of death with a functioning graft [10]. Patients with end-stage renal disease on dialysis have a 5-year survival of 60%, which improves to greater than 90% with kidney transplant. The small advantage seen in SHK may not justify removing that kidney from the organ pool where it will have a significantly greater impact in patients who require a kidney transplant alone [49].

Future initiatives must focus on universally agreed upon guidelines for eligibility of SHK and need to be defined by UNOS. Prioritization should continue to be given to those patients in urgent need, in whom SHK is the appropriate operation. Careful selection of candidates for SHK is needed, particularly when considering candidates not on dialysis who may do well with heart transplant alone. A "safety net" policy will effectively reprioritize kidney allocation to heart transplant alone recipients. Use of a staged approach with kidney transplant after heart transplant will increase utility while minimizing futility. Many SHK patients have worse kidney graft survival due to increased AKI incidence given the use of cardiopulmonary bypass, prolonged RV dysfunction, hemodynamic shifts, and vasopressor requirements. A "safety net" policy would extend allograft function, allow appropriate matching of donor-quality to recipient-characteristics, optimize equity and enhance allograft longevity, as intended by the Kidney Allocation System (KAS) [50].

Approach in Lung Transplant Patients

Lung transplantation (LT) is an established treatment for patients with end-stage lung disease but remains controversial in patients with significant multi-organ dysfunction. Patients with concomitant renal failure face unacceptably high mortality. Graft rejection prevention requires high doses of immunosuppression and the use of calcineurin inhibitors has been reported to cause significant post-transplant renal dysfunction.

Rationale, Eligibility, and Trends for CLK

Chronic kidney disease remains one of the most common complications in lung transplant patients and results in a four-fold increase in mortality [24]. At 5 years post-transplant, roughly 20% of patients will have significant CKD and 5% will be on maintenance dialysis. As in SHK transplant, CLK transplant eligibility criteria are not well-defined, and most centers have adopted similar criteria as are used in SHK transplants [51]. There have been relatively few CLK transplants, therefore survival estimates are limited. In 2019, only 13 CLK transplants were performed [52].

Outcomes, Controversies and Future Initiatives

Roughly 35% of patients undergoing CLK transplant were on dialysis pre-operatively, with the majority having ESRD as a consequence of CNI nephrotoxicity from a prior lung transplant alone. Overall survival for CLK compared to LT was comparable, with one year survival being 71% for CLK versus 81% for LT, and 5-year survival being 59% for CLK and 51% for LT, and median survival of 8 years. As expected, CLK survival rates were inferior to KTA (71% versus 95%) [53]. Many transplant centers recognize that kidney transplant immediately after lung transplant exposes the renal allograft to a nephrotoxic environment, due to hemodynamic instability, ECMO requirements, and medications [24]. Therefore, a staged approach to kidney transplant after lung transplant is growing in favor. Future initiatives, as in SHK, should focus on defining eligibility criteria for CLK, providing a "safety net" option for those lung transplant alone recipients with prolonged kidney dysfunction, and objective assessment of long-term data and outcomes.

ETHICAL CONSIDERATIONS IN MULTI-ORGAN TRANSPLANT

Historically, strong incentives for centers to perform MOT have existed. Under the current SRTR adjusted post-transplant outcome evaluations, only heart-lung and kidney - pancreas transplants are included. All other multi-organ transplants are excluded from the adjusted post-transplant survival calculations for kidney, heart, lung, and liver. Unadjusted post-transplant outcomes of MOTs are included in program-specific reports, but the center's mortality statistics are unaffected by negative outcomes. Historically, the SRTR excluded MOTs since they were rare, and reliable estimates of risk were not available. Therefore, centers often performed high risk MOTs without any consequence to outcome metrics.

Another incentive for centers performing MOT versus a single-organ alone transplant was the perception that MOT would avoid post-transplant complications, such as dialysis, that are costly and challenging. This led to a bias toward performing MOTs even when the individual recipient benefit was unclear.

Today, the numbers of MOTs are more substantial. In the most recent OPTN Policy Oversight Committee recommendations, Health Resources and Services Administration has encouraged SRTR to report MOT recipient outcomes in the transplant center metric. While it will take time for these models to be rebuilt with multi-organ inclusion, it is a step in the right direction to fully capture center outcomes and performance. Allowances for the high level of illness severity for these recipients should be given. This risk adjustment would promote transparency, accountability, and lead to a more equitable allocation policy.

The UNOS Ethics Committee has identified that allocation policies for MOT have the potential to create inequity in transplantation. Given the limited donor pool, both recipients awaiting MOT and single organ transplantation may face long waiting times [27]. Future initiatives must address equity and utility in MOT and consider the obligation to the kidney alone recipient. As stewards of a limited resource, these governing organizations, as well as the transplant community, must continue to strive for fairness and beneficence in organ allocation.

Conclusion

As the care of patients with chronic non-renal end organ failure has improved, the incidence of CKD and ESRD has increased. Patients awaiting non-renal, solid organ transplant with renal dysfunction are at risk of increased morbidity and mortality while on the waiting list. In addition, these patients have poorer post-transplant outcomes with non-renal solid organ transplant alone in the presence of renal dysfunction. An increasing indication for kidney transplantation is secondary kidney dysfunction in the setting of another severe organ dysfunction. Challenges exist in estimating the severity of renal dysfunction and predicting the degree of recovery of native kidney function that may occur after non-renal solid organ transplant alone. While MOT is increasingly performed, strict guidelines need to be established addressing MOT allocation policies, balancing urgency with utility and fairness .

References

[1] Ojo AO. Renal Disease in Recipients of Nonrenal Solid Organ Transplantation. *Semin Nephrol.* 2007;27(4):498–507.

[2] Inker LA, Astor BC, Fox CH, Isakova T, Lash JP, Peralta CA, et al. KDOQI US commentary on the 2012 KDIGO clinical practice guideline for the evaluation and management of CKD. *Am J Kidney Dis.* 2014;63(5):713–35.

[3] de Souza V, Hadj-Aissa A, Dolomanova O, Rabilloud M, Rognant N, Lemoine S, et al. Creatinine- versus cystatine C-based equations in assessing the renal function of candidates for liver transplant ation with cirrhosis. *Hepatology.* 2014;59(4):1522–31.

[4] Levey AS, Inker LA, Coresh J. GFR estimation: From physiology to public health. *Am J Kidney Dis*. 2014;63(5):820–34.

[5] Nickel NP, O'Leary JM, Brittain EL, Fessel JP, Zamanian RT, West JD, et al. Kidney dysfunction in patients with pulmonary arterial hypertension. *Pulm Circ.* 2017;7(1):38–54.

[6] Walther CP, Nambi V, Hanania NA, Navaneethan SD. Diagnosis and Management of Pulmonary Hypertension in Patients With CKD. *Am J Kidney Dis* 2020;75(6):935–45.

[7] Ross DW, Stevens GR, Wanchoo R, Majure DT, Jauhar S, Fernandez HA, et al. Left ventricular assist devices and the kidney. *Clin J Am Soc Nephrol.* 2018;13(2):348–55.

[8] Francoz C, Durand F, Kahn JA, Genyk YS, Nadim MK. Hepatorenal syndrome. *Clin J Am Soc Nephrol.* 2019;14(5):774–81.

[9] Bucsics T, Krones E. Renal dysfunction in cirrhosis: Acute kidney injury & the hepatorenal syndrome. *Gastroenterol Rep.* 2017;5(2):127–37.

[10] Stites E, Wiseman AC. Multiorgan transplantation. *Transplant Rev.* 2016;30(4):253–60.

[11] Miller BW. Chronic kidney disease in solid-organ transplantation. *Adv Chronic Kidney Dis.* 2006;13(1):29–34.

[12] Jagarlamudi N, Wong F. Acute kidney injury: prediction, prognostication and optimisation for liver transplant. *Hepatol Int.* 2020;14(2):167–79.

[13] Proulx NL, Akbari A, Garg AX, Rostom A, Jaffey J, Clark HD. Measured creatinine clearance from timed urine collections substantially overestimates glomerular filtration rate in patients with liver cirrhosis: A systematic review and individual patient meta-analysis. *Nephrol Dial Transplant.* 2005;20(8):1617–22.

[14] Petrucci I, Clementi A, Sessa C, Torrisi I MM. Ultrasound and color Doppler applications in chronic kidney disease. *J Nephrol.* 2018;6:863–79.

[15] Pham PTT, Slavov C, Pham PCT. Acute Kidney Injury After Liver, Heart, and Lung Transplants: Dialysis Modality, Predictors of Renal Function Recovery, and Impact on Survival. *Adv Chronic Kidney Dis* 2009;16(4):256–67.

[16] Baek SD, Jang M, Kim W, Yu H, Hwang S, Lee SG, et al. Benefits of Intraoperative Continuous Renal Replacement Therapy During Liver Transplantation in Patients With Renal Dysfunction. *Transplant Proc.* 2017;49(6):1344–50.

[17] Chawla LS, Bellomo R, Bihorac A, Goldstein SL, Siew ED, Bagshaw SM, et al. Acute kidney disease and renal recovery: Consensus report of the Acute Disease Quality Initiative (ADQI) 16 Workgroup. *Nat Rev Nephrol.* 2017;13(4):241–57.

[18] Rossi AP, Vella JP. Acute kidney disease after liver and heart transplantation. *Transplantation.* 2016;100(3):506–14.

[19] Thongprayoon C, Kaewput W, Thamcharoen N, Bathini T, Watthanasuntorn K, Lertjitbanjong P, et al. Incidence and Impact of Acute Kidney Injury after Liver Transplantation: A Meta-Analysis. *J Clin Med.* 2019;8(3):372.

[20] Kolsrud O, Karason K, Holmberg E, Ricksten SE, Felldin M, Samuelsson O, et al. Renal function and outcome after heart transplantation. *J Thorac Cardiovasc Surg.* 2018;155(4):1593-1604.e1.

[21] Thongprayoon C, Lertjitbanjong P, Hansrivijit P, Crisafio A, Mao M, Watthanasuntorn K, et al. Acute Kidney Injury in Patients Undergoing Cardiac Transplantation: A Meta-Analysis. *Medicines.* 2019;6(4):108.

[22] Thongprayoon C, Cheungpasitporn W, Lertjitbanjong P, Aeddula NR, Bathini T, Watthanasuntorn K, et al. Incidence and Impact of Acute Kidney Injury in Patients Receiving Extracorporeal Membrane Oxygenation: A Meta-Analysis. *J Clin Med.* 2019;8(7):981.

[23] Lertjitbanjong P, Thongprayoon C, Cheungpasitporn W, O'Corragain OA, Srivali N, Bathini T, et al. Acute Kidney Injury after Lung Transplantation: A Systematic Review and Meta-Analysis. *J Clin Med.* 2019;8(10):1713.

[24] Florens N, Dubourg L, Bitker L, Kalbacher E, Philit F, Mornex JF, et al. Measurement of glomerular filtration rate in lung transplant recipients highlights a dramatic loss of renal function after transplantation. *Clin Kidney J.* 2020;13(5):828–33.

[25] Srinivas TR, Stephany BR, Budev M, Mason DP, Starling RC, Miller C, et al. An emerging population: Kidney transplant candidates who are placed on the waiting list after liver, heart, and lung transplantation. *Clin J Am Soc Nephrol.* 2010;5(10):1881–6.

[26] Jackson KR, Covarrubias K, Holscher CM, Luo X, Chen J, Massie AB, et al. The national landscape of deceased donor kidney transplantation for the highly sensitized: Transplant rates, waitlist mortality, and posttransplant survival under KAS. *Am J Transplant.* 2019;19(4):1129–38.

[27] Fox A. Ethical Implications of Multi-Organ Transplants Ethical Implications of Multi-Organ Transplants. *OPTN Ethics Committee.* 2019;1–37.

[28] DHHS. *National Diabetes Statistics Report*, 2020 [Internet]. Centers for Disease Control and Prevention. National Diabetes Statistics Report: Estimates of Diabetes and Its Burden in the United States. 2020. p. 21. Available from: https://www.cdc.gov/diabetes /pdfs/data/statistics /national-diabetes-statistics-report.pdf.

[29] Hart A, Smith JM, Skeans MA, Gustafson SK, Wilk AR, Castro S, et al. OPTN/SRTR 2018 Annual Data Report: Kidney. *Am J Transplant.* 2020;20(s1):20–130.

[30] Kandaswamy R, Stock PG, Gustafson SK, Skeans MA, Urban R, Fox A, et al. OPTN/SRTR 2018 Annual Data Report: Pancreas. *Am J Transplant.* 2020;20(s1): 131–92.

[31] Robertson RP, Davis C, Larsen J, Stratta R, Sutherland DER. Pancreas transplantation for patients with type 1 diabetes. *Diabetes Care.* 2003;26(SUPPL. 1): 2003.

[32] Pancreas Allocation System [Internet]. *Organ Procurement and Transplantation Network.* 2018. Available from: https://optn.transplant .hrsa.gov/learn/professional-education /pancreas -allocation-system.

[33] Al-Qaoud TM, Odorico JS, Redfield RR. Pancreas transplantation in type 2 diabetes: Expanding the criteria. *Curr Opin Organ Transplant.* 2018;23(4):454–60.

[34] Lindahl JP, Hartmann A, Horneland R, Holdaas H, Reisæter A v., Midtvedt K, et al. Improved patient survival with simultaneous pancreas and kidney transplantation in recipients with diabetic end-stage renal disease. *Diabetologia.* 2013;56(6):1364–71.

[35] Dean PG, Kukla A, Stegall MD, Kudva YC. Pancreas transplantation. *BMJ* (Online). 2017;357:1–11.

[36] Simultaneous Liver Kidney (SLK) Allocation [Internet]. *Organ Procurement and Transplantation Network.* 2016. p. 1–12. Available from: https://optn.transplant . hrsa.gov/media /1888/kidney _policynotice_slk_201606.

[37] Eerhart MJ, Reyes JA, Leverson GE, Danobeitia JS, Blanton CL, Zitur LJ, et al. Kidney after Liver Transplantation Matched-pair Analysis: Are Kidneys Allocated to Appropriate Patients to Maximize Their Survival? *Transplantation.* 2020;104(4): 804–12.

[38] Choudhury RA, Reese PP, Goldberg DS, Bloom RD, Sawinski DL, Abt PL. A Paired Kidney Analysis of Multiorgan Transplantation: Implications for Allograft Survival. *Transplantation.* 2017;101(2):368–76.

[39] Cheng XS, Stedman MR, Chertow GM, Kim WR, Tan JC. Utility in treating kidney failure in end-stage liver disease with simultaneous liver-kidney transplantation. *Transplantation.* 2017;101(5):1111–9.

[40] Grant L, Tujios S, Singal AG. Outcomes of simultaneous liver -kidney transplantation. *Curr Opin Organ Transplant.* 2018;23(2):264–70.

[41] Lunsford KE, Agopian VG, Yi SG, Nguyen DTM, Graviss EA, Harlander-Locke MP, et al. Delayed implantation of pumped kidneys decreases renal allograft futility in combined liver -kidney transplantation. *Transplantation.* 2020;104(8):1591–603.

[42] Carubelli V, Metra M, Lund LH. Negotiating renal dysfunction when treating patients with heart failure. *Expert Rev Cardiovasc Ther*. 2018;16(2):113-122

[43] Shore S, Golbus JR, Aaronson KD, Nallamothu BK. Changes in the United States adult heart allocation policy: Challenges and opportunities. *Circ Cardiovasc Qual Outcomes.* 2020;(October):798–802.

[44] Habib PJ, Patel PC, Hodge D, Chimato N, Yip DS, Hosenpud JD, et al. Pre-orthotopic heart transplant estimated glomerular filtration rate predicts post-transplant mortality and renal outcomes: An analysis of the UNOS database. *J Heart Lung Transplant.* 2016;35(12):1471–9.

[45] Schaffer JM, Chiu P, Singh SK, Oyer PE, Reitz BA, Mallidi HR. Heart and combined heart-kidney transplantation in patients with concomitant renal insufficiency and end-stage heart failure. *Am J Transplant.* 2014;14(2):384–96.

[46] Savla J, Lin KY, Pradhan M, Ruebner RL, Rogers RS, Haskins SS, et al. Heart retransplant recipients have better survival with concurrent kidney transplant than with heart retransplant alone. *J Am Heart Assoc.* 2015;4(12):1–11.

[47] Chou AS, Habertheuer A, Chin AL, Sultan I, Vallabhajosyula P. Heart-Kidney and Heart-Liver Transplantation Provide Immunoprotection to the Cardiac Allograft. *Ann Thoracic Surg*. 2019;108(2):458–66.

[48] Cheng XS, Han J, Stedman MR, Chertow GM, Tan JC. And Then There Were Three: Effects of Pretransplant Dialysis on Multiorgan Transplantation. *Transplant Direct.* 2021;7(2): e657.

[49] Shaw BI, Sudan DL, Boulware LE, McElroy LM. Striking a balance in simultaneous heart kidney transplant: Optimizing outcomes for all wait-listed patients. *J Am Soc Nephrol.* 2020;31(8):1661–4.

[50] Cheng XS, Khush KK, Wiseman A, Teuteberg J, Tan JC. To kidney or not to kidney: Applying lessons learned from the simultaneous liver -kidney transplant policy to simultaneous heart-kidney transplantation. *Clin Transplant.* 2020;34(6):1–9.

[51] Ruderman I, Sevastos J, Anthony C, Ruygrok P, Chan W, Javorsky G, et al. Outcomes of simultaneous heart-kidney and lung-kidney transplantation s: The Australian and New Zealand experience. *Intern Med J.* 2015;45(12):1236–41.

[52] Aziz H, Kim J, Kwon YK. Current state of kidney utilization in multiorgan transplants. *Curr Opin Organ Transplant.* 2020;25(4):316–21.

[53] Reich HJ, Chan JL, Czer LSC, Mirocha J. *Combined Lung-Kidney Transplantation: An Analysis of the UNOS/OPTN Database.* 2013;1047–53.

In: Issues in Kidney Disease – Transplantation
Editors: B. V. R. Murthy and S. Z. Fadem

ISBN: 978-1-53619-960-4

Chapter 15

THE TRANSPLANT FAILURE – RETURN TO DIALYSIS, TRANSPLANT NEPHRECTOMY AND RE-TRANSPLANTATION

Medha Airy*, MD
Selzman Institute for Kidney Health, Section of Nephrology,
Baylor College of Medicine, Houston, TX, USA

ABSTRACT

Patients with failed renal transplants are clinically challenging to manage, and lack of guidelines makes it even more difficult. The prevalence of patients with a failed transplant has steadily increased over time, and their outcomes have been dismal compared to patients with chronic kidney disease approaching dialysis but had not yet received a transplant. The patient's acceptance of this diagnosis plays an important role in order to help manage his or her chronic condition(s) more effectively and efficiently. Decisions need to be made regarding choice of renal replacement therapy, management of immunosuppression, and management of the failed allograft, all of which are responsible for different patient outcomes. This chapter highlights the important aspects of management of patients with a failed transplant.

Keywords: transplant failure, transplant nephrectomy, re-transplantation, allosensitization

* Corresponding Author's Email: airy@bcm.edu.

INTRODUCTION

Tremendous progress has been made over the last two decades in immunosuppression management of kidney transplantation that improved the outcomes significantly in these patients. However, most of this improvement is observed in the first year after transplantation. Most recent United States Renal Data System (USRDS) Annual Data Report (ADR) was very encouraging with a 1-year graft survival rate of 93.7% for deceased donor kidney transplants (DDKT), and 96.7% for living donor kidney transplants (LDKT). However, 5-year graft survival rate falls to 76.7% and 85% for DDKT and LDKT, respectively (USRDS ADR 2015), and the 10-year graft survival rate to 49.7% and 65.2% for DDKT and LDKT, respectively (USRDS ADR 2013) [1]. Hence, approximately 35-50% patients lose their graft and return to dialysis or need a retransplant by 10 years after transplantation. The options that are available for these patients are discussed in this chapter.

RETURN TO DIALYSIS

Incidence of patients with failed transplants needing initiation on dialysis has increased globally, as evident from USRDS report [2, 3], as well as reports from Canada and Australia where patients with failed transplant constituted 2-3% of the incident population requiring dialysis initiation [4]. The options available for these patients include return to dialysis, relisting for another transplant, and need for a transplant nephrectomy. Main concerns when making such decisions revolve around the timing of initiation of renal replacement therapy, modality for renal replacement therapy (hemodialysis vs. peritoneal dialysis), management of immunosuppression, and decision for transplant nephrectomy, as they lose the kidney allograft function. These decisions are mostly physician-guided as no formal guidelines exist; moreover, the studies have been criticized for being small and observational in nature. Following sections discuss each of these concerns.

Timing of Initiation of Renal Replacement Therapy

As in transplant -naïve patients, the data for those with failed allografts regarding timing of initiation of dialysis is limited. Some studies in the past have supported the early initiation on dialysis in patients with End-Stage Kidney Disease [ESKD] [5, 6]. The results from the Initiating Dialysis Early and Late (IDEAL) study did not show significant difference in early vs. late initiation of dialysis (HR: 1.04, 95% CI 0.83-1.30, $p = 0.75$) [7]. These results did influence the guidelines, including the Kidney Disease Improving Global Outcomes (KDIGO) and the European Renal Association – European Dialysis and

Transplant Association (ERA -EDTA). Both KDIGO and ERA-EDTA have since indicated relying on symptomatology and biochemical markers when making decision on initiation of dialysis. For patients with failed allografts, a study by Gill et al. showed worse outcomes, with higher mortality rates in patients who initiated dialysis with the higher level of estimated glomerular filtration rate (eGFR) [8]. They reported a 4% higher risk of mortality with every 1 ml/min/1.73 m^2 increase in eGFR. Similar conclusions were drawn by Molnar and colleagues, who analyzed Scientific Registry of Transplant Recipients (SRTR) data and reported decreased survival especially in younger patients and in women initiating dialysis with a higher eGFR [9]. Based on these studies, the current recommendations for patients with failed allografts are similar to those with progressive chronic kidney disease (CKD). The decision of initiation remains contingent on clinical symptoms and biochemical markers than based on eGFR alone.

Modality of Renal Replacement Therapy

Patients with failed kidney transplants have the option of re-transplantation vs. choosing between hemodialysis or peritoneal dialysis (PD), similar to the transplant -naïve patients. Table 1 summarizes some of the studies available to compare the outcomes based on modality chosen by the patients upon returning to dialysis [10-18]. As highlighted in Table 1, most of the studies involve single-center experience and have a relatively small number of patients, hence results need to be interpreted accordingly. Most of the studies indicate no difference in the outcomes based on the modality chosen; however, the outcomes may be worse in patients who return to dialysis after transplant vs. transplant-naïve patients. Additionally, re-transplantation likely has better outcome compared to returning to dialysis [17]. Along with the single-center experience studies from the registry data, both the Canadian registry, as well as the USRDS data, have indicated similar outcomes with either modality [13, 14, 17]. Perl et al., analyzing the USRDS data, showed comparable overall outcomes with either modality, although an early survival advantage was observed with the use of PD [14]. Two studies using the Canadian Organ Replacement Register (CORR) one by Perl et al. [13], and another by Rao et al. [17], studying over 25,000 patients from different time periods, found similar outcomes in patients undergoing hemodialysis and PD. Hence, based on the available data, choice of dialysis modality does not affect the outcomes. Clinicians should discuss with the patient regarding both modalities; choice can be made based on feasibility and patient preference.

Table 1. Comparison of outcomes based on choice of modality on returning to dialysis after a failed transplant

Year	Author	Design	Intervention	Number of Patients	Results
2001	Davies	Single center, Prospective	Outcomes in patients returning to dialysis (HD and PD) from failed allograft and new dialysis patients	45	No survival difference between failed transplant patients starting HD vs. PD
2001	Sasal	Single center, Retrospective	Outcomes in failed transplant patients starting PD vs never transplanted patients	42	Late failed transplant patients had more complications and higher mortality compared to non-transplant patients.
2004	Duman	Single center, Retrospective	Outcomes in failed transplant patients starting PD vs never transplanted patients	34	Previous transplant did not adversely affect patient and technique survival
2005	Rao	Registry based, Canadian Organ Replacement register	Comparison of covariate adjusted mortality in five categories: transplant- naive dialysis, cadaveric primary renal transplant, living-donor primary renal transplant, failed transplant dialysis and retransplant	25632	Transplant- naive and failed transplant patients have equivalent mortality risk . Mortality is significantly reduced upon re-transplantation.
2006	Mujais	Case Control	Outcomes in patients starting PD after failed transplant vs patients new to renal replacement therapy or transitioning from HD to PD	494	Patients starting PD after failed transplant had similar patient and technique survival as controls.
2006	Dejonge	Single center retrospective	HD vs PD after failed transplant	60	No difference in survival curves in two groups. Rate of re-transplantation was higher in the PD group.
2011	Perl	Registry based, Canadian Organ Replacement Register	Patients initiating dialysis (HD or PD) after failed transplant	2110	PD compared with HD had similar early as well as overall survival.
2013	Perl	USRDS	Patients initiating dialysis (HD or PD) after failed transplant	16113	PD was associated with early survival advantage, inferior later survival and similar overall survival

TRANSPLANT NEPHRECTOMY

Transplant Nephrectomy (TN) procedure involves surgical removal of the failed allograft that can be done both in the early and late phase of allograft failure as well as for allograft complications. Numerous studies have examined the cumulative incidence of allograft failure TN, and reported it in the range from 4.5% to 84.4%, though these are difficult to compare due to variable follow up period[19]. TN was more common decades ago, before cyclosporine was introduced for immunosuppression as the number of patients with hyperacute rejection or symptomatic rejection was higher [20]. With decrease in acute rejection rates and significantly improved allograft survival with use of cyclosporine, early allograft nephrectomy rates were noted to decline [21-24]. While no widely accepted protocols or guidelines currently exist, indications for performing a TN in patients with a failed kidney allograft have included preemptive TN in asymptomatic patients [25, 26] or cause specific in patients who had clinical signs of rejection, unexplained hematuria, resistant infections, graft thrombosis causing pain, or malignancy [19, 21, 22, 27-29]. Preemptive nephrectomy allows quick and safe discontinuation of immunosuppression [19] as well as prevents a potential chronically inflamed state leading to complications such as erythropoietin resistance, endothelial dysfunction, and malnutrition [29]. Additionally, large observational studies have suggested a possibility of improved survival of patients who underwent TN. A study by Johnston et al. reviewed the USRDS data from 1995 to 2003 and reported a decreased adjusted mortality (HR = 0.89; 95% CI, 0.83-0.95) in patients who had TN for late allograft failure, defined as failure after 12 months of transplant [30]. However, TN after early allograft failure was associated with increased mortality (HR = 1.13; 95% CI; 1.01-1.26). In the study done by Ayus et al. using USRDS data as well for the period 1994-2004, reported an adjusted 32% lower all-cause mortality (95% CI, 26%-37%) for those undergoing allograft nephrectomy compared to those that did not [31] with benefit being present irrespective of the time from transplant failure. Higher success rates of receiving a second transplant were found in patients who had nephrectomy compared to those who did not. The difference in findings from the two studies could be attributed to the differences in the number of patients and the selection criteria used for the patients.

Irrespective of the benefits, there are also potential disadvantages of TN that need to be considered. Firstly, TN as a procedure, has significant morbidity and mortality. Commonly reported complications include bleeding, infections, injury to nerve or bowel, and formation of pseudo-aneurysms and lymphoceles [22, 24, 32-34]. Even though, in the earlier era, morbidity up to 40% [35] and mortality up to 7% [22] were reported, these complications have now been reduced drastically with advancement in surgical techniques as well as newer immunosuppression regimens. Additionally, there is an option to consider transplant emboli zation compared to surgical nephrectomy, which is associated with significantly reduced morbidity and mortality rate s. Secondly, there remains a concern that

TN is associated with a subsequent increase in panel-reactive antibody (PRA) levels [32, 43-36] which reduces the chance of finding a compatible donor and is associated with worse post-transplant outcomes [44]. The mechanism for this TN-associated sensitization has not been fully understood. It has been proposed that inflamed graft remnants left after surgery (i.e., ureteric stump) may elicit a strong immune response following immunosuppression withdrawal. An alternate explanation is that the failed transplant acts as a 'sink' sequestering anti-HLA antibodies out of the circulation. However, there have also been studies which did not show significant change in post-nephrectomy PRA level, and did not affect the rate of re-transplantation or outcomes in these patients [45]. Overall, the decision to proceed with the surgery remains center-specific, with most centers leaning towards TN for symptomatic indications. The risks of the procedure seem to outweigh the benefits for a routine TN. Hence, the rate of TN has significantly declined over the years.

Management of Immunosuppression

Patients with failed allograft function need adjustment for the immunosuppressive regimen based on the anticipated clinical course. A rapid reduction is often needed in cases of hyperacute or early rejection to avoid further complications such as graft rupture. For most of the other conditions, centers would continue low level immunosuppressive regimen if a retransplant is anticipated within a year or to maintain the residual renal function. However, if a patient needs transplant nephrectomy, or returns to dialysis and has no residual renal function, immunosuppression can be tapered off completely. In such cases, antimetabolites are the first ones to be discontinued, followed by reduction of the doses of calcineurin inhibitors (CNI) or mTOR (mammalian Target of Rapamycin) inhibitors, and lastly followed by steroid withdrawal. Although described by the British Transplantation Society in its guidelines in 2014 [46], this regimen has been widely practiced all over the world for a long time.

There may be a small benefit of continued immunosuppression in patients with failed allograft who return to PD. Jassal et al., using the USRDS data, showed an increase in life expectancy from 5.3 years to 5.8 years in patients with failed allografts maintained on immunosuppression after starting PD. This is possibly related to the preservation of residual renal function [47].

Another important concern is the risk of allosensitization upon complete discontinuation of immunosuppression. Studies have indicated lower sensitization rates, as indicated by PRA level and anti-HLA antibodies, in patients who were maintained on at least low level of immunosuppression [48, 49]. Sometimes these results get clouded by transfusions and TN making conclusion difficult on the sole effect of immunosuppression on allosensitization. While lower rates of sensitization and preservation of residual renal function seem advantageous because of continuing immunosuppression, this needs to be balanced against the adverse effects of prolonging immunosuppressed state, including the higher rates of opportunistic infections, cancer, and metabolic complications [50, 51].

RE-TRANSPLANTATION

It has been well established that kidney transplants offer best outcomes for patients with advanced chronic kidney disease needing replacement therapy [52]. Patients with failed transplants have the option of relisting for a deceased donor transplant or getting a living donation, similar to the transplant-naïve patients. According to the Annual Data Report of the US Organ Procurement and Transplantation Network (OPTN) and the Scientific Registry of Transplant Recipients (SRTR), patients needing retransplant constitutes 11.8% of the waiting list [53]. The advantages of re-transplant in those with failed transplant are similar to those who receive the transplant for the first time when compared to those returning to dialysis. In both groups (transplant naïve and re-transplant), a preemptive transplant has better outcomes compared to a transplant after starting dialysis. Important concerns with patients needing re-transplantation include increased sensitization and timing to second transplant, which additionally contribute to outcomes in these patients.

In a retrospective analysis using the USRDS data, Goldfarb et al., in 2006, suggested increased risk of allograft failure with Preemptive Second Kidney Transplant (PSKT) [54]. However, Johnston and colleagues, also analyzing USRDS data, in 2013, reported less acute rejections (12% vs. 16%, $p < 0.0001$), and a decreased rate of delayed graft function (8% vs. 23%, $p < 0.0001$) associated with PSKT compared to non-pre-emptive second transplantation [55]. Additionally, they reported decreased death with a functioning graft, with no difference in death censored graft survival [HR: 0.98, 95% C.I. (0.88-1.08)] among patients with PSKT. Girerd and colleagues depicted temporal trends and time-varying effects of PSKT on graft survival; they reported a significantly improved graft survival in the first 5 years with PSKT (94.1% vs 76.8%) compared to non-pre-emptive second transplantation. However, this effect seemed to diminish afterwards such that by 12 years post-transplant ation, there was no difference between the two groups [56]. Though a single-center analysis, this study had a long follow-up period, and hence merits a mention. Similar encouraging results were also noted from a Spanish study that reported PSKT as a feasible option with reduced comorbidities [57]. These studies suggest PSKT as a better option than non- pre-emptive second transplantation, whenever feasible. Furthermore, studies have also established that even 3rd and 4th transplants can be performed in patients needing retransplants with safe outcomes [58, 59].

Conclusion

Patients with failed transplants have options similar to transplant -naïve ESKD patients. Decisions on managing immunosuppression and failed allograft need special attention. Further research opportunities exist to crystallize management algorithms and to improve outcomes in these patients.

References

[1] United States Renal Data System. 2020 *USRDS Annual Data Report: Epidemiology of kidney disease in the United States.* National Institutes of Health, National Institute of Diabetes and Digestive and Kidney Diseases, Bethesda, MD, 2020.

[2] Brar A, Markell M, Stefanov DG, Timpo E, Jindal RM, Nee R, Sumrani N, John D, Tedla F, Salifu MO. Mortality after Renal Allograft Failure and Return to Dialysis. *Am J Nephrol.* 2017;45(2):180-186.

[3] Molnar MZ, Ichii H, Lineen J, Foster CE 3rd, Mathe Z, Schiff J, Kim SJ, Pahl MV, Amin AN, Kalantar-Zadeh K, Kovesdy CP. Timing of return to dialysis in patients with failing kidney transplants. *Semin Dial.* 2013;26(6):667-74.

[4] Perl J, Hasan O, Bargman JM, Jiang D, Na Y, Gill JS, Jassal SV: Impact of dialysis modality on survival after kidney transplant failure. *Clini J Am Soc Nephrol* 6:582–590, 2011.

[5] Beddhu S, Samore MH, Roberts MS, Stoddard GJ, Ramkumar N, Pappas LM, Cheung AK: Impact of timing of initiation of dialysis on mortality. *J Am Soc Nephrol* 14:2305–2312, 2003.

[6] Rosansky S, Glassock RJ, Clark WF: Early start of dialysis: a critical review. *Clin J Am Soc Nephrol* 6:1222–1228, 2011.

[7] Cooper BA, Branley P, Bulfone L, Collins JF, Craig JC, Fraenkel MB, Harris A, Johnson DW, Kesselhut J, Li JJ, Luxton G, Pilmore A, Tiller DJ, Harris DC, Pollock CA: A randomized, controlled trial of early versus late initiation of dialysis. *N Engl J Med* 363:609–619, 2010.

[8] Gill JS, Abichandani R, Kausz AT, Pereira BJ: Mortality after kidney transplant failure: the impact of non-immunologic factors. *Kidney Int* 62:1875–1883, 2002.

[9] Molnar MZ, Streja E, Kovesdy CP, Hoshino J, Hatamizadeh P, Glassock RJ, Ojo AO, Kalantar-Zadeh K: Estimated glomerular filtration rate at reinitiation of dialysis and mortality in failed kidney transplant recipients. *Nephrol Dial Transplant* 27:2913–2921, 2012.

[10] Davies SJ. Peritoneal dialysis in the patient with a failing renal allograft. *Perit Dial Int* 2001; 21: 280– 284.

[11] de Jonge H, Bammens B, Lemahieu W et al. Comparison of peritoneal dialysis and hemodialysis after renal transplant failure. *Nephrol Dial Transplant* 2006; 21: 1669–1674.

[12] Sasal J, Naimark D, Klassen J et al. Late renal transplant failure: an adverse prognostic factor at initiation of peritoneal dialysis. *Perit Dial Int* 2001; 21: 405–410.

[13] Perl J, Hasan O, Bargman JM, et al. Impact of dialysis modality on survival after kidney transplant failure. *Clin J Am Soc Nephrol* 2011; 6: 582–590.

[14] Perl J, Dong J, Rose C et al. Is dialysis modality a factor in the survival of patients initiating dialysis after kidney trans- plant failure? *Perit Dial Int* 2013; 33: 618–628.

[15] Salazar AM, Chavez CO, Alvarez TG et al. Returning to dialysis after kidney transplant failure. Does the dialysis treatment modality influence the survival prognosis ? *Transplantation* 2018; 102(7 Suppl 1): S537.

[16] Duman S, Asci G, Toz H, Ozkahya M, Ertilav M, Sezis M, Ok E: Patients with failed renal transplant may be suitable for peritoneal dialysis. *Int Urol Nephrol* 36:249–252, 2004.

[17] Rao PS, Schaubel DE, Saran R: Impact of graft failure on patient survival on dialysis: a comparison of transplant -naive and post-graft failure mortality rate s. *Nephrol Dial Transplant* 20:387–391, 2005.

[18] Mujais S, Story K: Patient and technique survival on peritoneal dialysis in patients with failed renal allograft: a case-control study. *Kidney Int Suppl* (103):S133–S137, 2006.

[19] Akoh JA. Transplant nephrectomy. *World J Transplant* 2011;1(1):4-12.

[20] Roberts CS, LaFond J, Fitts CT, et al. New patterns of transplant nephrectomy in the cyclosporine era. *J Am Coll Surg* 1994;178(1):59-64.

[21] Secin FP, Rovegno AR, del Rosario Brunet M, et al. Cumulative incidence, indications, morbidity and mortality of transplant nephrectomy and the most appropriate time for graft removal: only nonfunctioning transplants that cause intractable complications should be excised. *J Urol* 2003;169(4):1242-1246.

[22] Zargar MA, Kamali K. Reasons for transplant nephrectomy: a retrospective study of 60 cases. *Transplant Proc* 2001;33(5):2655-2656.

[23] Bonilla AJ, Alfaro AG, Henandez JP, et al. Review of a transplantectomy series. *Transplant Proc* 2015;47(1):81-83.

[24] Toth F, Zadori G, Fedor R, et al. A Single-center Experience of Allograft Nephrectomies Following Kidney Transplantation. *Transplant Proc* 2016;48 (7):2552-2554.

[25] Toledo-Pereyra LH, Gordon C, Kaufmann R, et al. Role of immediate versus delayed nephrectomy for failed renal transplants. *Am Surg* 1987;53(9):534-536.

[26] Ayus JC, Achinger SG. At the peril of dialysis patients: ignoring the failed transplant. *Semin Dial* 2005;18(3):180-184.

[27] Asch WS, Bia M. When should nephrectomy be performed for a failed renal transplant ? *Semin Dial* 2011;24(4):374-376.

[28] DiSesa VJ, Tilney NL. Conservative management of the failed renal allograft: indications for transplant nephrectomy. *Curr Surg* 1982;39(6):417-418.

[29] Mehrotra A, Tan JA, Ames SA. "Out of Sight, Out of Mind": The Failed Renal Allograft as a Cause of ESA Resistance. *Semin Dial* 2015;28(5):530-532.

[30] Johnston O, Rose C, Landsberg D, et al. Nephrectomy after transplant failure: current practice and outcomes. *Am J Transplant* 2007;7(8):1961-1967.

[31] Ayus JC, Achinger SG, Lee S, et al. Transplant nephrectomy improves survival following a failed renal allograft. *J Am Soc Nephrol* 2010;21(2):374-380.

[32] Del Bello A, Congy-Jolivet N, Sallusto F, et al. Donor-specific antibodies after ceasing immunosuppressive therapy, with or without an allograft nephrectomy. *Clin J Am Soc Nephrol* 2012;7(8):1310-1319.

[33] Del Bello A, Congy N, Sallusto F, et al. Anti-human leukocyte antigen immunization after early allograft nephrectomy. *Transplantation* 2012;93(9):936-941.

[34] Grochowiecki T, Szmidt J, Galazka Z, et al. Influence of timing of transplant nephrectomy on surgical complications. *Transplant Proc* 2000;32(6):1381.

[35] Noel C, Hazzan M, Boukelmoune M, et al. Indication for allograft nephrectomy after irreversible rejection: is there an ideal delay? *Transplant Proc* 1997;29(1-2):145-146.

[36] Khakhar AK, Shahinian VB, House AA, et al. The impact of allograft nephrectomy on percent panel reactive antibody and clinical outcome. *Transplant Proc* 2003;35(2):862-863.

[37] Sumrani N, Delaney V, Hong JH, et al. The influence of nephrectomy of the primary allograft on retransplant graft outcome in the cyclosporine era. *Transplantation* 1992;53(1):52-55.

[38] Helmrich D, Pisarski P, Offermann G, et al. Impact of transplant nephrectomy on peak PRA levels and outcome after kidney re-transplantation. *World J Transplant* 2014;4(2):141-147.

[39] Knight MG, Tiong HY, Li J, et al. Transplant nephrectomy after allograft failure is associated with allosensitization. *Urology* 2011;78(2):314-318.

[40] Schachtner T, Otto NM, Stein M, et al. Transplantectomy is associated with presensitization with donor-reactive T cells and graft failure after kidney retransplantation: a cohort study. *Nephrol Dial Transplant* 2018.

[41] Schleicher C, Wolters H, Kebschull L, et al. Impact of failed allograft nephrectomy on initial function and graft survival after kidney retransplantation. *Transpl Int* 2011;24(3):284-291.

[42] Rosenberg JC, Berri R, Jackowski M, et al. Multi-array antibody screening in detecting antibodies to mismatched HLA in patients awaiting a second transplant. *Transplant Proc* 2006;38(10):3393-3395.

[43] Ahmad N, Ahmed K, Mamode N. Does nephrectomy of failed allograft influence graft survival after re-transplantation ? *Nephrol Dial Transplant* 2009;24(2):639-642.

[44] Lefaucheur C, Loupy A, Hill GS, et al. Preexisting donor-specific HLA antibodies predict outcome in kidney transplantation. *J Am Soc Nephrol* 2010;21(8):1398-1406.

[45] Lucisano G, Brookes P, Santos-Nunez E et al. Allosensitization after transplant failure: the role of graft nephrectomy and immunosuppression – a retrospective study. *Transpl Int* 2019; 32: 949–959.

[46] Andrews PA; Standards Committee of the British Transplantation Society. Summary of the British Transplantation Society guidelines for management of the failing kidney transplant. *Transplantation* 2014; 98: 1130–1133.

[47] Jassal SV, Lok CE, Walele A, Bargman JM. Continued transplant immune-suppression may prolong survival after return to peritoneal dialysis: results of a decision analysis. *Am J Kidney Dis* 2002; 40: 178-83.

[48] Scornik JC, Kriesche H-U. Human leukocyte antigen sensitization after transplant loss: timing of antibody detection and implications for prevention. *Hum Immunol* 2011; 72: 398–401.

[49] Casey MJ, Wen X, Kayler LK et al. Prolonged immunosuppression preserves nonsensitization status after kidney transplant failure. *Transplantation* 2014; 98: 306–311.

[50] Smak Gregoor PJ, Zietse R, van Saase JL et al. Immunosuppression should be stopped in patients with renal allograft failure. *Clin Transplant* 2001; 15: 397–401.

[51] Vajdic CM, van Leeuwen MT, Webster AC et al. Cutaneous melanoma is related to immune suppression in kidney transplant recipients. *Cancer Epidemiol Biomarkers* Prev2009; 18: 2297–2303.

[52] Wolfe RA, Ashby VB, Milford EL, et al. Comparison of mortality in all patients on dialysis, patients on dialysis awaiting transplantation, and recipients of a first cadaveric transplant. *N Engl J Med* 1999; 341:1725e30.

[53] 2018 *Annual Data Report*. Scientific Registry of Transplant Recipients http://srtr.transplant .hrsa.gov/annual_reports/Default.aspx Accessed [22 Feb 2021].

[54] Goldfarb-Rumyantzev AS, Hurdle JF, Baird BC, et al. The role of pre-emptive re-transplant in graft and recipient outcome. *Nephrol Dial Transplant* 2006; 21:1355e64.

[55] Johnston O, Rose CL, Gill JS, Gill JS. Risks and benefits of preemptive second kidney transplantation. *Transplantation* 2013; 95:705e10.

[56] Girerd S, Girerd N, Aarnink A, Solimando E, Ladriere M, Kennel A, et al. Temporal trend and time-varying effect of pre- emptive second kidney transplantation on graft survival: a 30-year single-center cohort study. *Transplant Proc* 2016; 48:2663e8.

[57] Florit EA, Bennis S, Rodriguez E, et al. Pre-emptive retransplantation in patients with chronic kidney graft failure. *Transplant Proc* 2015; 47:2351e3.

[58] Izquierdo L, Peri L, Piqueras M et al. Third and fourth kidney transplant: still a reasonable option. *Transplant Proc* 2010; 42: 2498–2502.

[59] Loupy A, Anglicheau D, Timsit MO et al. Impact of surgical procedures and complications on outcomes of third and subsequent kidney transplants. *Transplantation* 2007; 83: 385–391.

In: Issues in Kidney Disease – Transplantation
Editors: B. V. R. Murthy and S. Z. Fadem
ISBN: 978-1-53619-960-4

Chapter 16

Psychosocial Aspects of Kidney Transplantation in Kidney Transplant Recipients and Living Donors

Angelina Edwards**, MD
Division of Kidney Diseases, Hypertension and Transplantation,
Department of Medicine, Houston Methodist Hospital, Houston, TX, USA

Abstract

Transplantation remains the optimal treatment for patients with end stage renal disease. In order to determine suitability for transplant, individuals must undergo thorough medical, surgical, and psychosocial evaluations. A successful transplant requires optimization of all three of these areas. Similarly, living kidney donors must undergo an equally robust assessment, with special emphasis on assessing the motivation for donation, lack of coercion, and a true state of voluntariness. For both transplant recipients and living donors, pre-existent psychosocial predictors can influence post-event outcomes. Therefore, the goal of the evaluation is to recognize candidates with risks and barriers requiring multidisciplinary interventions, both before and after transplantation or donation.

Keywords: psychosocial assessment, kidney transplant, living kidney donor

Introduction

The kidney transplant waiting list continues to grow [1]. Given the limited availability of organs, it is imperative that a thorough psychosocial assessment be performed to assure

* Corresponding Author's Email: aredwards@houstonmethodist.org.

the greatest success after transplant. The psychosocial issues around transplant impact the ultimate success of a transplant. Therefore, the psychosocial assessment is an essential component to a patient's candidacy.

Psychosocial Risk Factors and Post-Transplant Outcomes

Numerous studies have shown that psychosocial risk factors impact both medical and psychosocial transplant outcomes. Some of these factors, such as habitual medication nonadherence, may be a relative contraindication to transplantation while others may require pre-transplant interventions to assess readiness for transplant.

Social Support and Transplant Success

Inadequate social support has long been considered a contraindication for transplant. No guidelines clearly define social support, but it is assumed to encompass services, care and encouragement provided by the caregiver, usually the spouse, parent, child, sibling, and friends. Given the lack of specificity in defining a minimum threshold for support, variation exists within Transplant Programs. Using social support as determination of eligibility for transplant may disenfranchise certain patient populations, particularly those with complex social situations. Caregivers may be unable to commit to the requirements of the transplant team, given other obligations, such as limited ability to take off time from work, or financial hardship. It is these situations that require thoughtful consideration by the transplant program, to create circles of support around the patient and a community of helpers that may be able to step in at various times, during the evaluation, testing, and ultimate transplant period [2].

It is assumed that medication adherence and thus graft longevity are enhanced by adequate social support, but some studies have shown no consistent benefit [3]. Further studies are needed to determine the role that social support plays in post-transplant outcomes [4].

Medication and Treatment Nonadherence

In the end stage renal disease (ESRD) population, medication and treatment nonadherence is commonly encountered and results in poor health outcomes. Challenges with following fluid restriction, dietary restrictions, medications, and the dialysis regimen itself are common surrogates of nonadherence that are used by the evaluating transplant center [5]. In fact, the goal of obtaining a transplant is often a reason for motivating a patient to become compliant. Adherence in the transplant realm is commonly equated with medication and immunosuppression compliance, given the high stakes of allograft loss if this is lacking. However, transplant brings a need for other aspects of adherence, including lifestyle changes such as adequate fluid intake, attendance at lab and clinic appointments, and timely communication with the transplant team regarding changes in health status. Pre-transplant self-reported adherence, to either medications or treatment interventions, often predicts post-transplant outcomes [6]. Blatant nonadherence is a contraindication to transplant and remediation potential needs to be assessed. Often, non-adherent patients are given an opportunity to show improvement by adhering to steps outlined in a "compliance contract" or "behavioral contingency contract." Ensuring that patients understand the rationale behind each part of the medical regimen will increase the likelihood of adherence. Allowing patients to prove adherence may eventually lead to a patient becoming eligible and fostering a long-term relationship with the patient, built on communication and adherence [7].

Adherence to the post-transplant medication regimen plays a significant role in transplant outcomes, most notably patient and allograft longevity. There are several factors to consider in patients with medication nonadherence [8]. Table 1 highlights some of these factors. The transplant team should make every attempt to mitigate these issues, foster self-management skills, and work with the patient to ensure compliance for the preservation of the transplant.

Table 1. Themes of nonadherence in post-transplant kidney patients

Sociodemographic Factors	Patient Characteristics
• Adolescent/young adult	• Past non-adherence
• Minority ethnicity	• Psychological stress
• Low socioeconomic status	• Low health literacy
Condition Related Scenarios	• Cognitive Impairment
• Improved health status	Health Care/Provider Changes
• Longer time since transplant	• Pediatric transition to Adult Clinic
• Preemptive living donor transplant	• Insurance Status
Treatment Related Factors	• Provider/Patient Communication changes
• Greater total number of medications	
• More frequent dosing	
• Side effects	

Substance Use and Abuse

Alcohol and substance use is common in the ESRD population. It is imperative to screen for any active or past history of substance abuse during the transplant evaluation. Substance abuse has been linked to adverse outcomes post-transplant, including medication nonadherence and increased infection risk associated with illicit drugs. It is also associated with increased graft loss and death [9]. Therefore, patients with excess use of alcohol or illicit drugs are precluded from transplant until adequate rehabilitation has occurred and they are able to prove sustained periods of abstinence. The use of tobacco products is considered a relative contraindication to kidney transplant, given the cardiovascular risk that smoking portends [10].

Cannabis is categorized as a substance of abuse but legalization for medical reasons is rising. Patients with kidney failure may use medical or recreational cannabis to manage symptoms of nausea, vomiting, pruritus, poor appetite and chronic pain. Pre-transplant candidates who admit using or test positive for marijuana are declined by some centers, and only considered after a period of rehabilitation. Post-transplant concerns regarding cannabis use include infection risk (fungal pneumonia), variable drug levels, cognitive changes, and additional substance abuse [11]. Cannabis is known to affect motor coordination, short-term memory, neurocognitive function, and judgement and is associated with psychiatric conditions such as acute psychosis, schizophrenia, and depression. It is associated with increased allograft loss, increased risk of accidents, including motor vehicle collision and fractures, and death. For these reasons, it is important to continue to screen for substance abuse history in the post-transplant period, educate patients regarding the dangers of cannabis use and encourage continued abstinence [12].

Opioid analgesics serve as an important role in the management of acute and chronic pain. Up to 80% of patients with ESRD report chronic pain and are often prescribed opiates. Significant adverse outcomes are seen in dialysis patients on chronic opiates, including altered mental status, falls, and fractures. Given the high risk of abuse, overuse and misuse of opiates, along with the rising "epidemic " of overdose and death, opiate use should be assessed at the time of transplant evaluation [13]. All attempts should be made to evaluate the underlying cause of pain and refer to appropriate specialists prior to transplant. Many centers require patients to be under the care of a licensed pain management specialist, who will continue to care for their pain medication needs even after transplant. However, chronic pre- and post-transplant opiate dependence is linked to poor post-transplant outcomes, including death and graft failure. Therefore, a multidisciplinary approach to mitigate chronic opiate dependence is warranted should these patients be deemed eligible for transplantation [14].

Psychiatric Disorders and Predictors of Post-Transplant Challenges

The presence of pre-existent psychiatric disorders in the ESRD is high. Up to 38% of patients who require dialysis report severe psychological distress. Post-transplant, depression can persist, with an average prevalence of 27% [15]. Historically, patients are often under-diagnosed and under-treated. Screening tools specifically validated in the

ESRD population include the Beck Depression Inventory (BDI) and Patient Health Questionnaire-9 (PHQ-9), with recommendations for social workers to perform depression screens at the time of dialysis initiation, and biannually [16, 17]. Patient scores of 14 or higher on the BDI and/or 10 or higher on the PHQ-9 warrant additional referral to a Psychiatrist for therapeutic intervention [18]. In addition to pharmacotherapy, recent studies have highlighted the beneficial effects of cognitive behavioral therapy, exercise, and relaxation techniques on quality of life and depressive symptoms in dialysis patients [19].

Anxiety is also common amongst ESRD patients, with presentations varying from 12-58% depending on the screening tool used, and can co-exist with other psychiatric disorder s, including depression, post-traumatic stress, and obsessive-compulsive disorder. Women are more affected than men and symptoms can manifest as restlessness, irritability, withdrawal from social activities, rumination, difficulty concentrating, muscle tension, and sleep disturbance s. Anxiety may manifest at different times and in different ways for dialysis patients. Assessment using the Generalized Anxiety Disorder Scale (GAD-7) has been validated in dialysis patients [20]. Screening is recommended at the time of dialysis initiation, annual mental health assessment, at major life events or losses, and if disruptive behavior, such as missed treatments or stopping treatments early, is observed. Patient scores of 10 or greater on the GAD-7 scale warrant referral to Psychiatry. Patients with anxiety must be screened for concomitant depression, suicidal ideation, and substance abuse [21].

Psychopathology is not an absolute contraindication for transplant. Patients with established psychiatric diagnoses should be evaluated for psychiatric stability by their established provider and may benefit from assessment by the Transplant Psychiatrist. Utilization of the above screens at the time of transplant evaluation can alert the team of high-risk patients who require in depth psychological intervention and repeat assessment to determine the impact of the intervention. Once deemed stable from their psychiatric illness, patients should be assessed to ensure that they are capable of giving informed consent and adhering to therapy, before being listed for transplantation .

It is common for patients to experience psychological stress during the transplant evaluation. Uncertainty of the future, stress of testing, declining health while on the waitlist, and thoughts of death can hasten depression and anxiety. Therefore, it is important that assessment and screening be a constant part of transplant preparation and readiness.

Cognitive Impairment and Transplant Outcomes

Patients with chronic kidney disease treated with dialysis have impaired cognitive function compared to the general population. Incidence varies from 10-30% of young and middle age patients to 30-55% in the elderly. Neurocognitive dysfunction is poorly recognized and underreported. Its association with dialysis may be due to the uremic milieu, chronic inflammation, and dialysis-related hypotension leading to cerebral hypoxia. Specific areas of deficiency in dialysis-dependent patients include poor attention, executive function, and orientation [22]. Cognitive impairment is increasingly recognized as a risk factor for adverse outcomes, hospitalizations, and all-cause mortality. Specifically in transplant, established dementia and Alzheimer's are contraindications to transplant, given the concern for worsening neurotoxic effects of immunosuppression and established graft loss [23]. Most transplant centers do not consider mild cognitive impairment as an absolute contraindication to transplant, as long as informed consent is ensured, and a support system is in place to ensure adherence and patient safety. However, growing evidence links graft loss and all-cause mortality with pre-transplant neurocognitive dysfunction [24]. Therefore, incorporation of neurocognitive assessment, by qualified psychologists or geriatricians, using the Mini Mental Status Examination to assess global function and the validated Kidney Disease Quality of Life Cognitive Function scale will help identify high-risk patients [25]. Further studies are needed to detect if pre-transplant interventions on neurocognitive preservation strategies yield beneficial results post-transplant.

Racial Disparity and Access to Transplant

The Department of Health and Human Services mandate that organ allocation be equitable. However, it has long been observed that blacks are less likely to be referred, evaluated, listed, and successfully transplanted compared to white ESRD [26]. Listed Hispanic patients have also had historically lower transplant rates. Reasons for this inequity are a combination of factors, including distance to transplant centers, insurance status, financial limitations, referral bias, and organ allocation inequities. The Kidney Allocation System (KAS), implemented by the United Network of Organ Sharing (UNOS) set out to balance equity and utility in organ allocation by 1) calculating waiting time from the start of dialysis rather than the date of waitlisting; 2) prioritizing highly sensitized patients with elevated panel reactive antibodies; and 3) increasing access to blood group B patients. Post-KAS results showed improvement in transplant rates of highly sensitized patients, who historically are non-white ethnic minorities [27]. However, waitlisting and racial disparity continue to exist [28, 29]. Opportunities to lessen the disparities include improved access to care, enhanced practice-level cultural sensitivity, earlier referral, and research to assess effects of environment and genetics on health outcomes. Future directives must focus on policy changes that can address these disparities and improve access to transplant.

Sociocultural Perspective and Patient Perception of Transplant

Sociocultural perspective is the awareness of circumstances surrounding individuals and how their behaviors and beliefs are impacted by surroundings, social, and cultural factors. Studies show that patients with ESRD have a high level of medical mistrust that may impact their desire for a transplant, despite the life-transforming and life-sustaining benefits it provides. Patient mistrust about where kidney donors come from, barriers to access, miscommunication between the nephrologist and the transplant team can create a thread of mistrust that leads to ambivalence about transplant. This ambivalence is often misinterpreted as a lack of interest in transplant; therefore, these patients may not be continuously pursued by the Transplant Center [30]. Associations between sociocultural factors and transplant evaluation initiation have been studied amongst certain transplant centers. Results show that high level of medical mistrust, perceived racism, and experiencing discrimination in healthcare were significantly associated with lower likelihood of initiating evaluation. These associations were independent of clinical and socioeconomic characteristics. Therefore, evaluating racial disparity in the context of these sociocultural factors allows future direction to address and reduce these disparities and reassure patients of the benefits of transplant [31].

Health Literacy

Health literacy is defined as the degree that individuals are able to understand the health information necessary to make appropriate health decisions. Limited health literacy is common in the United States, with roughly a third of adult patients facing difficulty navigating a complex health system and understanding medical jargon. High educational attainment does not correlate with high health literacy. Limited health literacy leads to increased hospital admissions, higher annual care costs, and more complex chronic disease management [32]. Various tools are used to assess health literacy, with several being utilized in kidney transplant candidates [33–35]. Lower health literacy has been linked to reduced likelihood of being placed on the kidney transplant waitlist. Given the lengthy nature of a kidney transplant evaluation, the multiple steps required before listing may prove difficult for those who lack adequate literacy. Similarly, low health literacy is associated with increased mortality on the waitlist, identifying these patients as medically fragile and requiring additional close monitoring to overcome the complexities of their chronic disease state [36]. Providers of patients with low health literacy should make a concerted effort to identify these individuals and offer tailored education and other provisions to assist this vulnerable population navigate the rigors of the transplant evaluation [37].

Self-Management Post Transplant and Health Promotion Predictors

According to the Institute of Medicine, self-management is a task that individuals with chronic conditions must perform to live well. These tasks include having the confidence to navigate medical management, role management, and emotional management of their conditions. Recognizing that patients cannot do this alone, the Institute of Medicine (IOM) defined self-management support as the systematic provision of education and supportive interventions by health care staff to increase patients' skills and confidence in managing their health problems. These interventions include regular assessment of progress and problems, goal setting, and problem-solving support [38]. Following kidney transplant, patients are expected to take an active role in health promotion. Recipients and caregivers must adapt to new medication and lifestyle regimens, frequent laboratory and clinic follow-up, and cope with the emotional responsibility of caring for the new organ. The role of the Transplant team, particularly the Transplant Nurse Coordinator and Social Worker, is to help facilitate a smooth transition and adaptation to transplant self-management. Table 2 outlines health promotion practices that can help recipients navigate challenges and promote self-management [39].

Table 2. Steps to enhance self-management

Self-Management Task	Self-Management Challenges	Types of Support Needs	Transplant Team Interventions	Care Giver Interventions
Medical Management	• Becoming a Professional Patient • Establishing a medical regimen in daily life	• Instrumental Support • Reorganize daily life structures & find new routines	• Providing knowledge & instruction • Discuss how to reorganize daily life structures and establish a routine	• Offer practical support in daily life • Understand the medical consequences to the recipient
Emotion Management	• Emotions related to transplant • Dealing with body image	• Psychosocial Support	• Recognize the emotional impact of kidney transplant • Proactively asking about recipients' emotions • Provide feedback and encouragement	• Offering empathetic listening • Encouraging self-confidence and empowerment

Patients can strengthen their capacity of self-management by mastering tasks and maintaining a sense of accountability to the doctors and transplant team. Factors that diminish self-management include fear of potential consequences of immunosuppression, forgetfulness and contradictory advice. Motivators of self-management, such as prevention of rejection or recurrence of original kidney disease, may inspire vigilance but can lead to extreme anxiety and fear if not kept in the right medical perspective. The clinical team plays a vital role in promoting autonomy through clear recommendations, shared decision-making, and early effective interventions [40].

Financial Resources and Insurance Coverage

Given the high cost of immunosuppression therapy, dedicated assessment by a financial counselor is a key component to the transplant evaluation. Financial resources and insurance coverage should be thoroughly assessed for each candidate, both at the time of evaluation and subsequent follow-up appointments. Potential financial barriers should be addressed prior to transplant, with determination of whether transplant is feasible. Costs of travel and stay close to the transplant program should be considered and community resources explored.

Most dialysis patients gain entitlement to Medicare with an ESRD diagnosis. Medicare benefits end three years after the kidney transplant for those who are younger than age 65 and do not carry another disability diagnosis. Recipients impacted by this are more often young, African Americans with limited financial resources. Patients are encouraged to return to work after transplant in order to secure ongoing insurance benefits but often are unable and lose the Medicare coverage. This loss of immunosuppression drug coverage often results in graft failure and return to dialysis [41].

Recently, the Comprehensive Immunosuppressive Drug Coverage for Kidney Transplant Patients Act of 2019 was passed, which indefinitely extends Medicare coverage of immunosuppressive drugs for kidney transplant recipients for individuals who do not have other coverage [42].

Regardless of the type of insurance, ensuring ongoing access will aide in the longevity of the allograft.

Psychometric Tools for Transplant Assessment

Various tools have been implemented to assess areas of psychosocial vulnerability and predict psychosocial and medical outcomes post-transplant. Although no standard guidelines exist, there are several tools that have empirically been used in solid organ transplants [43]. Examples include the Stanford Integrated Psychosocial Assessment for Transplantation (SIPAT) or the Transplant Evaluation and Rating Scale (TERS). The Stanford Integrated Psychosocial Assessment for Transplant (SIPAT) is a newer tool that offers a comprehensive standardization of information collected during the psychosocial evaluation; it has high inter-rater reliability and is predictive of transplant psychosocial outcomes [44]. Future initiatives should focus on standardization of these tools and assessing the predictive validity of such tools in large cohorts of transplant patients.

LIVING DONORS

Introduction

With the increasing disparity of supply and demand for a deceased donor transplant, living kidney donation and transplantation is an acceptable and beneficial alternative to dialysis. Despite these benefits, it remains a complex medical, moral, and ethical issue [45]. Guidance and requirements for living donor candidates comes from Centers for Medicare and Medicaid Services (CMS) Conditions for Transplant Center Participation and interpretive guidelines and Policy 14 from the Organ Procurement and Transplantation Network (OPTN) [46, 47]. The evaluation and determination of living donor candidates is based on a comprehensive medical screen but more importantly, the ethical precept of "do no harm." Assessing capacity, psychological status, motivation, ability for informed consent, and financial suitability are required components of the psychosocial evaluation of a living kidney donor [48] The United Network of Organ Sharing (UNOS) mandates a minimum follow-up period of 2 years post-donation, to assess the medical, emotional and financial impact of donation.

Evaluation

It is the duty of the Transplant Team to ensure that a donor is free from coercion or financial gain and to educate the donor about the alternatives to donation, the expected outcome to donation and the short- and long-term consequences of donation. A multidisciplinary team of physicians, surgeons, dieticians, social workers, psychiatrists and living donor advocates work together to assess the living donor physical wellbeing and candidacy. Written instruction of all elements of the evaluation and copies of educational material in a format that is easy to understand must be provided. If possible, the donor team is usually independent of the recipient team to minimize conflict of interest and ensure a balanced evaluation.

Medical and Surgical Assessment

The most recent Kidney Disease: Improving Global Outcomes (KDIGO) Clinical Practice Guideline on the Evaluation and Care of Living Kidney Donors provides a comprehensive approach and guides analysis for focuses on the medical and psychosocial risk assessment. It creates an objective framework that transplant programs can build upon to determine an acceptable risk [49]. Since living donation is the only procedure that provides no medical benefit to the patient, a comprehensive risk assessment comprised of detailed history and testing guides shared decision-making between the donor and the program. The donor medical, family and surgical history is reviewed, with attention to health characteristics, genetic predispositions and life-style habits that may increase the development of chronic kidney disease. Living donors should be fully aware of the perioperative and long-term risks of donation. Table 3 details elements of risk that must be shared to comply with informed consent. Despite the uncertainty of predicting risk following donation, the overall risk of donation remains acceptably low. Several meta-analysis and systematic reviews have focused on health-risks for living kidney donors, and attempted to objectively quantify that risk [45, 49–52]. When compared with the non-donor population, living donors have no increased risk of all-cause mortality or major chronic disease states such as systolic hypertension, type 2 diabetes, cancer, or cardiovascular disease. As expected, they do have lower renal function and an increased risk of developing ESRD post-donation. However, the absolute risk remains low at a rate of 1 case out of 1000 person-years [45]. Overall, continued thoughtful and stringent screening of donors, with appropriate post-donation follow-up can mitigate future medical complications. A more extensive review of the medical aspects of living donation is discussed in the chapter on "Evaluation of the Living Donor" in this book.

Table 3. Disclosure of the following transient or permanent risks as a part of informed consent [46]

Risk Associated with the Evaluation	• Discovery of serious medical conditions, requiring further testing, referral to other specialists, and treatment, all of which will be the financial responsibility of the donor. • Discovery of reportable infectious diseases • Discovery of genetic disease s, previously unknown to the donor candidate • Unintentional discovery of misattributed biologic relationship through blood group or immune incompatibility • Radiation exposure • Possible allergic reaction to contrast
Medical Risk	• Expected post-donation reduction in renal function • Possible acute kidney injury requiring dialysis during the immediate post-donation period • Impact of CKD and ESRD development in the future and prioritization of kidney donors on the organ allocation list • Female donors of child-bearing age are at increased risk of gestational hypertension and preeclampsia
Surgical Risk	• Death, bleeding, post-surgical infections • Abdominal symptoms: bloating, pain, nausea, vomiting, or bowel obstruction • Post-operative fatigue, pain, nerve injury, blood clots, hernia

Psychosocial Assessment

Key aspects of the living donor evaluation include assessment of eligibility and readiness for donation, education, and post-donation planning and care-giver support. Per UNOS guidance, the evaluation should be done in-person, by a licensed social worker, psychiatrist or psychologist familiar with the transplant process, yet separate from the recipient team. A dedicated psychiatry assessment may also be carried out in those with current or prior psychiatric disorder s. Most programs have adopted a succinct and standard set of questions to address these components guided by OPTN Policy. Given the lack of concrete evidence -based studies, each transplant center establishes its own set format. The current KDIGO Clinical Practice Guideline on the Evaluation and Care of Living Kidney Donors captures several of the recurring elements [49]. Table 4 provides a guide for the psychosocial evaluation.

Table 4. Key components of the psychosocial evaluation [46, 48, 49, 53]

Eligibility and Readiness	• Background and Current Status: *standard information covering areas of educational level, living situation, cultural background, religious beliefs and practices, significant relationships, community and leisure activities, employment, legal offense history, citizenship* • Relationship with the Recipient: *nature and degree of closeness, how did the relationship develop, expectations of the outcomes of donation and how it will impact the relationship* • Motivation: *elucidate patterns of altruism; explore the rationale and reason for donation, ensure voluntariness, and the lack of coercion, inducements, or ulterior motives (i.e., to atone, to gain approval, to remedy psychological malady, to reinforce self-image)* • History of current or previous psychiatric disorders • History of current or past substance dependence or abuse • Risk of donor transmission of an infectious disease to the recipient, based on U.S Public Health Service Guideline [54]
Education and Readiness	• Knowledge: *awareness of potential short-and long-term risks for surgical complications and health outcomes, of both recipient and donor* • Education: *Assess medical, emotional and financial impacts of donation; accessing and applying for financial resources and Family Leave and Medical Act (FMLA); information on advance directive and living will* • Understanding: *acceptance that exact risk prediction is difficult to objectively quantify given the limitations of long-term data tailored to specific demographics and health factors* • Capacity: *assess understanding and the process of informed consent* • Readiness for the medical implications of donation • Readiness for the psychosocial impact of donation • Readiness for the physical activity limitations following donation • Readiness for the financial implications of donation: *impact on wages and employment, expenses for travel, dependent care and medical expenses; impact on health and life insurance policies* • Responsibility to maintain future health and future donor-follow-up
Support	• *Evaluate current and future support networks; assess availability both during the donor's recovery and an ongoing basis* • *Plan for any psychosocial risks and determine how these can be managed*

Unlike the recipient evaluation, transplant centers exhibit a wide array of protocols for the psychosocial assessment of living donors. Most centers are guided by the policies of the OPTN. Given the lack of a standardized approach, attempts have been made to create a valid and reliable screening tool. The Live Donor Assessment Tool provides a semi-structured process to quantify the appropriateness versus the risks to potential donors. By incorporating the guidelines specified by the OPTN, the Living Donor Assessment Tool (LDAT) creates a rubric score from the following nine domains: donor motivation, knowledge of donation, feelings regarding donation, closeness to the donor, support available to the donor, stability in life, expectations post-donation, psychiatric issues and history of substance abuse [55]. Higher scores predict greater psychosocial appropriateness for donation while lower scores may identify donors who would require additional pre-donation counseling and post-donation psychosocial intervention [56]. Regardless of the format, each transplant program should follow a predetermined protocol for the psychosocial assessment. Pre-donation characteristics that portend poor post-donation psychosocial outcomes include ambivalence, compromised mental health, limited financial resources, and a strained recipient-donor relationship. Assessing these issues will help inform the transplant center as to how best to intervene to limit post-donation challenges. Future studies are needed to compare various evaluation approaches, acceptance criteria and how well post-donation outcomes can be predicted.

Assessing Psychiatric Disorders

Pre-existing psychiatric conditions or un-diagnosed psychiatric disorders may impair the donor's ability to make an informed decision, understand the risks, or cope with potential complications after living donor surgery [46]. Prolonged grief responses or post-partum depression may also place candidates at a greater risk for post-donation depression or exacerbation of an underlying psychiatric condition. In the absence of strict criteria, transplant centers adopt their own criteria to trigger psychiatry evaluation of donors. Table 5 outlines broad scenarios for dedicated Psychiatric Evaluation adopted by centers in order to determine suitability for donation and inform the donor team. While most centers agree on most of these criteria, differences exist in some of these between centers.

Table 5. Triggers for psychiatry evaluation [56]

• History of mental health disorder	• Donors with questionable relationship
• History of chemical dependence/abuse	• Altruistic or non-directed donors
• Cognitive concerns	• Social media donors
• Donors displaying ambivalence	• Kidney Paired Donation (KPD) Donors
• Suspicion of secondary gain	• Donor under the age of 21

Elements of Informed Consent

Living donors represent a unique population, who are willing to undergo an elective procedure with no medical benefit to themselves. Therefore, informed consent is an ethical prerequisite and is required under US regulation. Following education and thorough assessment of capacity, the Transplant Program is mandated to accurately assess the candidate's ability to consent for living donation. To ensure voluntarism, the signed consent should be obtained in the absence of the intended recipient and other family members or persons who could influence the decision to donate. The donor candidate must acknowledge the risks and benefits associated with donation and be given adequate time to consider the ramifications of donation and whether they wish to donate. Donors must be presented the other alternatives available to the recipient if they were not to donate, including transplantation via a deceased donor or receiving renal replacement therapy in the form of hemodialysis or peritoneal dialysis. As a part of the discussion, living donors are reminded that it is a federal crime to accept any payment for organs donated, whether it be cash, vacations or anything of value under the National Organ Transplant Act of 1984.

The living donor program is required to document informed consent in the living donor medical record. The living donor's signature on the document ensures that the donor is: 1) willing to donate, 2) free of coercion or inducement from the transplant recipient, family member or medical team, 3) informed that he or she can decline donation at any time. The decision to withdraw from donation must be kept confidential and the donor should be supported and assisted with communicating this to the recipient.

The Role of the Independent Living Donor Advocate (ILDA)

Since 2007, CMS and OPTN requires living-donor recovery hospitals to designate and provide each donor candidate with an ILDA who is not involved with the potential recipient evaluation and is independent of the decision to transplant the potential recipient. The ILDA is either one person or a team with a key contact. They must have adequate qualification and training requirements regarding knowledge of living organ donation, transplantation, medical ethics, informed consent, and the potential impact of family or other external pressure on the living donor's decision about whether to donate. They also review whether the living donor has received information on each of the following areas: informed consent, the evaluation process, the surgical procedure, medical and psychosocial risks, right to withdraw, and follow-up requirements [53].

As time has passed, the role of the ILDA has evolved beyond the original requirements stipulated by CMS and OPTN. The American Society of Transplantation Live Donor Community of Practice and the ILDA workgroup provide further guidance on the role of ILDA. Some of the key recommendations focus on the ILDA's skill set and knowledge base, assessment of informed consent, involvement throughout the continuum of the donation and reporting structure outside of the transplant center. Since the role is relatively new, on-going research efforts will focus on identifying knowledge gaps and pursuing evidence -based best practices [57].

Psychosocial Outcomes Post-Donation

The OPTN has mandated a minimum of two-year post-donation follow-up for all living kidney donors in order to assess the physical, psychological, emotional and financial effect of donation. The majority of donors view donation in a positive light with significant psychosocial benefit and improved dynamics of the recipient-donor relationship. Most find the experience to be a positive one and feel that their donation was the right decision [58, 59]. Reassuringly, most donors do not regret their decision to donate, show no remorse and would undergo the process again, even in the rare circumstance that the recipient experiences a bad outcome. Donors may experience a small decrease in health -related quality of life in the post-donation period but return to their baseline and are equivalent to the general population in the long term [59]. Additional studies have shown that donors experience minimal to no dysfunction in mood, body image, or life satisfaction during the post-donation period [60].

However, some donors may experience significant challenges [52]. A minority of donors will experience post-donation depression, anxiety, and stress, usually in those with pre-existent psychiatric challenges. Recipient graft loss and death have been associated with increased risk of post-donation depression, particularly among non-spouse, unrelated donors [61]. Although most donors experience no depression, it is important to address this small but significant post-donation complication and be vigilant for any early signs or manifestations.

Another post-donation challenge can be changes in the recipient-donor relationship. Unresolved angst, unintentional neglect, and overprotectiveness may emerge after donation. Some recipients may feel inclined to a perpetual demonstration of gratitude to the donor, leading to a sense of duty and obligation. The donor may experience a warped sense of ownership of the kidney, ensuring that the recipient is "taking care" of the organ. Siblings may experience neglect, particularly if donation occurs at a younger age and if more of the caregiver focus is on the recipient [62]. Unrelated donors may experience resentment, particularly if the donor experiences prolonged recovery or fatigue [63]. Preparing the donor, establishing realistic expectations and offering close post-donation follow-up can help mitigate some of the dynamic changes that may occur in the recipient-donor relationship.

In regard to the financial challenges of donation, donors often suffer lost-wages, unpaid leave, and return to work before feeling fully rehabilitated [64]. The National Living Donor Assistance Center (NLDAC), under the auspices of the Health Resources and Services Administration, operates the reimbursement of travel and subsistence expenses, incurred by the living donor during the evaluation and donation period. Attempts to remove financial barriers of living donation have recently resulted in expansion of the NLDAC funds under the Advancing American Kidney Health Act. Additional support will now include coverage of lost wages, child-care and elder-care incurred by the donor [65]. Future initiatives to create financial neutrality will help to promote living donation and mitigate post-donation financial risk.

Conclusion

Kidney Transplantation is the optimal option for treatment of ESRD, and transplant with a living donor provides the best long-term medical outcomes. Suitability for candidacy is built on a thorough psychosocial assessment. Identifying psychosocial challenges and enacting steps for remediation preserves equity in the transplant process. Ultimately the success of transplant and donation depend upon the ability for both recipients and donors to navigate the rigors of the psychosocial evaluation.

References

[1] Hart A, Smith JM, Skeans MA, Gustafson SK, Wilk AR, Castro S, et al. OPTN/SRTR 2017 Annual Data Report: Kidney. *Am J Transplant* 2019;19:19–123.

[2] Ladin K, Emerson J, Berry K, Butt Z, Gordon EJ, Daniels N, et al. Excluding patients from transplant due to social support: Results from a national survey of transplant providers. *Am J Transplant.* 2019;19(1):193–203.

[3] Ladin K, Emerson J, Butt Z, Gordon EJ, Hanto DW, Perloff J, et al. How important is social support in determining patients' suitability for transplantation ? Results from a National Survey of Transplant Clinicians. *J Med Ethics.* 2018 Oct;44(10):666–74.

[4] Ladin K, Daniels A, Osani M, Bannuru RR. Is social support associated with post-transplant medication adherence and outcomes? A systematic review and meta-analysis. Vol. 32, *Transplant Rev.* 2018. p. 16–28.

[5] Murali KM, Mullan J, Roodenrys S, Hassan HC, Lambert K, Lonergan M. Strategies to improve dietary, fluid, dialysis or medication adherence in patients with end stage kidney disease on dialysis: A systematic review and meta-analysis of randomized intervention trials. *PLoS ONE.* 2019;14(1):1–27.

[6] Dobbels F, Vanhaecke J, Dupont L, Nevens F, Verleden G, Pirenne J, et al. Pretransplant predictors of posttransplant adherence and clinical outcome: An evidence base for pretransplant psychosocial screening. *Transplantation.* 2009;87(10):1497–504.

[7] Kuntz K, Weinland SR, Butt Z. Psychosocial Challenges in Solid Organ Transplantation. *J Clin Psychol Med Settings.* 2015;22(2–3):122–35.

[8] Nevins TE, Nickerson PW, Dew MA. Understanding medication nonadherence after kidney transplant. *J Am Soc Nephrol.* 2017;28(8):2290–301.

[9] Parker R, Armstrong MJ, Corbett C, Day EJ, Neuberger JM. Alcohol and substance abuse in solid-organ transplant recipients. *Transplantation.* 2013;96(12):1015–24.

[10] Weinrauch LA, Claggett B, Liu J, Finn P v., Weir MR, Weiner DE, et al. Smoking and outcomes in kidney transplant recipients: A post hoc survival analysis of the FAVORIT trial. *Int J Nephrol Renovasc Dis.* 2018;11:155–64.

[11] Rai HS, Winder GS. Marijuana Use and Organ Transplantation: a Review and Implications for Clinical Practice. *Curr Psychiatry Rep.* 2017;19(11).

[12] Alhamad T, Koraishy FM, Lam NN, Katari S, Naik AS, Schnitzler MA, et al. Cannabis Dependence or Abuse in Kidney Transplantation: Implications for Posttransplant Outcomes. *Transplantation.* 2019;103(11):2373–82.

[13] Ishida JH, McCulloch CE, Steinman MA, Grimes BA, Johansen KL. Opioid analgesics and adverse outcomes among hemodialysis patients. *Clin J Am Soc.* 2018;13(5):746–53.

[14] Lentine KL, Lam NN, Naik AS, Axelrod DA, Zhang Z, Dharnidharka VR, et al. Prescription opioid use before and after kidney transplant: Implications for posttransplant outcomes. *Am J Transplant.* 2018;18(12):2987–99.

[15] Palmer S, Vecchio M, Craig JC, Tonelli M, Johnson DW, Nicolucci A, et al. Prevalence of depression in chronic kidney disease: Systematic review and meta-analysis of observational studies. *Kidney Int* 2013;84(1):179–91.

[16] Watnick S, Wang PL, Demadura T, Ganzini L. Validation of 2 depression screening tools in dialysis patients. *Am J Kidney Dis.* 2005;46(5):919–24.

[17] K/DOQI Workgroup. K/DOQI clinical practice guidelines for cardiovascular disease in dialysis patients. *Am J Kidney Dis.* 2005; Apr;45(4 Suppl 3): S1-153.

[18] King-Wing Ma T, Kam-Tao Li P. Depression in dialysis patients. *Nephrology.* 2016;21(8):639–46.

[19] Natale P, Sc P, Ruospo M, Vm S, Ks R, Gfm S, et al. Psychosocial interventions for preventing and treating depression in dialysis patients. *Cochrane Database of Systematic Reviews.* 2019;12(CD004542.).

[20] Chilcot J, Hudson JL, Moss-Morris R, Carroll A, Game D, Simpson A, et al. Screening for psychological distress using the Patient Health Questionnaire Anxiety and Depression Scale (PHQ-ADS): Initial validation of structural validity in dialysis patients. *Gen Hosp Psychiatry* 2018;50:15–9.

[21] Cohen SD, Cukor D, Kimmel PL. Anxiety in patients treated with hemodialysis. *Clin J Am Soc Nephrol.* 2016;11(12):2250–5.

[22] O'Lone E, Connors M, Masson P, Wu S, Kelly PJ, Gillespie D, et al. Cognition in people with end-stage kidney disease treated with hemodialysis: A systematic review and meta-analysis. *Am J Kidney Dis.* 2016;67(6):925–35.

[23] McAdams-DeMarco MA, Bae S, Chu N, Gross AL, Brown CH, Oh E, et al. Dementia and Alzheimer's disease among older kidney transplant recipients. *J Am Soc Nephrol.* 2017;28(5):1575–83.

[24] Thomas AG, Ruck JM, Shaffer AA, Haugen CE, Ying H, Warsame F, et al. Kidney transplant outcomes in recipients with cognitive impairment: A national registry and prospective cohort study. *Transplantation.* 2019;103(7):1504–13.

[25] Kurella M, Luan J, Yaffe K, Chertow GM. Validation of the Kidney Disease Quality of Life (KDQOL) Cognitive Function subscale. *Kidney Int.* 2004;66(6):2361–7.

[26] Schold JD, Gregg JA, Harman JS, Hall AG, Patton PR, Meier-Kriesche HU. Barriers to evaluation and wait listing for kidney transplantation. *Clin J Am Soc Nephrol.* 2011;6(7):1760–7.

[27] Jackson KR, Covarrubias K, Holscher CM, Luo X, Chen J, Massie AB, et al. The national landscape of deceased donor kidney transplantation for the highly sensitized: Transplant rates, waitlist mortality, and posttransplant survival under KAS. *Am J Transplant.* 2019;19(4):1129–38.

[28] Zhang X, Melanson TA, Plantinga LC, Basu M, Pastan SO, Mohan S, et al. Racial/ethnic disparities in waitlisting for deceased donor kidney transplantation 1 year after implementation of the new national kidney allocation system. *Am J Transplant.* 2018;18(8):1936–46.

[29] Harding K, Mersha TB, Pham PT, Waterman AD, Webb FJ, Vassalotti JA, et al. Health Disparities in Kidney Transplantation for African Americans. *Am J Nephrol.* 2017;46(2):165–75.

[30] Wachterman MW, McCarthy EP, Marcantonio ER, Ersek M. Mistrust, misperceptions, and miscommunication: A qualitative study of preferences about kidney transplantation among African Americans. Vol. 47, *Transplant Proc.* 2015. p. 240–6.

[31] Hamoda RE, McPherson LJ, Lipford K, Jacob Arriola K, Plantinga L, Gander JC, et al. Association of sociocultural factors with initiation of the kidney transplant evaluation process. *Am J Transplant.* 2020;20(1):190–203.

[32] Nielsen-Bohlman L, Panzer AM, Kindig DA editors. Institute of Medicine (US) Committee on Health Literacy. *Health Literacy: A Prescription to End Confusion.* Washington (DC): National Academies Press (US). 2004;

[33] Paasche-Orlow M. *Health Literacy Tool She*d .[cited 2021 Sep 30]. Available from: https://healthliteracy.bu.edu.

[34] Kazley AS, Jordan J, Simpson KN, Chavin K, Rodrigue J, Baliga P. Development and Testing of a Disease-Specific Health Literacy Measure in Kidney Transplant Patients. *Prog Transplant.* 2014;24(3):263–70.

[35] Gordon E, Wolf M. Health literacy skills of kidney transplant recipients. *Prog Transplant.* 2009;19(1):25–34.

[36] Warsame F, Haugen CE, Ying H, Garonzik-Wang JM, Desai NM, Hall RK, et al. Limited health literacy and adverse outcomes among kidney transplant candidates. Vol. 19, *Am J Transplant.* 2019;19: 457–65.

[37] Jones J, Rosaasen N, Taylor J, Mainra R, Shoker A, Blackburn D, et al. Health Literacy, Knowledge, and Patient Satisfaction Before Kidney Transplantation. Vol. 48, *Transplantation Proc.* 2016;48:2608-14

[38] Adams K, Greiner AC, Corrigan JM Eds. *The 1st Annual Crossing the Quality Chasm Summit: A Focus on Communities*. Washington, National Academic Press. 2004. 176. Available from: https://doi.org/10.17226/11085.

[39] Been-Dahmen JMJ, Grijpma JW, Ista E, Dwarswaard J, Maasdam L, Weimar W, et al. Self-management challenges and support needs among kidney transplant recipients: A qualitative study. *J Adv Nurs.* 2018;74(10):2393–405.

[40] Jamieson NJ, Hanson CS, Josephson MA, Gordon EJ, Craig JC, Halleck F, et al. Motivations, challenges, and attitudes to self-management in kidney transplant recipients: A systematic review of qualitative studies. *Am J Kindey Dis.* 2016;67(3):461–78.

[41] Hart A, Gustafson SK, Wey A, Salkowski N, Snyder JJ, Kasiske BL, et al. The association between loss of Medicare, immunosuppressive medication use, and kidney transplant outcomes. *Am J Transplant.* 2019;19(7):1964–71.

[42] H.R.5534 - Comprehensive Immunosuppressive Drug Coverage for Kidney Transplant Patients Act of 2020 .116th Congress (2019-2020). [cited 2021 Nov 30]. Available from: https://www.congress .gov/bill/116th-congress/house-bill/5534.

[43] Nghiem DM, Gomez J, Gloston GF, Torres DS, Marek RJ. Psychological Assessment Instruments for Use in Liver and Kidney Transplant Evaluations: Scarcity of Evidence and Recommendations. *J Pers Assess.* .2020;102(2):183–95.

[44] Chen G, Bell CS, Loughhead P, Ibeche B, Bynon JS, Hall DR, et al. Exploration of the Stanford Integrated Psychosocial Assessment for Transplantation With Psychosocial and Medical Outcomes in Kidney and Kidney–Pancreas Transplant Recipients. *Prog Transplant.* 2019;29(3):230–8

[45] O'keeffe LM, Ramond A, Oliver-Williams C, Willeit P, Paige E, Trotter P, et al. Mid-And long-Term health risks in living kidney donors: A systematic review and meta-Analysis. *Ann Int Med.* 2018;168(4):276–84.

[46] *Organ Procurement and Transplantation Network (OPTN)* Policy 14 : Living Donation. 279–98. Available from: https://optn.transplant .hrsa.gov/media /1200/ optn_policies.pdf.

[47] Programs OT. *State Operations Manual Appendix X – Guidance to Surveyors : Organ Transplant Programs Part I* – The Standard Organ Transplant Program Survey Protocol. 2–21.

[48] Dew MA, Jacobs CL, Jowsey SG, Hanto R, Miller C, Delmonico FL. Guidelines for the Psychosocial Evaluation of Living Unrelated Kidney Donors in the United States. *Am J Transplant.* 2007;7:1047-54.

[49] Lentine KL, Kasiske BL, Levey AS, Adams PL, Alberú J, Bakr MA, et al. KDIGO Clinical Practice Guideline on the Evaluation and Care of Living Kidney Donors. *Transplantation*. 2017;101(8S):1–109.

[50] Grams ME, Sang Y, Levey AS, Matsushita K, Ballew S, Chang AR, et al. Kidney-Failure Risk Projection for the Living Kidney-Donor Candidate. *N Engl J Med.* 2016;374(5):411–21.

[51] Ibrahim HN, Foley RN, Reule SA, Spong R, Kukla A, Issa N, et al. Renal function profile in white kidney donors: The first 4 decades. *J Am Soc Nephrol.* 2016;27(9): 2885–93.

[52] Lentine KL, Lam NN, Segev DL. Risks of living kidney donation: Current state of knowledge on outcomes important to donors. *Clin J Am Soc Nephrol*. 2019;14(4): 597–608.

[53] LaPointe Rudow D, Swartz K, Phillips C, Hollenberger J, Schmick T, Steel J. The Psychosocial and Independent Living Donor Advocate Evaluation and Post-Surgery Care of Living Donors Living Donor Transplantation. *J Clin Psych Med Settings.* 2015; 22:136–49.

[54] Jones JM, Kracalik I, Levi ME, Bowman JS, Berger JJ, Bixler D, et al. Assessing Solid Organ Donors and Monitoring Transplant Recipients for Human Immunodeficiency Virus, Hepatitis B Virus, and Hepatitis C Virus Infection - U.S. Public Health Service Guideline, 2020. MMWR Recommendations and reports: *Morbid Mortal Wkly Rep*. 2020;69(4):1–16.

[55] Iacoviello BM, Shenoy A, Braoude J, Jennings T, Vaidya S, Brouwer J, et al. The Live Donor Assessment Tool: A Psychosocial Assessment Tool for Live Organ Donors. *Psychosomatics*. 2015;56(3):254–61

[56] Kook Y won A, Shenoy A, Hunt J, Desrosiers F, Gordon-Elliott JS, Jowsey-Gregoire S, et al. Multicenter investigation of the reliability and validity of the live donor assessment tool as an enhancement to the psychosocial evaluation of living donors. *Am J Transplant*. 2019;19(4):1119–28.

[57] Hays RE, LaPointe Rudow D, Dew MA, Taler SJ, Spicer H, Mandelbrot DA. The independent living donor advocate: A guidance document from the american society of transplantation 's living donor community of practice (AST LDCOP). *Am J Transplant.* 2015;15(2):518–25.

[58] Jacobs CL, Gross CR, Messersmith EE, Hong BA, Gillespie BW, Hill-Callahan P, et al. Article Emotional and Financial Experiences of Kidney Donors over the Past 50 Years: The RELIVE Study. *Clin J Am Soc Nephrol* .2015; 10:2221–31. Available from: www.cjasn.org.

[59] Wirken L, van Middendorp H, Hooghof CW, Rovers MM, Hoitsma AJ, Hilbrands LB, et al. The course and predictors of health -related quality of life in living kidney donors: A systematic review and meta-analysis. *Am J Transplant.* 2015;15(12):3041–54.

[60] Rodrigue JR, Schold JD, Morrissey P, Whiting J, Vella J, Kayler LK, et al. Mood, body image, fear of kidney failure, life satisfaction, and decisional stability following living kidney donation: Findings from the KDOC study. *Am J Transplant.* 2018;18(6):1397–407.

[61] Lentine KL, Schnitzler MA, Xiao H, Axelrod D, Davis CL, McCabe M, et al. Depression diagnoses after living kidney donation: Linking U.S. Registry data and administrative claims. *Transplantation.* 2012;94(1):77–83.

[62] Ralph AF, Butow P, Hanson CS, Chadban SJ, Chapman JR, Craig JC, et al. Donor and Recipient Views on Their Relationship in Living Kidney Donation: Thematic Synthesis of Qualitative Studies. *Am J Kidney Dis*. 2017;69(5):602–16.

[63] Rodrigue JR, Fleishman A, Schold JD, Morrissey P, Whiting J, Vella J, et al. Patterns and predictors of fatigue following living donor nephrectomy: Findings from the KDOC Study. *Am J Transplant.* 2020;20(1):181–9.

[64] Larson DB, Wiseman JF, Vock DM, Berglund DM, Roman AM, Ibrahim HN, et al. Financial burden associated with time to return to work after living kidney donation. *Am J Transplant.* 2019;19(1):204–7.

[65] DHHS. Federal Register, V Federal Register, V. Vol. 85, Department of Health and Human Services: Removing Financial Disincentives to Living Organ. *Fed Regist.* 2020: 59438–44.

In: Issues in Kidney Disease – Transplantation
Editors: B. V. R. Murthy and S. Z. Fadem
ISBN: 978-1-53619-960-4

Chapter 17

ETHICS IN RENAL TRANSPLANTATION

Charles T. Van Buren*, MD
Department of Surgery, McGovern School of Medicine, University of Texas Health, Houston, TX, USA

ABSTRACT

The development of the surgical technique and the means of preventing rejection of a transplanted kidney from a deceased or living donor heralded a new era in the treatment of the previously fatal clinic diagnosis of chronic renal failure. As the success of this new discipline has grown, an ethical means of determining who might access the life-saving technology has posed a challenge for physicians in the field. The major issue is how to increase the supply of transplantable kidneys and who should have priority for this resource. This chapter addresses the ethical challenges posed by these important medical questions.

Keywords: ethics, renal transplantation, equity, commerce

INTRODUCTION

From the development of dialysis for the clinical management of end-stage chronic renal failure and the later use of renal transplantation to restore lost renal function, the treatment of these patients has served as a microcosm of the challenges faced by physicians to deliver adequate medical care. The treatments are expensive, the resources inadequate to treat all patients, and decisions must be made about the fair allocation of these limited resources. Guidelines were needed for equitable allocation of these organs. While the

* Corresponding Author's Email: chasvb@sbcglobal.net.

criteria of brain death and brain-stem death were established and accepted by the scientific community, for the wider acceptance by the society, overcoming religious barriers needed to be addressed for organ donation to become a reality. Also, the access to transplantation is not uniform among sections of society. Ethical challenges have also cropped up with regard to commercialization in transplantation, particularly with living donation. This chapter describes the efforts of the medical community, the governments, and the society to overcome some of these ethical challenges, and the areas where these efforts still fall short in meeting these demands.

ETHICAL CHALLENGES IN KIDNEY TRANSPLANTATION

The first hemodialysis in a chronic kidney patient was performed in 1960. It was not long afterwards that this therapy became an effective means to prolong life in patients with kidney failure. However, resources were not available, and a system to optimize care was the need of the hour. To determine who would receive treatment prior to having a funding source for dialysis therapy, a panel was initially established in Seattle to choose the best patients to treat who would most benefit from the lifesaving therapy [1]. When the choices of the screening panel were analyzed, the patients chosen resembled both economically and demographically the members of the panel. This experience warned that more equitable methods needed to be found to assign treatment for end stage renal disease (ESRD) .

In 1972, in the US, patients who otherwise met the work history requirement for Medicare but were not yet 65 years old became eligible for coverage of dialysis by Medicare, thus eliminating financial barriers for most patients for dialysis; this facility was also extended to renal transplantation [2]. Initially there was not that great a demand for renal transplantation from deceased donor kidneys. While living related renal transplants were successful with one-year graft survival of approximately 80% for one haplotype matches, the one-year success of cadaver donor renal allografts ranged from 35-50%, with patient mortality approaching 20% [3]. Older patients or those with significant medical problems were deemed medically unsuitable for transplantation from deceased donors. Once cyclosporine emerged as an effective immunosuppressant, the risk of death or transplant failure decreased significantly, and the demand for kidney transplantation grew, outstripping the supply of available donor kidneys [4]. Most of the ethical issues in transplantation have arisen from this mismatch of supply and demand. The challenges have been twofold: 1) how to increase available transplantable kidneys; and 2) how to fairly distribute the limited supplies of deceased donor kidneys.

The country with the best in the world organ donation rate per million population is Spain. This country has legislated presumed consent: if a family member is confirmed to be brain dead, the patient will be an organ donor unless the family specifically denies permission for donation [5]. This law has led to development of an aggressive medical system to resuscitate patients with clinically grave neurologic injuries to increase organ donation. What is remarkable is how Spain is really the only Western country that has achieved this level of success. Many of the other European countries with national health care systems have much poorer organ donation rates. The problem of a national system of presumed consent in the United States is the largely state -determined jurisdictions to certify brain death and to determine organ donation policy. Few Organ Procurement Organizations (OPO) in the United States have advocated presumed consent because of the lack of apparent political support for such a policy and the risk of being drawn into a political morass over what would certainly be a contentious issue. There are few religious proscriptions against organ donation. Protestant sects, Roman Catholicism, Islam, Judaism, and Buddhism all regard organ donation as an act of generosity and kindness which they regard as good. They do leave the final decision to the individual families [6]. Only Shintoism might prove an impediment to the generalized support of organ donation.

An alternative approach would be to provide financial incentives for donation of a deceased relative's organ. While there has been support for this approach from some organ transplant physicians, there are questions of whether this would actually increase donation rates. The only individuals this practice might convince to donate would be those who are poor and/or young, since the financial incentives discussed have been modest. The first problem with this approach is that it currently contradicts the specifications of the 1986 National Organ Transplant Act (NOTA) prohibiting the commercialization of donor organs [7]. Virtually all the national and international transplant organizations state that organ donation should be financially neutral; no financial gain should be derived from organ donation, according to these guidelines [8]. The problem is that the entire concept of organ donation is based upon the trust of the donor family that the professionals involved with OPOs will be good stewards of this precious gift. During a federal collaborative to increase organ donation, some of the highest consent rates for donation were in the public hospitals of the leading OPOs, because of the skill of the requestors in articulating the needs of the local community [9]. It has long been recognized that poorer communities are more generous in altruistic giving than many wealthy communities [10]. Commodifying the gift of organ donation forfeits this trust, making the donation primarily a financial transaction. Furthermore, it may raise doubts of how vigorously the now brain -dead patient was resuscitated, potentially leading to a decrease in donation rates.

Providing a financial incentive for living unrelated donation has been proposed to increase kidney donation rates. A former President of the American Society of Transplant Surgeons (ASTS), in remarks after a symposium discussing financial incentives for organ donation, advocated a government sponsored provision of $40-80K, to individuals willing to donate [11]. He further justified this by the observation that other altruistic actions, such as military service, were rewarded by government-provided college tuition support and health care. An important distinction is that military recruits are not entering the service knowing for certain they will sustain an injury. In contrast, living kidney donors all suffer pain postoperatively and infrequent complications, such as incisional hernias and even a rare risk of developing ESRD. Moreover, all the physicians and nurses performing the surgery would be coerced into injuring this patient to facilitate the exchange of the organ for the financial remuneration, a violation of the principle of "above all, do no harm" [7]. Finally, in the public surveys about paid organ donation, the majority of the public oppose the concept, with only 25% favoring it; only 5% state they would be willing to donate an organ for this incentive, raising real questions about what increase in donation would be affected by this morally debatable policy [12]. Further complicating the question of expanding living kidney donation rates are the risks to the donors themselves. By reviewing Center for Medicare and Medicaid Services (CMS) data as well as those from the Organ Procurement and Transplantation Network (OPTN), Wainwright and her co-authors identified 218 living kidney donors who developed ESRD after donation [13]. The average time from donation until development of ESRD was just over 11 years. Males, older age whites, and younger age blacks all had significantly increased risks of ESRD compared to the overall population. As a recognition of this risk factor UNOS has placed prior kidney donors near the top of the priority list for receiving deceased donor kidneys .

The practice of commercial transplantation has been condemned by the international groups that support transplantation activities worldwide. The Palermo Protocol, the Council of Europe, and the Declaration of the Istanbul Custodial group all condemn commercialization of transplantation based upon paid living donors [14]. Nevertheless, the practice continues in many Eastern and South America n countries. The outcomes are difficult to discern. Recipients who succumb prior to returning to their home countries are not included in the data collected. The paid donors often suffer from decreased ability to perform manual labor. The recipient outcomes vary from comparable to non-commercial living donors to significantly lower transplant success rates and higher post-transplant infection rates [15].

An entirely separate issue is the use of organs from executed donors to perform transplants. Interestingly, this was the source for some of the first cadaveric donor renal transplants performed before immunosuppression was developed. Charles Dubost and Marceau Sevelle performed cadaver donor renal transplants using kidneys from individuals who consented to this donation following execution by guillotine [16]. This was a very different era, with transplantation itself an experimental procedure with a failed kidney allograft days or weeks afterward due to rejection. The Chinese used organs from executed donors as their primary source for deceased donor organ transplants; under pressure from medical and professional transplantation societies, this practice of using organs from executed prisoners ceased in 2015 [17].

The one initiative that increased organ donation rates by 22.5% was the federal collaborative [18]. This effort was led by leaders in the OPO community and was a successful effort to spread best organ donation practices to all OPOs. There remains a large gap between the most productive OPOs and those whose performance significantly trails their peers. Part of this stems from an evaluation tool the federal government uses to evaluate OPO performance. It is based on process, and the data presented to the government on suitable donors is not standardized, varying from one OPO to another [19]. The United States is an outlier in this regard; all other countries report organ donation rates using externally verifiable metrics. Fortunately, there is a federal initiative to adopt externally verifiable metrics to evaluate OPO performance [20].

A final problem in the use of deceased donor kidneys is the criteria the federal government uses to evaluate kidney transplant programs. In contrast with the criteria used to evaluate OPO performance, these are hard metrics, focusing on one- and three-year transplant patient and kidney allograft survival figures. While one cannot debate optimizing patient survival, the challenges posed by achieving over 90% deceased donor allograft survival are significant. One cannot transplant higher risk patients such as those with high percentage of HLA -directed antibodies and the presence of donor specific antibodies (DSA); these patients are passed over to the less complicated transplant patients, despite the patient who had DSA being higher on the list. Moreover, there are less than perfect kidneys that are certainly usable if the outcomes could be 80% one-year graft survival, thus removing more patients from dialysis. The donor assessment criteria are not granular enough to truly assess the risk adjustment needed to predict outcomes of these organs, and consequently many transplantable organs are discarded. No one wants to risk survival of his or her transplant program to transplant a few more patients.

Evaluation of patients and determining who is to be listed for transplantation is the first step of organ allocation. When screening patients for suitability of receiving a deceased organ transplant, transplant programs in the 1970s and early 1980s often excluded diabetic patients from deceased donor renal transplantation because of the likelihood of recurrence of the disease in the transplants. The University of Minnesota, led by John Najarian, realized the injustice of this policy, since the time until the initial recurrence of the diabetic nephropathy would minimally be 12-15 years, whereas the half-life survival of kidney transplants from cadaver donors was only 1-3 years in the pre-cyclosporine era [21]. Even after the advent of cyclosporine immunosuppression, the half-life increased to 11 years [22]. By pioneering the transplantation of diabetics, the University of Minnesota expanded access to transplant to a group of patients that now comprise 37% of the waiting list [23].

While there are clearly improvements that can be made in the supply and use of transplantable kidneys, the allocation of these precious resources also needs to be examined. The system for allocation and distribution of deceased donor organs is managed for the federal government by a private contractor, the United Network for Organ Sharing (UNOS). This organization defines the policies for distribution of donated organs. UNOS has focused on the efficient utilization of these organs over an equitable distribution. Since its inception, the national organ allocation system was based upon using human leukocyte antigen (HLA) matching to assign priority for receiving deceased donor kidneys, based upon the presumption that well-matched kidneys had better graft survival. The problem with this system was that African American (AA) patients, who comprised nearly one third of the patients on the waiting list, had a different HLA phenotype than white patients. Since most donors in the U.S. are white, using HLA matching was racially discriminatory. This was noticed in 1988 [24]. UNOS was successfully petitioned in 1992 to allow one OPO to avoid using HLA matching for locally distributed kidneys, to avoid this racial discrimination. This resulted in this OPO having a significantly shorter waiting time for AA patients to be transplanted than the national difference of nearly 100% longer for AA patients to be transplanted than white patients [25]. In 1994, Held and others documented that the benefit of HLA matching in survival was entirely due to the mandated national sharing of 6 antigen HLA matched kidneys, and that the benefit of greater access for AA patients far exceeded any decrease in allograft survival [26]. Despite this data, UNOS did not eliminate use of HLA Class I antigen matching until 2012, over 2 decades after it granted a variance to an OPO to use precisely this policy. The reason for this persistence in an unjust allocation policy is difficult to decipher. Interest in improving success of transplant outcomes cannot be the justification. Highly sensitized patients, multiple organ transplant recipients, and adolescents are all given priority over unsensitized patients receiving a deceased donor kidney, and yet all these patients have significantly worse kidney allograft outcomes [27]. Whatever the justifications, the harm caused to AA patients awaiting transplant was real.

The recently described difference in HLA antigen distribution leads AA patients to be more likely to be sensitized following blood transfusion [28]. Consequently, on the UNOS waiting list there are disproportionately a larger number of highly sensitized AA patients who have been waiting longer for a transplant. A 2014 UNOS policy change which gave national priority to transplant patients with antibody to 98-100% of HLA antibodies would theoretically give advantage to those patients with these characteristics, since they would be drawing from a national rather than a local donor pool [29]. Instead, AA patients with a calculated panel of reactive antibody (cPRA) of 98-100% had a statistically significantly lower likelihood to be transplanted than AA patients with 80-97% cPRA, who could only be transplanted from local donors. The same was not observed for either Hispanic or non-Hispanic whites. Non-Hispanic whites with 98-100% cPRA were transplanted at a higher rate than the same ethnic group with 80-97% cPRA, indicating the policy did function as intended for them [30]. The explanation for these unexpected findings for AA patients with cPRA 98-100% can be explained by the fact that transplant programs must designate what antigens are unacceptable for these highly sensitized patients, to avoid shipping kidneys that would not be acceptable for the intended recipient. This is termed a virtual crossmatch. There is no national system to determine the measurement threshold for defining what is or is not an unacceptable HLA antigen for a sensitized patient. More importantly, DSA correlates poorly with a positive crossmatch, which is a contraindication to transplantation. It would stand to reason that if HLA matching for Class I antigens is racially discriminatory, then ruling out patients based on the presence of DSA against HLA antigens would also be racially discriminatory, perhaps accounting for the decreased access for 98-100% cPRA AA patients compared to AA patients with lower cPRA who can only draw from the local donor pool but can have an actual cytotoxic crossmatch rather than a virtual crossmatch.

This phenomenon associated with virtual crossmatches disadvantages a relatively small number of patients, since only 4-5% of total donor kidneys nationally are shared for these high cPRA patients. However, a UNOS policy change enacted in 2019 (implemented in 2021) no longer distributes deceased donor kidneys initially in the local OPO but distributes them outside the OPO initially over a 250 nautical mile radius [31]. The problem with this policy is that patients with high cPRA are at the top of the list. Kidneys distributed outside of the OPO will be distributed based upon virtual crossmatches. Thus 100% of the donor kidneys in the U.S. will potentially be distributed without the benefit of crossmatch, disadvantaging sensitized AA patients. UNOS has the potential of recreating the discriminatory system disadvantaging AA patients it thought it had eliminated.

These are some, but certainly not all, ethical issues arising in the field of transplantation. The problems are not unique to transplantation, or even medicine. Resources are frequently inadequate to meet the needs of all who need services. The means of addressing these problems are to increase the supply of resources and, at the same time, find the fairest means of determining whose needs will be met first.

CONCLUSION

The ethical challenges in transplantation have arisen due to its success. As the demand for renal transplants has grown since both the risk of transplantation as well as the rate of acute kidney rejection has decreased, the ethical conflicts have arisen from a desire to increase transplant organ donor supply in addition to determining an equitable means of distributing the limited supply of available kidneys. In the attempts to increase supply, some countries have turned to using organs from executed prisoners; recent efforts by transplantation organizations to stop this practice have been successful. Condemnation of paid living donors for commercial use of the purchased kidneys has limited but not eliminated this practice yet. The attempts to balance efficiency with equity in allocating deceased donor kidneys in the United States had led to inadequate access to this altruistic gift for African Americans. Policy changes finally effected to address this issue have improved access to renal transplantation for African Americans. However, recent changes to distribution regulation by UNOS have raised the questions of yet another disadvantage for this group of patients. Meaningful improvements in transplantation access for all patients will depend upon improving performance of local organ banks as well as decreasing the loss of organs due to chronic rejection.

REFERENCES

[1] Childress, JA. Who Shall Live When Not All Can Live? *Soundings* 1970;43(4););:339-362.

[2] Eggers PW. Medicare 's End Stage Renal Disease Program. *Health Care Financ Rev.* 2000; 22: 55–60.

[3] Tilney NL, Strom TB, Vineyard GC, Merrill JP. Factors contributing to the declining mortality rate in renal transplantation. *N Engl J Med.* 1978; 299: 1321–25.

[4] Kahan BD. Cyclosporine: a powerful addition to the immunosuppressive armamentarium. *Am J Kidney Dis.* 1984; 3: 444–55.

[5] Matesanz R, Domínguez-Gil B, Coll E, Mahíllo B, Marazuela R. How Spain Reached 40 Deceased Organ Donors per Million Population. *Am J Transplant.* 2017; 17: 1447–54.

[6] Da Silva IR, Frontera JA. Worldwide barriers to organ donation. *JAMA Neurol.* 2015; 72: 112–18.

[7] Caplan A. Bioethics of organ transplantation. *Cold Spring Harb Perspect Med.* 2014; 4: a015685.

[8] Capron AM, Delmonico FL, Danovitch GM. Financial Neutrality in Organ Donation. *J Am Soc Nephrol.* 2020; 31: 229–30.

[9] Shafer T, Wood RP, Van Buren C, et al. An in-house coordinator program to increase organ donation in public trauma hospitals. *J Transpl Coord.* 1998; 8: 82–87.

[10] Côté S, House J, Willer R. High economic inequality leads higher-income individuals to be less generous. *Proc Natl Acad Sci USA.* 2015; 112: 15838–43.

[11] Monaco AP. Rewards for organ donation: the time has come. *Kidney Int.* 2006; 69: 955–57.

[12] Kranenburg L, Schram A, Zuidema W, et al. Public survey of financial incentives for kidney donation. *Nephrol Dial Transplant.* 2008; 23: 1039–42.

[13] Wainright JL, Robinson AM, Wilk AR, Klassen DK, Cherikh WS, Stewart DE. Risk of ESRD in prior living kidney donors. *Am J Transplant.* 2018 May;18:1129-39.

[14] Chapman JR, Delmonico FL. Buyer beware transplantation. *Kidney Int.* 2016; 89: 983–85.

[15] Sajjad I, Baines LS, Patel P, Salifu MO, Jindal RM. Commercialization of kidney transplants: a systematic review of outcomes in recipients and donors. *Am J Nephrol.* 2008;28:744-54.

[16] Schultheiss D, Jardin A. René Küss (1913-2006)-a transplant pioneer in Paris. *Transplant Proc.* 2013; 45: 1220–23..

[17] Anonymous. Weaning China off Organs from Executed Prisoners. *Lancet*, 2015;385 (9962):1-1.

[18] Shafer TJ, Wagner D, Chessare J, et al. US organ donation breakthrough collaborative increases organ donation. *Crit Care Nurs Q.* 2008; 31: 190–210.

[19] DeRoos LJ, Zhou Y, Marrero WJ, et al. Assessment of National Organ Donation Rates and Organ Procurement Organization Metrics. *JAMA Surg.* 2021; 156: 173–80.

[20] Organ Procurement Organizations Condiitons for Coverage. *Fed Regist.* 2019;84(246):70628-70710. https://www.govinfo.gov/content/pkg/FR-2019-12-23/pdf/2019-27418.pdf

[21] Kizilisik AT, Ray JB, Nylander WA, Langone AJ, Helderman JH, Shaffer D. Kidney transplantation in a veterans administration medical center: 40 years' experience. *Exp Clin Transplant.* 2004; 2: 238–41.

[22] Opelz G, Döhler B. Cyclosporine and long-term kidney graft survival. *Transplantation.* 2001; 72: 1267–73.

[23] *UNOS* website – https://unos.org - 2021.

[24] Kahan, B; Van Buren, C; Kerman, R; Lewis, R. Exchanging Donor Kidneys. *N Engl J Med* 1988;319: 1092-1094.

[25] Van Buren, C; Shafer, T. Does Kidney Allocation Based on HLA Matching Adversely Affect Minority Access to Transplantation? *Am J Transplant Suppl 1, 2001*, Abs #885: 318.

[26] Held PJ, Kahan BD, Hunsicker LG, et al. The impact of HLA mismatches on the survival of first cadaveric kidney transplants. *N Engl J Med.* 1994; 331: 765–70.

[27] Hart A, Smith JM, Skeans MA, et al. OPTN/SRTR 2017 Annual Data Report: Kidney. *Am J Transplant* 2019; 19 (*Suppl 2*): 19–123. [28]

[28] Kerman RH, Kimball PM, Van Buren CT, et al. Influence of race on crossmatch outcome and recipient eligibility for transplantation. *Transplantation.* 1992; 53: 64–67.

[29] Keith DS, Vranic GM. Approach to the Highly Sensitized Kidney Transplant Candidate. *Clin J Am Soc Nephrol.* 2016 Apr 7;11: 684-93

[30] Jindra P, Murthy BV, Van Buren CT, Virtual XMatch Adversely Affects Access for Highly Sensitized African Americans to Renal Transplantation. *Am J Transplant* 2020 (*Suppl 3*); *Abs* # 235: 418–19.

[31] Addressing medically urgent candidates in new kidney allocation policy. 2020; - https://optn.transplant .hrsa.gov/media /3840/2020-06_kid_med_urgency_policy_notice.pdf

INDEX

D

E

F

G

H

I

K

L

M

N

O

P

R

S

T

V